Bipolar, Recovery and NLP

I0127408

The Trilogy by jason Pegler

Bipolar, Recovery and NLP

Bipolar, Recovery and NLP

"A Can of Madness does what it says in the... er can. A brilliant memoir of mania; all the pain, humour, fear and despair is chronicled here in prose of clarity and distinction. Unforgettable and important" **- Stephen Fry**

"This book will help people to understand one of the greatest issues of our time, how to treat those who are mentally disturbed, as human beings" **– Rt. Hon. Tony Benn MP**

"A Can of Madness takes you as close to the manic experience as you can get, it makes 'Prozac Nation' look like a walk in the park." **– The Big Issue**

He's got guts, he's got heart and he's got vision. That's why people like him – and his new book – are essential for the mental health movement. - **Dolly Sen, author, poet and mental health activist.**

"Jason Pegler has written a work of huge importance to all of Society. He provides a unique insight into the sometimes calamitous world of those with mental health challenges and into the delightful and beneficial creativity of these minds. In doing so he provides those of us with a tenuous grasp on 'sanity' the much needed opportunity to develop understanding, compassion and a new way to look at the world and ourselves. Above all he postulates that the perception of mental illness exists as much in the minds of the observer as it does in those said to be suffering."

Paul Brandwood - Chairman of the Chipmunka Foundation.

Bipolar, Recovery and NLP

Bipolar, Recovery and NLP

The trilogy within this paperback

A Can of Madness

A Can of Madness is Jason's autobiography up until the age of 27. He was born in 1975 and lives in London. He intends to direct A Can of Madness as a blockbuster movie and then work on the inside of Hollywood to change the way the world thinks about mental health thus reducing the pain, suffering and humiliation that people with mental health issues experience on a daily basis.

Curing Madness

Curing Madness is a compilation of selected works written by Jason Pegler from the age of 19 to 29. Jason Pegler which details the thought processes he used to understand the history of madness, living with a diagnosis of manic depression and using writing and NLP (neuro linguistic programming) to cure himself. It includes a couple of excellent scripts about his experiences of manic depression, rap lyrics, an essay that examines madness in Greek Mythology and a personal account of what happened to him after he published his seminal book 'A Can of Madness'.

The Ultimate Guide To Well Being

Jason Pegler has been medication since the end of 2004. 'The Ultimate Guide to Well Being' is Jason Pegler's third book. The goal of the book is to achieve 100% ultimate well being by going through the tasks and exercises included and to have fun whilst doing it. Jason reveals the benefits of Neuro-Linguistic Programming, social entrepreneurship and harnessing creativity to the general public and people affected by mental health issues. Topics discussed in the book include; having a healthy mind, body and soul; knowing what is crucial to your happiness; inspiring yourself and having time for other people; how you can make the world a better place; connecting spiritually and making the impossible possible. Read this book and pass on the techniques and actions to save and improve lives.

Bipolar, Recovery and NLP

Bipolar, Recovery and NLP

Chipmunkapublishing

In 2002 Jason Pegler and Andrew Latchford set up Chipmunkapublishing, which quickly became a social phenomenon helping thousands of people with mental health problems worldwide. A new generation of mental health sufferers could now force the world to listen to their plight and therefore accommodate them in a humane manner just like Martin Luther King had led black Americans to equality in the United States of America. As Chipmunkapublishing grew it reached out to carers, the medical profession, the media, politicians, celebrities and society. The Chipmunka vision illustrates that we are in a transitional period in history where mental health will essentially be "normalised" and broken down as a taboo. This is inevitable in a world where mental health suffering is on the increase. As global communication improves in the consumerist generation of the 21st Century it is inevitable that we will all be more sensitive to the mental health of others.

Chipmunkapublishing is a social enterprise that drives its resources back into the community.

Bipolar, Recovery and NLP

Bipolar, Recovery and NLP

About the author

Jason Pegler is a social entrepreneur, inspirational speaker, writer and rap artist. He is CEO of Chipmunkapublishing and also the Co Founder and driving force behind the Chipmunka Foundation and the Chipmunka Group. The Chipmunka Foundation was set up in August 2004 to further the Chipmunka vision and become the world's largest most effective health charity. For more details please go to www.chipmunkapublishing.com. Jason has been off his medication since the end of 2004 and has become one of the world's foremost experts on mental health. He now dedicates his life to helping others afflicted by mental illness.

Bipolar, Recovery and NLP

Bipolar, Recovery and NLP

A Can of Madness

By Jason Pegler

Bipolar, Recovery and NLP

Published by
Chipmunkapublishing
PO Box 6872
Brentwood
Essex
CM13 1ZT
United Kingdom

www.chipmunkapublishing.com

A record of this book is in the British Library

Bipolar, Recovery and NLP

Love to my family and friends and everyone who cares about the mental health of others.

Bipolar, Recovery and NLP

Bipolar, Recovery and NLP

This book is dedicated to Tom Robertson and Ali Priestly

Bipolar, Recovery and NLP

Bipolar, Recovery and NLP

Foreword

This is a strong book: full of strong language. But the hard words are not just the superfluous, value-added expletives of gangster rap there to make the writer feel hard. These are the natural expressions of a young man trying to make sense of experiences that can only be fully understood from within. They resonate with anger, sometimes with bewilderment and, always, with knowledge and understanding. By grounding his descriptions of madness in the emerging story of his life, Jason Pegler makes his story accessible to anyone with hopes, fears and compassion.

Jason's story draws frankly on his childhood, upbringing and experiences at school; it marks his intellectual and physical developments; and it acclaims his passions and desires. In common with many young and talented people, Jason's story mixes the conventional, socially desirable successes and achievements – examinations, rugby matches, university – with the risky and audacious exploits of youth: booze, brawls and sex. But the central theme is his battle with his personal madness, and the humiliations with which this brings him in contact.

For those of us who work in the healthcare system, many of Jason's descriptions should be a warning; this is not the way it should be. His recurring experiences of lack of time, lack of training and, worst of all, lack of compassion on the part of healthcare staff provide a mirror in which we must hope *we* are not reflected. For people who share some of Jason's experiences, and for their friends and families, the book is hopeful that its message, that seemingly devastating circumstances can be overcome, helps.

This is a strong book. Read it and gain strength.

Teifion Davies

Senior Lecturer, editor of *The ABC of mental health* and Consultant Psychiatrist at St Thomas' Hospital, Lambeth, London, United Kingdom.

Bipolar, Recovery and NLP

Bipolar, Recovery and NLP

Preface

What follows is intended to help people understand the condition of manic depression and similar mental illnesses. And I hope that sufferers, their families and friends will gain an enormous amount of strength from reading it. My own experience is that it's possible to emerge at the other end of adversity and live a decent life. Admittedly you may have to make changes in your life and behaviour, but that's a small sacrifice compared with the alternatives.

The first step is to accept that you've got a problem, or rather, that there *is* a problem, the exact cause(s) of which, more often than not, will forever remain unknown. The second is to deal with it, and the sooner the better.

When writing this book, I often thought back to how long it took me to accept my own illness. I have discovered that I have helped many people cope with their illness better than I did. This alone makes the pain of writing it and talking about it worthwhile.

Prepare for a journey that will take you close to the edge as you read the most honest account written about manic depression that you have ever seen. For those of you who find it a page turner read on and once you have finished telling people about it encourage them to be more open about their own mental health. For those who may be offended I apologise beforehand and urge you to read on.

Writing this book made me a better person as I got all the pain out of my system. To make it more politically correct at this stage I would feel like I am not being true to myself as the words you are about to read explain exactly how I felt at that moment in time. 'Writing about my experiences saved my life and publishing the work of others has enabled me to help more people'.

Bipolar, Recovery and NLP

Bipolar, Recovery and NLP

Chapter 1 – In the beginning...

As I was being driven off in the back of a police van in a space suit, I thought I was Donovan Bad Boy Smith being driven to a rave. I could hear music in my head and flashed back to another night at the Brunel Rooms in Swindon. *The Brunel Rooms, a hardcore Mecca for druggies from Gloucester and surrounding areas in the early to mid-nineties.* Donovan was so hard core when I saw him there that he'd refused to turn off his set at 3am. He'd carried on until 3.30am when someone finally turned off the electricity mid flow.

Talking of flows (as opposed to stable mindsets), just how the fuck do you live with a mental illness? Don't ask me, I'm still trying to find out now. After all, it's not something you plan let alone something you'd ever expect to have. As we all say: it won't happen to me. But it can. And in this case, it did.

And if Hercules and Ajax couldn't hack it, how the hell could I? Unsurprisingly, I didn't – and that's why I wallowed in self-pity for so long.

So, do you want to know what it's like to be crazy, mad, and loopy? Well, I'm about to tell you. I'm also going to tell you how it feels to be suicidal for months on end – the fate of the manic. One thing, however, is for sure: the sooner you kill mania the better because you're a danger to yourself and other people when you don't know what you're doing. The longer mania is allowed to continue the longer and more severe the inevitable depression will be.

The problem is that mania is a unique and sometimes beautiful experience, even though its genius is flawed and must be quelled. The irony is that it draws strength from imperfection. Think of the Mona Lisa without her eyebrows. She's more appealing because there's something that's not quite right. She is in some way different, contrary to the norm, and thus fascinates the observer.

I also draw strength from Van Gogh, as I imagine him painting just down the road from me in Stockwell. Slipping in and out of consciousness when writing, I try to summon up his 'madness'.

Finally, I take comfort from the poet and composer, Ivor Gurney. Like me he was manic, and like me he came from Gloucester and moved to South London. Apparently, he would often walk from one to the other, singing folk music and sleeping in barns along the way.

...

Hucclecote, one of the more pleasant areas of Gloucester (although still with its fair share of pingheads and run-of-the-mill crims loitering outside the Wagon and the shops), is about a mile, mile and a half outside the town centre on the Cheltenham side. We moved there because my parents were keen that my brother, Harvey, and I did well at school – Hucclecote is a bike ride away from the renowned grammar school, Sir Thomas Rich's, in Longlevens. The plan was that we would each would pass our Eleven Plus and get in.

Green Lane, where I lived, was quiet, (lower-) middle class and had a huge green at the end of it. Because it's right on Hucclecote Road, access to either Gloucester, or its more upmarket neighbour Cheltenham located only seven miles away, is easy. But that's enough on Gloucester for now. Let's meet the family.

My dad. A senior fireman, often under stress, worked extremely hard all his life (saving two lives in the process) and was the best snooker player in the district for the best part of his life, as well as a pretty good golfer. In fact, he still is. My mum. More maternal than perhaps is the norm, liked staying at home (although always had a part-time job) tidying up and drinking tea. Imaginative and strangely fond of teddy bears. Harvey. More complex – see below.

...

When I was seven, my parents were advised to put me up a year as I was streets ahead of everyone else. I didn't want to because I was scared of being bullied. There again, at the same time, two boys were bullying me in my own year so what the hell – they'd pick on me when the rest of the class were in orchestra and insult me by calling me *brainy*. They'd also hit me and once, when I kicked one of them in retaliation, I missed all my lunchtimes for a week because I was too scared to tell the headmistress that I was provoked. The timing was ironic because, the very same morning she'd reprimanded me, she'd made an announcement in assembly that there was to be no kicking in the school. As things turned out, my parents were undecided as to whether to put me up a year (they were unable to discuss anything rationally) so I stayed put.

When I was nine, I won the Gloucester Chess Congress – out of 243 entrants. I won all eight of my games which, as far as I know, was and still is a record despite most of the competition being a year older than me. I also had the highest reading age throughout my school years and when everyone else was struggling with their 1-12 times tables I had already finished my 12-20s. I finished the year's maths cards in about four weeks so they forced me to do comprehension for the rest of the year. That was after I'd completed another load of maths cards ordered specially for me. In hindsight, there was little to keep my buzzing brain occupied. A pity, because I loved learning. But not only at school.

When I was little, I enjoyed playing the map game with my dad. He'd place a big wooden map on the floor and I'd learn every capital in the world. He would then test me not only on capitals, but on flags too. I even learnt all the American states in alphabetical order.

And when sport was on the TV, or when he'd tuck me in, he also used to pretend he was the greatest sportsman in the world at everything. Which to many, it seemed he was: he had about a hundred trophies for sports but wouldn't display them in the lounge. He was reserved, certainly no show off; a man of action, not of words who slogged his guts out providing for his family. This was my dad and I was proud of him. He would always work overtime or play golf, volleyball or snooker. He was extremely competitive and a perfectionist in everything he did. I knew I possessed his natural doggedness in competition with my success at football, chess and rugby.

My greatest achievements had been winning the County Under- 11, 15, 18 and Southwest Under-16 Chess Championships. This was my life and it was unique. It would become more and more unique but unfortunately not in the way that I had once envisaged.

I had some very unhappy moments in junior school. This was largely because the other kids were jealous of my intelligence. I didn't feel very popular although I discovered that the best looking girl in the school fancied me after I dropped a Valentine's card round her house. My mum drove me round there and I placed it in the letterbox then darted off as if I had just stolen someone's bag from a pub. Eventually, I ended up 'smooching' with her at the junior disco only to ruin things by proceeding to beat up another kid who interfered. That was not how the junior school social clique led by Cheryl Long worked, and once I'd blown it there was no way back in.

When I was nine our school went away on camp. I won a moonie competition with two other boys in my class. We were trying to shock the girls and I won hands down as I went one step further than my classmates, showing the four prettiest girls in the school my cock in private. In return they agreed to let me see their bare arses – they didn't let me down. Not a bad day's work, all the more so for the fact that nobody else had had that privilege, at least as far as I knew. However, one of them said my dick looked like a sausage and for the rest of the excursion proceeded to sing "Moonie Addict" at me in place of "Sister Addict".

I spent the last two nights of that particular holiday experiencing my first "breakdown". I spoke to one of the teachers in charge of us who had never taught me. Mrs. Knight was a scary looking woman with black curly hair and always wore funny scarves that made her look older than she was. She had a reputation for being strict but was quite sympathetic with my situation. I told her that my parents were separated. My mum was living round my Nan's and they were going to get a divorce. They were also planning to drag my older brother and me through the courts. She understood and said something like: "Unfortunately it's something that happens, but I'm sure the worst is over ... Just hold on tight, and everything will be OK. You'll see my dear." I told her that I didn't mind if they got divorced. In fact, I wanted them to. I was just sick of the arguing and sick of being used as a go between. I was fed up with being dragged through shit.

There were psychologically traumatising incidents at school. The other boys didn't like me because I would score more goals than everyone else put together in every football match – during breaks and for the school team. I beat them all at chess, spelling, reading, writing, and even Top Trumps – I had a photographic memory for learning numbers so knew which category to pick on each card.

Bipolar, Recovery and NLP

One week, however, they got their own back on me. Because I was a Man U supporter, every lunch and break time they paraded round the school singing: "We all hate Man United, they're not gonna win the league, and we'll really shake them up when they lose the FA Cup 'cause United are the crappest football team." They would follow me round whenever I was in the playground and some of them would push me. Sometimes this made me cry; at other times it made me angry but the chanting would continue irrespectively.

The experience reminded me of my first day in junior school when kids from the upper year picked on me because my brother and his mates had picked on them in their previous years. Now, though, he had left and was at a different school unable to protect me. As for the bullies in my year, I was stronger than they were individually but not collectively – although with one exception: a boy from Canada who marched on his own singing. He supported Norwich City. Now that took guts and stupidity. It got to me so much that I told the teacher who rounded the ringleaders up. He went ape shit and, with the whole year in a specially arranged meeting, demanded that they all apologise to me. They did, but the scars are still there somewhere in my subconscious. One teacher used to make me come in early at lunchtimes because I sweated so much. *Fucking bitch. I'd slit her throat if I ever saw her again. Who the fuck did she think she was? Was she some kind of Dominatrix or something? Now that would have been more interesting.*

One consolation for the unhappy moments in my childhood was my dog, Ben. I'd asked for a dog when I was nine and for once my dad caved in. When we took him home, he stank of shit so my mum and dad gave him a bath. The first night, he shat all over the house and whined incessantly. My dad wanted to take him back the next morning so I slept with him the next night to try and keep him quiet. He stayed in our house by the skin of his canine teeth and everyone eventually came to love him. He was so cute as a puppy with his big head and his big paws. We'd take him for walks down the green and he was dead happy running around, chasing balls and sticks, and wagging his tail. He became very loyal and my mum and I took him to training classes. He finally became house trained and a good guard dog. He was part of the family and stayed with dad, Harvey and me when mum left.

For various reasons, he fell into my mum's hands in 1995 and she projected her love for everyone else onto him. Ultimately, though, he was still my dog and acknowledged that with the look he sometimes gave me. The last time I saw him as a manic I made him head police dog of the world to stomp out crime, once and for all. His back legs weakened and grey fur appeared round his face as he reached old age. His acceptance into the family seemed to symbolise my parents staying together until I was 15. Then my mum left home and, after moving out of her mother's went to live with Michael, now my step dad. I liked him a lot and made a speech supporting them at their wedding. The only wedding I have ever been to is my mum's. Michael would always be the joker and liked rugby. Once he watched me play and I scored the only try of the game. He had taken my mum to Wales and I didn't think I minded because she was happy.

My grandfather died when I was 14. His was the first dead body I ever saw. He died of angina in 1989. I kissed his cold forehead on my Nan's request in the funeral parlour and watched my brother do the same. It was a peculiar moment. I tried to comfort myself by thinking of an afterlife but was beaten by what I saw: he was dead. What was more distressing was the way my Nan was behaving: "Doesn't he look nice and smart in that suit? He was always smart, Colin, his hair and his clothes; always immaculate." My Nan started to cry and I hugged her tightly as she cracked up.

Aware of her devastation, I cried too. They had been happily married for 52 years and now she was alone: nobody to cook for, or to snuggle up with by the fire during cold, wet and windy nights; nobody to make those special cups of tea; nobody to talk to when she was happy and nobody to talk to when she was sad; nobody to cuddle and, worst of all, nobody to sleep with at night. That's if my Nan would ever be able to go to sleep again. For six months after his death she slept downstairs in the lounge, too scared to sleep upstairs without him, and lived in that big house alone. He had provided for her, paid the bills, protected her and given her life a purpose. He had given her everything.

All that remained were memories of the time they had spent together, objects they had obtained over the years and photographs they had taken of one another. Today, a picture stands in the lounge of my granddad when he was young. My Nan always shows it to new visitors and has told me a thousand times that I have the same eyes as him and that I am as kind as he was. Well, I'm happy for my Nan to recognise a likeness between us but I know that I'm not as kind as he was.

He was a bit of a saint. Everyone liked him. For 25 years, he worked for Morses and was the top local salesman. If people couldn't afford what they had ordered, but he could, he would pay for them out of his own wages so they wouldn't get into trouble. What's more, he would never ask for the money back. As the vicar said at his funeral: "I didn't know Colin personally, but I am struck today by what a special person everyone I have spoken to says he was."

The only time I ever saw him angry was when it came to my dad. Let's just say they didn't get on. Despite this, he still let my dad boss my mum around when he could have easily stepped in. If I was in his shoes, I know I would have.

He was passive; a true gentleman. He was the sort of man who would not speak during dinner because it was rude. He was no coward but someone who did things by the book. He was the youngest of 13 brothers and sisters and times were hard when he grew up. They would have to ration their food and yet he managed to break away, find a steady job and pay off a mortgage. He had bettered himself and was content. My saddest memory of his life is that he never went abroad. He always wanted to but my Nan was scared of flying so they never did. He didn't want to upset her so that was the end of that.

I never had the opportunity to talk with him at great length: he was always ill when I was growing up and couldn't speak very well either because of chronic bronchitis or a sore throat. He was no intellectual but would read detective novels every evening by the fire. The only practical things I learned from him were not to have gravy on a Sunday lunch and not to smoke like he had. Through him, though, I learnt something very important: that it's OK for a man to have a sensitive side, especially with a woman –

and that most women actually prefer it.

...

I had experienced violence in my life but never saw myself as a violent person, except for the odd bit of vandalism when I'd drunk too much. There again, I was always fighting on the rugby field and was banned for two months when I was 16. However, although this was aggression, at least it was in a controlled environment. As for fights on the street, I never started any of them, I just seemed to be in the wrong place at the wrong time. I was also never a bully, and would even stick up for the geek in my year at school. He used to be tormented for peeing his pants and I stopped him from being kicked and teased on several occasions. Strangely enough – or not as the case may be – he went to Oxford and read biochemistry.

Anyway, back to the rugby. I played rugby for Gloucester Under-16s, when even the fantastic England hooker Phil Greening didn't make the team. Mind you, he was a year younger than everyone else at the trial. I reckon I could have gone far if someone had taken me under their wing. One of the teachers at school, Mr Goddard, wanted me to play for Berry Hill and be captain of a team he was coaching. If I'd taken the weights more seriously and stayed off the drink I could have made it. I don't need anybody else to tell me that. From the age of 15 I was playing for Old Richian's Colts who were one of the best Under-19 teams in the country. In the three seasons I played for them, we won 58 games, drew one and lost one. I scored loads of tries and would often have write-ups in The Citizen, Gloucester's paper.

...

Despite having freckles and some fairly bad acne I always seemed to attract girls. When I was 16 I had a girlfriend for a few months but we never had sex. I tried to at my mum's house one time but I was drunk, had taken speed and magic mushrooms, and couldn't get it up. Our relationship was absurd – she never said a word. We two-timed each other and eventually split up. A few weeks later, though, I heard she still fancied me so I asked her out again with the sole intention of dumping her to get revenge. It worked but I still never fucked her. I mean, what was the problem?

Bipolar, Recovery and NLP

I also remember having an aching hard-on with several naked girls when I was 14 but they wouldn't let me have sex with them – either because they didn't want to get pregnant or because they didn't want to be called slags. There again, I did manage to push it in to one of them but she wriggled off. In the event, I started fucking one who had passed out but she woke up barfing on my shoe. Her friends broke in and gave her a bath to sober her up.

It was frustrating. When I was 14 I started getting drunk and was forever snogging girls. It was easy. Then it became more difficult. I think I got a bad reputation for drinking a lot – perhaps some girls had heard that I didn't finish the job off properly; or maybe I was getting ugly, unlucky or turning into a homosexual.

The first time I came in a pussy I was 15. It was with this really sexy French brunette. She screamed a lot and kept saying "Oui", obviously enjoying it, which was exciting, but at the same time rather vacuous. My problem was that I was too proud. For example, when I was 14 a girl I had been getting off with who was older than me asked if I was a virgin. I tried to be cool and said no. Her reaction was to think I would be unfaithful to her if we had sex. I'd made the wrong decision and would see my first shag put back for a while.

By the age of 14 I'd been to my first rave but I didn't go regularly until I was 16 or 17. Fantasia was the most successful legalised rave in 1993, and I went to one at Castle Donnington. Twenty-eight thousand people were there and I had three rhubarb and custards. After all, I hadn't had any tea. I didn't have a ticket but told the bouncers that a gang in the queue had stole mine. The second security guard I told this story to must have bought it or at least admired my audacity as he gave me a ticket. Two girls who were friends of my brother drove me there and I didn't see them until seven the next morning. I spent 11 hours walking around hiding my t-shirt which had a huge "E" on it under my jacket – a raver too terrified to dance in case anybody laughed at him for being the worst "mover" there. Thing is, I knew I was a great dancer. That's how paranoid pills can make you. Every hour I'd go to meet my friend Peach at the fairground, but he wasn't there as we'd arranged. I found out later that a group from the rock- head tent had mugged him.

The only people I saw who I knew I steered clear of including

Bipolar, Recovery and NLP

MC Al'n and his posse. He was a dodgy bloke who sold fake acid and walked off with people's cash. Mind you, he'd always been all right to me. I also saw DJ Spider who was a major drug dealer in the Forest of Dean. I'd taken my first E at the age of 15 when I was round his house. I also saw this huge guy called Steve, who I had beaten up previously, with his crew. This was seven months before my manic depression first surfaced.

Steve exemplified what I hated about Gloucester. It was full of small-minded people who would judge you without reason. There was no reason for him to fight except for his rotten ego. I was outside Fifth Avenue with my brother, Dom and his sister Tara when Steve approached us with an accomplice.

"What are you doing here? Get off my fucking road. I'm going down this alley and if you're still here when I get back, I'm going to kick the shit out of you – all of you."

My brother and Dom were sat cross-legged wearing headbands. They said that they didn't want any trouble and were ready to leave. I wasn't, I was sick of being bossed around. I mean I might have let my parents, the bullies when I was little, and some hard nuts in the past bully me, but nobody else. No way. I had to make a stand. Steve returned from the alley and I had just about convinced everyone to stay put.

"What, you still here?"

"Who do you think you are?" I calmly replied.

I could feel butterflies in my stomach. I was 6'3" and 14 stone but this guy was 6'5" and 18 stone. We stood opposite each other, and I couldn't resist it when he took a swing at me. I dodged out of the way and swung my hips giving him a right hook to the side of his head. He dropped straight to the floor. As I kicked him in the head a few times, Dom prevented his friend from intervening and Tara urged me to stop. The fat slob on the deck eventually managed to get back up. He put his arm round me and congratulated me saying that he had wanted a pop at me since he met me at a party a few years back. He said he had a knife in his pocket and that he could have killed me.

I remained quiet as he left praying for some more action. But what for? This was one of so many fights that I had and so minor in comparison to others I had already had and would have in the future. Believe me, the great brawl scene in Scorsese's *Mean*

Bipolar, Recovery and NLP

Streets was a weekly occurrence in Gloucester. It was a rugby town where everyone thought that they were bigger and better than they were. Small-minded and arrogant locals drank shit-loads of booze after a mind numbingly boring week. That's how they let themselves go, by picking on some poor sod or group of sods. To make things worse, they were never held accountable for anything, the police were often too scared to intervene. Meanwhile, less than a mile from where I decked Steve, Fred West was rearranging his house and proudly adding to his collection of dead bodies. I wasn't surprised when the story broke out because I always felt there was something odd and perverse about Gloucester – a sinister undercurrent if you like.

...

On the subject of oddness, mad people in Gloucester were sent, for recuperative purposes, to Coney Hill hospital – the butt of much local humour. I'd never known anyone who had gone there despite the fact that there was a history of mental instability in my family. I knew that my Grandma's brother had killed himself just after World War II, thinking the Germans were still after him. I also knew she had been institutionalised herself before. She'd attempted suicide by filling the house with gas and putting her head in the oven. Her ex-husband, my Uncle Tom, had returned to find her unconscious and took her to hospital.

My grandmother would always tell me a story about her conquering her mental breakdown and compare it to how she had given up smoking. The thing is, years later, she started smoking again. The story goes something like this.

"I tried to kill myself twice – not once, but twice. The first time, I was depressed because my ex-husband Tom had left me. He'd been having an affair. Anyway, I don't want to talk about that. It won't cheer you up. No, listen to this ... (Prodding my forearm with her finger and then sipping some gin.) I let gas off all over my kitchen and stuck my head in the oven. Somebody called for the ambulance and I was barely conscious. Lucky to be alive, I can tell you, at least that's what the nurse at the hospital told me afterwards (laughs, gulps down some more gin then regains her composure). They took me to a mental hospital and it looked like hell on earth. Remember, suicide, or rather attempted suicide, was illegal in those days so they could have arrested me... I could have been arrested. Anyway, back to what happened. As soon as I saw the state of the patients in there ... the poor sods ... I immediately decided that I was not going to stay there and demanded to see the doctor. I remember the doctor; he was a lovely man. I told him that I wasn't mad and wasn't staying with those people in there. They weren't well and I wasn't going to feel any better by being there.

The doctor held me by the hand and said: 'What you did, Mrs. Best, wasn't a cry for help. You really meant it didn't you?'

"You bet I did. By God, I meant it. I wanted to end my life. "'Well, that's a very brave thing you did Mrs. Best,' he agreed. You know, Jason my darling (reaching for my hand and squeezing it), that same man, the doctor – I can't remember his name – told me that I was one of the most intelligent people he had ever met. You see kid, that's where you get your intelligence from – not your mother or your father or your Nana. It's me kid.

"You see, Jason, that was the first and only time that I have been in a mental hospital. From that moment on I decided that I would never go into one again. It was as simple as that. I suffered depression for years after that, mind you. But I will never go back to a place like that. Only to see you, and I don't want to see you in a place like that again dear boy."

One or both of us would cry when she told me this story although the more senile she became the more she repeated it and the more disillusioned I would get. If she told it to me when I was really depressed I would think that I was a weaker person than she was ... If she told it me at any other time I would think she misunderstood my situation. No two circumstances were the same and I thought my illness was clearly worse than hers ever was. It had been diagnosed and she had never had to experience mania or the coming to terms with it. Although she cared a great deal in her own way, she could only offer comfort on the rare occasion when I was so depressed that I would have believed anything she said. In those states of mind, I would even have listened to a vicar.

That was the version of being mentally ill my grandmother told me when she was drunk. When she was sober, it was a less dramatic but more detailed story. You see, she was depressed whenever she was sober unless she was playing scrabble with her friends or touring round the Lake District. Her sober narration

Bipolar, Recovery and NLP

went something like this.

"In 1953 or 1954 (I can't remember which) I was admitted to Lancaster Moor Hospital. My name was Mrs. Crichton then. The Doctor summoned me and offered me coffee. Now, that was unheard of in those days. He told me never to allow anybody to tell me that I was mentally ill, and that just because I was in for the so-called 17-day section, didn't mean I was crazy.

However, I wished I was dead. I was in love with a married man named Bobby, but he said that he would never divorce his wife. He was a farmer. He had fourteen farms and three slaughterhouses. Farmers didn't want to divorce in those days because they didn't want to split the land. Divorce was a dirty word, I can tell you. I became really depressed and got a chopper from the kitchen in my house in Barrow and breathed in gas out of the hole I made in the tube. I can't remember anything else. All the doors were locked. The next thing I remember was your Great Nana sat on top of me pumping my arms up and down. I never wanted to be saved and wished – and still do wish – that I was dead. An ambulance and doctor came and took me off to Lancaster Moore Mental Hospital. It took 40 minutes. I arrived at nine and that morning was like an unending desert of time. They gave me some aspirins, which I'm allergic to, and some other drugs – I can't remember their name.

"I kept myself to myself and always sat by a window. I always wanted to see outside. Bobby came to see me out of guilt and gave me 200 Players cigarettes. I had known him five years.

"My mother was very cruel to me. She'd even thrown my father, Joseph Henry, out when I was nine and my brother, Jack, eight. I hate her for that. He was a man who loved his children and was nicknamed "Snowy" because of his silver white hair. He worked for Vickers. They were in Barrow and built warships, submarines and cruisers. He'd fought in the World War I – which was enough to drive any man mad. The last time I saw him was in court. My mother had taken him there for non-payment of rent which didn't really affect her because I paid most of it anyway. She just did it out of spite.

"Your Great Nana, that's my mother, was always jealous of all of my friends. She was always away when I grew up. I lived with my Auntie Nellie from the age of 11 until I was 16 or 17, I can't remember exactly. I didn't see much of her when I was growing up and it was upsetting to see her jealous. She even became jealous of Auntie Nellie. I mean, I loved Auntie Nellie but that never compared to the love I had for my mother. I mean, that was different. Everyone knows that. One other thing, Jason, simple people don't go mad. Brainy people do. Remember that, Jason my darling. Come and give your Grandma a big hug. There, there."

I asked my grandmother about two other members of our family that had suffered from mental illness and was disturbed by some of the things she told me. I knew about her brother and thought I'd leave that until last so I asked her first of all about Auntie Ethel Thomson. My grandmother was a great storyteller.

"My Auntie, Ethel Thomson, killed herself in 1932, maybe three or even four, I can't remember. She was a depressive. She was terribly sad. Now, I was born in Barrow-in-Furness, on 29 December, 1919 so I was about 14 when it happened. The poor woman. She was better off for doing it though, I can tell you. She was always crying, and ran a corner shop with her mother. Hospitals were very strict in those days. She had an illegitimate child. This was seen as a terrible thing to do back then. They wouldn't let her out of the hospital, but somehow she managed to get out and she ran under the railway line and flung herself under a train. This was in February. They found her foot a mile down the line. They found her head stuck to the end of the train. They left patients in there for years and years. Some of them were in there for the rest of their lives. They didn't know what to do with them then; there was no treatment for it.

"It was my Jack who told me that Ethel had killed herself on a Sunday morning. I used to visit her in there. It was at Lancaster Moor Hospital – the same one that Jack and I were in. People used to jeer at them and make fun of them but it wasn't their fault that they were ill. That's not right. They were still human beings just like you and me."

I saved talking about Jack in detail until last because I knew it would upset my grandmother the most. "Jack Crichton Thompson, my brother, God bless him, was born on 14 October, 1917. He worked on a machine in Vickers in Barrow. It was semi-skilled factory work that concentrated mostly on shipbuilding. He suffered from severe depression and used to cry all the time. It struck him

Bipolar, Recovery and NLP

in his late 20s or early 30s, I can't remember exactly. Before then, we'd always be joking and laughing not like all the miserable sods today. In 1936, King Edward V11 gave up the throne. Your Great Nana and I had a fish and chip shop.

"Jack was very popular. He would go for a drink with other young lads at the Plaza in 1936. They went ballroom dancing. Oh, there was less crime then; the world was less violent. People fought the enemy then, not each other. At the age of 22, he was married with three children. He kept working somehow and joined the army of occupation in 1944, in Belgium.

"I moved to Gloucester, and sometime after that, Renée, my brother's wife, wrote to me and told me that Jack was unwell. She explained how he had sat on the wall in Cavendish Square in Barrow laughing to himself. Then Renée threw Jack out. They split up sometime between 1960 and 1964. Jack probably knew that she was having an affair but nobody else found out until later on. He worked for a few more months but was finally admitted to Lancaster Moor hospital. I went up and spoke to the psychiatrist. Jack was so sad. I gave him a sandwich and he wolfed it down. I took him back to Gloucester to the wine shop with me for a few days. I remember that his face lit up when I said that I was going to take him out of that horrible place. Soon after, I decided to take him out for good and look after him.

"Tom was wonderful with him. Jack went off and Tom went looking for him.

"Jack had a funny appetite. He didn't eat. He couldn't walk. He badly needed treatment and we didn't know what to do with him so, as a last measure, we took him to hospital in Gloucester on a Sunday. Jack wandered off and moved to live with your Great Nana on Stanley Road. I had my own shop where the big Debenhams is now. It was a wine shop at 15 St Aldgate Street. I paid the rent for the wine shop and the rent for your Great Nana's mortgage. Tom was the meanest man in the world when it came to money. Jack lived at Stanley Road for a year. He saw doctors and took pills. He was on medication.

"A week after he died a man came in the shop. I was Mrs. Pegler then. The doctor said that he would have killed himself if he was in the same situation and his words gave, and still give, me great comfort whenever I think about your uncle Jack, and my brother, God bless him. Jack was taking pills, you see, and had overdosed. All that day, I remember as if it were yesterday. I had been extremely worried. I was manager of the shop and couldn't leave it, but I wish I had. By God, I wish I had. Your Great Nana and I watched him die in hospital. It was a relief. He couldn't suffer any more pain that way. He had suffered enough, you see.

"He had schizophrenia not manic depression like you. It was down on his record. He would hallucinate. He would open curtains an inch and see thousands of soldiers in the street thinking they were coming for him. He was terrified. I would go along with it. I didn't want him to feel that he was on his own, you see. 'Don't worry, they're nothing to do with us,' I would say. 'They're from the council,' or something like that, I would say. I used to make it up as I went along. One of the symptoms of his illness was suspicion. I made sure never to contradict him. Oh my poor brother. He missed his children."

I was very touched by what my grandmother had told me about members of our family and their illnesses. I felt sorry for the fact that she'd witnessed so much suffering in her life. I knew that she would have been very good working with the mentally ill. She understood them and empathised with them, you see. I know my mum would be good at that too – especially now she's experienced so much of what it is like with me. It takes special people to be good mental health nurses and there should be certain additional prerequisites to qualify. For example empathy, understanding, a specifically trained knowledge of mental illnesses, and the social skills necessary for this type of care.

I asked my Grandmother to think of one happy memory of her brother and she immediately mentioned one time when he had come home on leave from the army. "He'd put on weight, looked fit – like a proper soldier – and said that he would have loved to have been in the army for the rest of his life." That made me feel more at ease when I put my pen down after our heart to heart. At least we'd ended on a positive note.

I had a bit of a headache, felt a bit anxious and thought of how my Grandma told me that she loved nothing more than walking across Walney beach in Barrow with the wind on her face. She loved the wind and the freedom of the lakes and, despite her depression, idiosyncrasies and unpopularity within the family, was

Bipolar, Recovery and NLP

actually a remarkable woman. I hoped that I would always remember her as that. A remarkable woman who had worked until she was well into her seventies and who had led an interesting life travelling all over the world.

Thing is, there had been a lot of problems in my family life and a lot of people felt that she was to blame for them. She had helped my mum and dad out of debts when they were younger and paid for my dad to go to America where he met my step mum Clare, but she always wanted something in return. She was an interfering woman but cooked me a lot of meals after my mum left and gave me a lot of money to go out with my friends. After I left for university, it would upset me seeing her. She had senile dementia and I couldn't handle her mood swings. Maybe she was a manic-depressive – I didn't know and most of the time I didn't want to think about it. If she wasn't then she was a moaner. Always moaning about what she had given people and that she had got nothing in return. She wasn't making herself any happier by moaning about everything but she could never snap out of it, and that was the most tragic thing in her life. Not that she had tried to kill herself, or that Bobby never left his wife, or that she was unpopular but that she was unable to forget about things and move forward. If she could have done that she'd have been a lot happier, as would have everybody she came into contact with. Because of her, other members of the family had to try harder to get along.

However, I am very grateful to her and always will be for a number of reasons – for example she supported me emotionally when mum left, and took me on my first aeroplane. I was 12 and Harvey was 16. The three of us went to Greece on a historic tour. We went to Athens, Corinth, Olympia and Delphi. It gave me a unique insight into the classical world. I stood on running tracks at the awesome amphitheatres and imagined the competitors in the ancient Olympiads. I stared out from under the Acropolis in the intense heat with a sense of nostalgia that I had never had before. I would always remember the amazing view of the Gulf of Corinth. The classical world was closer to me than it had ever been and led me to study classical civilisation at A-level.

Bipolar, Recovery and NLP

Chapter 2 – I've lost it

My first episode occurred when I was 17 – possibly a result of drugs – and hospitalised me for six months. There were no warning signs before the avalanche of mental illness engulfed me although certain factors doubtless played a role: unhappy marriage, divorced parents, domestic violence, heavy alcohol intake and, of course, cannabis, LSD, speed and ecstasy.

This was nothing out of the ordinary, though, and was standard for someone growing up in the 1990s. Take my brother. He was studying a philosophy degree in London and took drugs for "intellectual reasons", as he put it. For example he wanted to know what it was like to listen to Sgt. Pepper on LSD. He did that and was proud of that. I was just as curious about taking drugs as he was, that's why I took acid before he did, but the fact was that everyone was doing it. Meanwhile, I was becoming obsessed with the rave scene. I would steal from my father and sell drugs at school to feed my habits for amphetamine and alcohol. The pleasant rural area that I lived in was notorious for pingheads residing in various squats. These special-brew addicts would do anything for a bag of billy. They just loved cooking up and, while this repulsed me, I actually thought they were quite cool. Now I just feel sorry for them.

A part of me regrets getting ill so soon as I never got round to taking as many drugs as my friends. I loved to go raving. I loved dancing to the hardcore. I loved the rush and the way the girls danced. It really turned me on. The whole movement gave me an identity during my adolescence.

I first "officially" went mad – experienced the unexplainable phenomenon of mania – in Gloucester in November 1993, aged 17. It's impossible to say when it started exactly, it may have just surfaced then, but nobody can prove that is wasn't there all along. Just because I was diagnosed then didn't mean that I didn't have it before. As I remember it, I'd gone to stay with my best friend, Dominic, at the university in Swansea and we went to a few clubs. He's medium height, pretty stocky, has dark hair, extremely intelligent, has a sick sense of humour like me and always looks a bit worried except when he's laughing.

I took a White Calais and a Pink New Yorker in this hardcore

Bipolar, Recovery and NLP

club called Martha's on the Kingsway. That night, DJ Lomas was making a special appearance. I stomped around until ten in the morning but seemed to get higher and higher for the next two weeks. One minute I was an aspiring clubber along with my friend and his acquaintances; the next minute things had got completely out of control.

I first remember completely losing the plot at school in an English A-level lesson. We had a double lesson on Ursula Fanthorpe and her poetry. This lesbian had inspired our overweight but raunchy English teacher into reaffirming her feminism. My mind was racing far quicker than it could do in a sane state. I wouldn't let anybody voice their opinions. I recall being drawn into one poem as it mentioned Lechlade. Only a few weeks before there had been an illegal rave there that the police had been unable to stop. Twenty-five thousand people turned up and in my confusion I thought the revolution had come. As Lechlade wasn't far from Gloucester perhaps I was needed to front it? A madman makes links in this way and in the early stages of mania can have extraordinary confidence.

After having informed the class what it had been like to be at Lechlade, I proclaimed and repeated several times that everything was a paradox. Nobody, outwardly at least, disagreed with me. Either they were in shock or they were scared to be sparked out by a psycho. When I was asked to define the word "paradox" my immediate response was to say that the question was a paradox in itself. Alas, the mania only had its own internal logic you see. One eccentric member of the class who had been put forward to sit the Oxford entrance exam with me interrupted my Virginia Woolf-like stream of consciousness monologue, to which I responded: "Shut up Mr. Lockwood", which he did straight away.

My mind had been bordering on the absurd since I'd stayed, along with my English class, in the middle of the Yorkshire Moors a couple of weeks previously. The night before I had gone to a rave club and spent the entire night paranoid and lunched out on three trips. I had had no sleep and was fucked for the next four days. I hardly said a word on the five hour minibus journey and was just as paranoid with my classmates as I had been in the club. I remember the trip extremely well. We were studying the novel Wuthering Heights and spent the weekend at a grand and beautiful cottage. It was completely isolated just like the two houses in the novel *Wuthering Heights* and *Thrushcross Grange*. The weekend turned out to be a pilgrimage into the world of the Brontës and each of us recorded the events in a diary as they happened. We went to the Brontë museum, saw Peniston Crags where Heathcliff and Cathy professed their love for each other, and even walked through the graveyard where Emily Brontë is buried. I found the latter disturbing and remember the weather being particularly foggy.

After having a fucking strong Lebanese joint that I had picked up from a traveller the previous week I told my entire life story to a member of the class, Chris. He was black, very kind and intelligent, and his dad was a lawyer. He also knew a lot about the rave scene so I had respect for him. Once, he sent me a Christmas card with a poem he'd written about Mciing and getting off his head – and this guy was drug free. Now that was the sign of a tough cookie. I admired that. All his friends were on drugs and most of them dealt, but he was clean.

I was totally off my head as we sat on a fence in those bucolic surroundings and ranted on about everything that had gone wrong in my life. He would listen and on the odd occasion give words of advice. Sometimes in life he said it is "good to take three steps forward and then a step back". I thought of his interesting words but it was already too late. I had stepped too far forward and my legs would soon buckle under the pressure and be scarred forever.

In the club, two of my friends, Dom and Tim, were just as paranoid as I was. We sat cross-legged in the chill out room too scared to dance and too afraid to talk to each other. I broke the silence by asking someone to give me some Vicks Vaporub. He took the nasal stick out of the tube and rubbed it around my eyes. I sat down blinded, fearing that I would never be able to see again. One of my friends asked me what I had been talking about. My only response was to say that there was a guy in Swindon who had taken over 500 ecstasy tablets so far that year, 1993. My heart rate increased, and I struggled to handle a dozen Es. I felt weak psychologically as there was a simple philosophy in club life: the more Es, coke and ketamine you've taken the cooler you are perceived to be. It was a mad week which started with 15000 watts of hardcore pumping out and it took its toll, but it was nothing compared to the madness which had started to poison me during that English lesson. The only surprise was that I hadn't gone mad during a lesson on the manic-depressive Sylvia Plath's *Bell Jar* whose text I was also studying at the time.

My mind became more and more complex. My English teacher asked to see me after school on the day I lost it in her lessons. As I walked in to greet her I felt on top of the world. For whatever reason, although possibly because I felt secure in the knowledge that I was top of the class, I confessed everything about my drug taking to her. I was satisfied in the knowledge that I would form a sexual relationship with her although I anticipated that I would be the submissive one.

"Jason, before you say anything come and sit next to me and tell me what's going on." I replied in what I thought was an assured manner.

"There's going to be a nuclear war and I'm going to stop it. Look at these books… It all makes sense…"

"Are you on drugs?"

I was proud to inform her of my previous antics. "I've been smoking hash since I was 14, and have had speed, acid and ecstasy loads of times. Some of it's mixed with coke, smack and ketamine (that's a tranquilliser used on horses). I've had opium as well but never injected anything. Some of my mates do that, down the squat. (Mrs. Barnes proceeded to burst out in buckets of tears.)

"Oh you poor dear. Drugs are bad for you (now holding my hand). Don't you realise that? You've got to stop taking them. Will you promise to stop taking them for me?"

"Yes, miss."

"That's a good boy. Is anyone else taking drugs in the school?"

"At the end of the fifth year, 40 of my year had taken acid. There's a few in our form now, Chris, Nick, Ali, Paul, Mark, Gary and Emma, but none of them have taken as much as me. There's a few on acid in the fourth year, like Hanks, and they're all good recruits in helping to stop the nuclear war… I'm setting out a plan… got to succeed…"

"No more outbreaks in class, Ok? Go home and get some rest. Try to get some sleep tonight. Promise."

"Promise."

Meanwhile, I was positioning myself to be head of the

Bipolar, Recovery and NLP

European Hard core Committee. I mean, what the fuck was that? My intention was to create world peace by having everybody take drugs and dance as "one family". What a crock of shit. All I had done was take a rave anthem and attributed grandiose thoughts to it. I might as well have been one of the pingheads down the squat jabbering their heads off on billy. I wasn't changing the world. I wasn't making any difference whatsoever. Yes, I could have been staring out of a window at a tree for four hours without moving a muscle as one of my friends told me he had done. I would realise several months later that my thoughts were on a different level. At least when cooking up, you know when to expect the hit. I was permanently buzzing on another level.

I became fascinated by my untheorised theory that a nuclear war was imminent and proceeded to inform my friends of the phenomenon. First, I visited my good friend Brad (he was a pinghead so was therefore definitely on the level). We knew each other so well he would understand. He told me that he would buy me any reading material if it would help prevent the war. In my manic state, I manoeuvred everything in my room into a strategic position planning an unplanned course of action.

I set about organising a trip to Cheltenham to see Macbeth ... I wanted to reserve 12 seats and sit people in particular positions so they could discuss in detail which role they would take in my anti-nuclear war alliance. I rode round to see friends who showed apparent interest, but before the performance intense paranoia had set in. My closest friend was actually my worst enemy ... Everybody in Gloucester was plotting against me and I had to get out ... The only escape was to stay with another friend at Littledean in the Forest of Dean ...

My father's girlfriend, Claire, drove me to Gloucester bus station although I felt as if I was in a space shuttle ... From there I took the bus. The bus journey was ludicrous. I spent 25 minutes on the top deck of the double decker, at the back, speaking to a 14 year-old about my mission. *In my rucksack I had 30 or so books all of which were of significance and could be placed in strategic orders, coloured pencils, and several hardcore tapes each of which contained messages of prophecy* ... I told the boy that I was going to stop a nuclear war and that he should thank me ... I talked about rave culture and how it was taking over the world. During

Bipolar, Recovery and NLP

the entire journey he watched me intently but didn't utter a word. In hindsight, I think he was probably scared out of his wits and thought I was crazy. At the time, I thought he knew the score. I thought he was hard core and understood my mission. Maybe I should have listened to my brother who always said that repetitive music melts your brain and classical music enhances it. This is an intriguing point with some scientific evidence. Nevertheless, it was too late for me as the mania was too strong.

…

On arriving in Littledean, I was greeted with a cup of tea and a spliff and told to stop talking bollocks by my hippy and magic mushroom-selling friend, Ashley. This was the same person who I had comforted for hours on the phone several times when he was scared he had astroprojected into another world. Maybe he did have an outer body experience or maybe he just couldn't handle his acid. He went to sleep while I went downstairs. The old house was dark and quiet. His hippie mother and father were asleep as was his 13 year-old sister.

I performed some kind of manic ritual in the kitchen taking all my clothes off and rolling my wrist around very quickly while keeping my thumb forward. This was a habit that I had acquired having taken four grams of speed when dancing to hardcore at a club called Brunel Rooms in Swindon. I stared at the digital time on the microwave and intelligently waited until 4.44am… Then I could transport myself into the future… My paranoia had turned into ecstasy, or so I thought.

In my eyes, my friend's mother was the healer of the world and it was my duty to make Stoic love to her… Then I would have prevented Armageddon and been initiated as head of the European Hard Core Committee by her husband… I thought back to those times when he let me pick magic mushrooms from his land. I looked back with pride on the day he chose me. This was when he asked me, in his kitchen, how many magic mushrooms I had picked. He had an endearing smile on his face with a sense of natural goodness, honour and integrity.

Now it was time to act on my manic impulses and bring about my destiny… I walked around the house entirely relaxed and stepped into the young daughter's room. She saw me naked and yawned in what seemed like a totally relaxed and expectant manner. I left with a feeling that I had conquered the world and given this Virgin Mary what she had been waiting for... I rested in the spare room feeling a cross between a king and Little Red Riding Hood ... I opened the window expecting the wolf to come and was prepared to give it a beating. The monster would be followed by one of my many new female servants who would perform the sexual gratification that their master desired...

These rambling thoughts are typical of any manic episode and can never be properly understood unless you've experienced mania first hand. There are so many and they are so frequent that it is only possible to mention and recall a few of them. From the dominant master, I then focused on turning myself into an abject slave. I now took the line held by my English teacher. The first cultures were matriarchal and I sacrificed my mind, body and soul for the goodness of women and therefore mankind.

I can remember performing a ritual for my new mistress. I took a metal pole about two feet long out of the fireplace and placed it on the little finger of my right hand. There was some metal cord attached to it that I tied around my finger several times. As I did this, I relented my eternal craving and became the abject slave of a domineering woman.

By morning, I was still naked and from where he was feeding the horses her husband could see me in the spare room. In a firm manner he told me to get dressed. My friend saw the pole on my hand and told me to put it back before his mother got angry. I coyly replaced it and several minutes later I was watching television downstairs when my mistress asked me if I wanted some honey on toast. I was delighted – all the other times I'd stayed round there she had never offered me anything. I thought back to Jacques Lacan – live the language of your dreams. Therefore, in my mind, as soon as she uttered those words I had fucked her. I would never tell anyone as I feared my punishment for hubris would be too great... My imagination decided that her son and I would be treated like kings and would be given a different beautiful girl every night to copulate with... *Through this household world peace would begin to spread ...*

Her husband drove me home safely and quickly. Neither of us uttered a word. He arrived at my house, spoke to my father and left thick mud all over the carpet. Then I thought it was a compliment … Now I know it was a sign of disrespect.

Soon after, two of my friends asked me to come out and smoke some spliff. I declined on my dad's advice. I think deep down I knew that something was wrong with me as I usually ignored what my father said. To this day I do not know what my father's conversation with the old hippie was about and am still too embarrassed to ask.

I tore up magazines and displayed them on the two single beds in my room. Some of them were pornographic, and I organised material thinking that I was a sexual guru ... The sister of my friend in Swansea was my next conquest ... I read her a love ode from Horace over the phone when she asked for my brother. I could tell she was turned on although she didn't admit it ... After all, she was still just about seeing my brother and I was four years younger than them.

She was a woman and according to my interpretation of Lacan I had made love to her along with every other woman on the planet. The only difference was that I had given this one special treatment.

I went to the bathroom and realised another part of my destiny. Unfortunately, I wasn't to be an Aeneas founding Troy but would settle for being the Head of English at Balliol College, Oxford. I was also destined to be the most respected poet in Britain. I searched through a Sylvia Plath book and noticed that I had bookmarked a page. It was the poem entitled "The Graduate". My rediscovery of this marking meant that I was going to graduate with flying colours and I had not even applied for university at this stage.

This elation was similar to an epiphany I had experienced while I had been on ecstasy the previous week. The lemon and lime I had consumed was mixed with ketamine, smack and acid. I was in a nightclub with my best mates, Brad who was pinging up speed at the time, and Dominic. We all necked one along with a virgin E taker who disappeared and later told us amazingly that he did not feel a thing except for the alcohol he was drinking. I was higher than a kite within half an hour and after five minutes of insane dancing I decided to watch the dance floor telling Dom that I would be the greatest writer in the world.

Bipolar, Recovery and NLP

He was so off his box that he kept nodding his head and raising his eyebrows. The three of us walked home, and the ketamine made me feel five years old. Or was it the smack? Even now I don't know, I never mixed it whatever it was – but it was mind boggling. Dom walked home. Later, to my great surprise, he told me that he had gone straight to sleep. Brad and I talked until 9.00am about life, people, relationships, the universe and how we were going to pack the next spliff even more full of gear than the last one. We were stood in the local public toilets which were a common meeting point for pingheads. We shared the same cubicle once in a while taking it in turns to sit on the toilet seat. This was a crazy night, and I'd probably had the strongest pill I'd ever taken. There again, it's sweet fuck-all compared to mania.

Things were becoming more and more blurred. Somewhere in between my conscious and subconscious I believed that I had passed the next day's Oxford entrance exam without even sitting it. The exam was due the day I went into hospital and I was in no state to sit it. Despite correctly anticipating that Hardy's poems, and not his prose, were to be discussed, another manic realisation would be in vain.

I was to experience a journey that was to be way beyond the realms of normal consciousness. The indescribable and extraordinary links occurred more frequently and became more severe. By morning, I had demolished my room pushing all my books and everything else off the shelves. My dad heard me yelling from the garden. He saw me planning to throw my electric guitar out onto the patio from the first floor and urged me to put it down. In a sudden flash, I became jealous that I couldn't play the guitar as well as Hendrix and hurled it through the window.

My father shrieked "no" in despair. What had caused this outrage? Drugs no doubt. I find it hard to think about although I do recall an incident that had occurred earlier in that week with my brother. I interrupted his revision for the same entrance exam that I had missed in fits of tears. I had read *Wide Sargasso Sea* by Jean Rhys and had broken down. Was it that I cared too much about the human race and took it upon myself to endure the suffering of others? Was I hyper-intelligent? Was I genetically inferior to others? The answer was probably a combination of all three.

I told my brother that it was not fair that black people had

Bipolar, Recovery and NLP

suffered so much, but at least, I continued, the problem was being dealt with. He agreed and I thought once again about the happy black raver at school, Chris, who had showed me some dance moves, didn't take drugs at all and danced for Fantasia.

After I had thrown the guitar out the window in my manic state my dad sent my grandmother into my room to try and calm me down. She asked me if I wanted some honey on toast. I gleefully accepted it as if it were some kind of reward for being her precious grandson. When she returned she said that my brother wanted to see me. I asked my brother to listen to the tape that I was playing. It was Phantasy and SS, Fantasia Summertime 1992. The MCs, Joe Peng and Robbie Dee, were fucking intense.

"To those of you who know the score ... how's about a little bit of hardcore ... Speaker box climbers get off the stage - you are distressing it for everyone ... Get off the speakers ... For the last time get, off the speakers."

Instead of reacting and trying to comfort me by putting his arm round me my brother, who was eccentric at the sanest of times, stepped on my bed and started dancing. I shouted for him to get down. My dad came down and hearing my plea told him to do the same. As soon as he did I head-butted him. It was badly misplaced, and my brother dragged me to the floor putting me into the same stranglehold that he put my dad in when he threatened to hit my mum several years previously. Eventually my dad persuaded him to let go after crying out that we were brothers and that we shouldn't be doing this to each other.

Within five minutes my dad had called the police and an ambulance. Because my brother didn't want to press charges they said whether or not I went with the ambulance was down to me. Meanwhile, I thought this was all a test, perhaps part of the Oxford entrance exam, and that I still was destined for a life of psychological, emotional and physical ecstasy. I chose the ambulance and started to fantasise again. This time I was to meet the heartthrob of my youth, Alena Campbell. We had been close from the age of 14–16. Her brother went to my school and was tragically run over on his bicycle. We had been friends ever since. I was convinced that I would soon meet up with her and be the only man in a never ending mass eternal orgy of which she would be the head. I was destined to escape from an everyday life that

47

always had a sad edge to it.

I sat in the ambulance alone and was quite excited about my forthcoming adventure ... They took me to the hospital and lay me down on a bed. They asked me my name and a few other questions and gave me a brain scan. I thought that the 20 or so staff who were watching me believed that I was the most intelligent person in the world and that they were examining a brain which had worked out the way to bring world peace and happiness... (They were all dressed up as if they were going to perform an operation. This is no bullshit.) I thought I was going to be ruler of the world and that this was a historic moment... Jesus was my son and I was God ... I was on top of the world...

The ambulance then drove me to the police station. I thought that I was being kept in a safe haven as it wasn't yet the time to deliver the news to everyone. Everything seemed to make sense. Even the policeman who offered me a cigarette in the car park of the police station seemed to have a perfect cameo role... He was a clone of my stepbrother Paul... His spirit belonged to a family that had given my mother a happier life. He was a member of a family that had healed one of the suffering. In the reception at *Bearland* I thought I was playing the Commodore 64 computer game *Footballer of the Year*. Now even someone on heroin couldn't have a thought as fucked up as that. If they ever have, I can only offer my condolences – not my sympathy. You see, I never needed to put a needle in my arm to become manic and get suicidal afterwards. I had no choice. That's the difference between them and me. They can go to rehab and get off. Whatever pills I take, or relapse prevention work I go through, I'm stuck with it and that's the difference. They're more fortunate in that they don't get a life sentence. Sure, bad luck and unforeseen circumstances may have driven them to it, but everyone goes through shit at some point in their lives and most people carry on regardless. Sometimes it just boils down to a battle of will-power. That's what settles many differences between people – along with luck and opportunities or a lack of them. Ultimately, a drug addict or addict of anything becomes an addict by choice. Not me. I had no choice and I still have no choice. I fight every day to conquer my affliction and the best I can do is to minimise its effect or postpone the inevitable. It was not the experience itself that was always the most disturbing

Bipolar, Recovery and NLP

but the coming to terms with it afterwards.

At the police station I was taken to a cell and locked up. There was graffiti scratched all over the cell. I immediately noticed the rapper's name, Ice Cube, that had been carved on the door. I then started to think I was Ice Cube and that I was *Amerikkka's Most Wanted* ... I proceeded to kick the cell doors and walls for four hours. Soon I was smashing the cell window as hard as I could. This really hurt as my forehead was catching the top of the steel door.

There was only one interruption. A policeman entered with a cup of tea and placed it on the bed. Nothing registered, he might as well have poured it over my head. He must have noticed my new bruising but left without giving a fuck. What sort of inhumane treatment was this? By the time I saw another copper I had a bruise on my head the size of a melon. I continued to bang my

Head   on   the   steel   door   and   scream AAAAAAHHHGGGGGHHHH for a good half an hour. A pig came in and led me to an open room. He told me to get undressed and put the shower on for me. Taking my clothes he left a white suit for me to put on and walked off. I happily had a shower and thought that all the pain and suffering was over. I thought that I had to endure twice the pain that Christ did, as I was God ...

After my shower, I was locked in the room and started to plan my escape. I sat on the floor in the break dance position for a back spin and, in various yoga poses, worked out how I was going to climb the ceiling. I thought of DJ Spider and how I had my first E round his house – a White Calais. I had felt great. My eyes saw different things, everything sparkling, glimmering. I remembered that I had seen him at Fantasia. I remembered how I had not danced at Universe when I went with Brad the year before. I tried dancing for 10 seconds but felt so uncoordinated on the acid that I sat down in an even more paranoid state than I had been in before. We had a trip, two grams of billy and two and a half E's each. Brad was dancing all the time while I was lunched out and chain smoking, furious that I didn't have the courage to dance and bring the Ribena raver posse together as I had done so well in the Brunel Rooms before.

As I positioned myself to climb the wall, I revelled in the fact that the whole world was waiting for me to dance ... All these DJs

Bipolar, Recovery and NLP

were just waiting for somebody who knew the score ... A messiah, a prophet, a bringer of peace – and that was me, who would have believed it, a 17 year-old from Gloucester.

I'm not sure to this day how far I climbed. I seemed to have got suspended on the side of the wall somehow when my dad and stepmother approached looking at me through the clear door. In my naked state I felt proud and proceeded to put the white body suit on.

Now, the French psychoanalyst Jacques Lacan had taught me how to conquer my stepmother. At that time, she was the last woman on earth that I had to conquer. She had seen me naked and that was enough. I thought back to how, the previous night, I had woken her up when my dad was on nights. I had entered their bedroom wearing my father's fire uniform – fully equipped with his boots, waterproofs, jacket, helmet and gas mask. She screamed as I turned the light on. What happened after that I fail to remember. Maybe one day, if our relationship improves sufficiently, I will ask her.

My dad told me that he was going to take me to a place where they would take care of me. This was great, and was all in line with my theory. I found his tears comforting. It must have been a very emotional experience to realise that he was the father of God ... I mean, that is a pretty important role in life. I felt unique in the body suit.

As he left, he said that he loved me. This was the first time that I remember hearing those words from a father who I had always respected for his hard work and sporting expertise.

As I was being driven off in the back of a police van in a space suit, I thought I was Donovan Bad Boy Smith being driven to a rave. I could hear music in my head and flashed back to another night at the Brunel Rooms in Swindon. *The Brunel Rooms, a hardcore Mecca for druggies from Gloucester and surrounding areas in the early to mid nineties.* Donovan was so hard core when I saw him there that he'd refused to turn off his set at 3am. He'd carried on until 3.30am when someone finally turned off the electricity mid flow.

...

I arrived at Coney Hill mental hospital very late at night. A

50

Bipolar, Recovery and NLP

nurse greeted me with what I interpreted as open arms. I thought that she was a subservient witch who was going to join the aforementioned orgy. She gave me some pills to swallow. Pretty quickly I began to feel hazy. I went to the toilet in my pyjamas and started to cry when I attempted to urinate. The pain was excruciating – as though Satan himself was inflicting pain on my penis.

In bed I studied my book on Ursula Fanthorpe's poetry, scribbling all over it. I was still convinced that I was destined for stardom in some way and was comforted from the presence of what I believed to be an old school friend snoring in the bed opposite. It was Adam Rimmer, the only member of my year who had psyched me out. We were once very close until, when quizzed, I told his girlfriend that he had got off with another girl. A fight ensued that was pretty even but he made me think he was harder by threatening to get his mate Linden to beat me up. Linden was a few years older and was clearly harder than both of us, but lying in that bed I felt that Adam had forgiven me.

There were about 20 patients in all. I went round calling staff, patients and visitors alike different DJ names, while quoting the words of MCs. The ward consisted of a large lounge with a dining area, a small hall with a phone, a quiet room for visitors to see the person they were visiting in private, and a staff room strictly out of bounds to the patients. There were also two lock-up rooms at the end of the corridor.

Eventually, my mania began to wane. This was due to the drugs that had been administered, in particular the anal injection of Haliperidol that I had received on my arrival. For years, I was furious with these people for curbing those moments of internal magic. Mania had given me something in life that others could only strive for. I was perfectly happy. It didn't matter that I wasn't actually making any sense. I knew afterwards that it didn't last forever and that depression always ensued. I would long to have those moments of mania back, but instead I had to realise that I was actually in a mental asylum. I was living in a place that was meant for other people not for a chess champion and Gloucester rugby representative, and especially not for the person who believed he was the most intelligent pupil in his grammar school. This was not the life that a talented, but essentially normal, person

51

Bipolar, Recovery and NLP

should be leading.

I was surrounded by patients who were far older than me. I could see why some of them belonged there, but to me it didn't make any sense at all. I used to speculate on what I had done wrong. If I could find out, I would know never to make the same mistakes again. There were too many things to cope with: returning to sanity, realising that all my thoughts were incoherent, putting up with the humiliation of being in there, seeing how it affected the people around me and most of all being so unstable that I suffered from fits of rage and depression.

After a month, they released me from Section 1 and discharged me. I had calmed down and was somewhat depressed although this, apparently, was to be expected given what had happened. On Christmas Eve, my mum drove me to her house for the "festive" period. I didn't sleep and had her up all night writing poetry. Christmas day arrived, and to avoid ruining it my stepfather, brother and mum put up with my mania. They drove me back to hospital on Boxing Day. As we went down one empty road I tried to climb out of the back window.

I was admitted back into the ward and given some drugs, notably Benzotropine, that had an adverse effect. This period marked a black hole in my life. From 27 December, 1992 to 1 February, 1993 I suffered from complete amnesia. On 1 February, I remember standing on a bed and urinating on top of some newspapers when my mum walked in, similar to a scene in the film *Made in Britain*. I noticed that I now had my own room. My mum told me that I had been given the only individual room so that the staff could keep an eye on me because I was particularly ill. My mum cleaned up the newspaper by going to the toilet and returning with lots of tissue. To this day my parents, who visited frequently, have told me little about my behaviour during that period. My mum told me how I threw a chair through the common room window when I caught sight of my dad visiting. Dad proceeded to tell me that they then put me in a straight jacket. I presume that was because I threw the chair. My mum said that it took a group of five male nurses to restrain me. It was a shock to have no recollection of such a violent incident.

The depression of my first episode remains confusing. The experience was new and it's still hard to quantify. Above all, I was numb – sleeping all the time, avoiding any kind of social contact, lacking any kind of motivation to do anything. Nothing made me happy – whether seeing my friends, family or even playing music. You could have given me a million pounds and, although it would have registered, it would have meant fuck all to me at the time. It's hard to describe. You just have to fucking sit and wait or kill yourself if you can't hack it. Thing is, killing yourself takes thought and effort, and when people are massively depressed they lack motivation to do anything except perform natural acts like breathing, pissing and shitting.

I feel really shit. There's no future. I'm so unhappy and I'll never be happy again so I'll fucking kill myself. I'll jump off a building. That would kill me. Thing is, I'm too depressed to even fucking stand up let alone walk, and walk all the way up a fucking tall building. You must be fucking joking. I could get a lift but I don't want to see anyone. They'd only be wankers anyway and they wouldn't understand the shit I'm going through. I'll have another cigarette and kill myself that way. Shit, that's too slow. If I had some pills now I'd take a fucking overdose. I don't give a fuck. Thing is, I don't know what would kill me and I'm too depressed to go anywhere. Just want to stay here and feel like fucking shit. There's no future anyway so it doesn't fucking matter.

The thing about feeling suicidal is that it lasts for fucking ages. The thought process above repeats itself endlessly, and often on different levels. During the low parts of an episode, you think of all the possible ways of killing yourself: hanging yourself, shooting yourself, running in front of a tube (the latter has often been a very tempting one for me). The list goes on: drowning yourself, slitting your wrists, beating yourself to death, poisoning yourself, getting someone to shoot you, etc.

In hospital, I have seen lots of people who have tried committing suicide. Some were readmitted to stop another attempt, some were let out and tried it so came back in again, and others had tried it in the past. Some do it because they crave attention. These ones aren't really attempting suicide. Like my friend from uni, Roger, they merely inflict pain on themselves. If someone knows that they tried to kill themselves, they'll feel sorry for them, and that will give the attention seeker someone to talk to.

It's hard to spot the difference between a genuine suicide

attempt and a cry for help, although if anything, the ones who are quiet about it are usually more serious. It's a personal thing and not something you usually go bragging about to other patients.

The saddest thing is that the staff don't seem to give a fuck about it. I mean, they detach themselves from it. I guess they have to though – otherwise the daily routine would be too hard to bear. Also, if they always discussed it, wards would be more like uni philosophy tutorials on ethics. Sometimes though – and it really pains me to say it – they're not properly trained in these matters. A lot of them seem more interested in reading the fucking sport in the paper and bossing people around – quoting what patients are not allowed to do and shit like that. They don't give a fuck. Sometimes I wish the strictest and unemotional ones – because there is the occasional caring staff member – could swap places with a suicide candidate for life. They wouldn't be so fucking insensitive then, would they? No, they'd be curled up on the floor of the corridor like those other poor fuckers you see in the mental hospital trying to talk about their problems, or completely avoiding social contact with anybody and sleeping all the time. Some may be OK one minute and fucked the next, especially if they're receiving ECT (electro convulsive treatment) i.e. electroshock therapy.

When I first told my family that I felt like killing myself there were different reactions. My grandmother's was the most comforting. She would cry and say: "You poor little boy. I've felt like that you know. Just like that. And it's a terrible thing. It's a bloody terrible thing. But I don't feel like that anymore. You've gotta fight through it kid." My brother would either analyse why I felt like I did by interviewing me with carefully thought out questions or, if that failed, to make me feel better would tell me that it was a selfish act. It would be selfish because it would affect the rest of the family and he would be unhappy if I wasn't around at Christmas time. My dad would simply say: "Oh, bloody hell" in disbelief and then give me a slap on the head, telling me that he was there for me at any time of the day or night if I wanted to talk.

As for my mum, I think that it affected her the most. Her first response would be to try and snap me out of it by saying that "things will get better. The worst is nearly over now. You've got plenty of time to get well." When that didn't work, she would say:

Bipolar, Recovery and NLP

"I feel like that sometimes." She would often repeat this and would wonder what she'd done wrong when bringing me up. When I sensed this, I would become less self-obsessed and think of how terrible her life would be if I killed myself. Maybe it was a selfish act. I think the only reason why I haven't killed myself in the past is that I would feel guilty if I killed myself: guilty for hurting those close to me, especially my mum, dad and brother.

I'm lucky that I've never heard voices. Schizophrenics put up with a level of shit most of us could never imagine. They really have to get their stuff together and exert their willpower to reconnect with society. Take Winnie, for example, a black girl in Coney Hill. She was forever hearing voices that instructed her to kill people. She was a very strong-minded and caring individual and insisted that everyone read the bible and love each other – although for many people on the ward who were almost catatonic, along with the staff, she was the most disruptive patient there. She had been brainwashed by somebody or something and was now preaching the bible. One day, she was alone in the lock up room as she had been noisy on the ward. She kept on asking me to save her but I couldn't. She told me to stay strong and said that she loved me. I said that I loved her and I did, in a funny sort of way, but I also knew that she was the most disruptive patient there.

My strangest memory of assessing my manic state in Coney Hill was when I went for a brain scan. The nurse on duty told me that I was going to have a haircut. I still believed her when wires were being stuck to my head and a machine placed over my head and everywhere. What a nutter.

Routines exist even in mental hospitals. In hospital, there are the morning, afternoon and evening calls for medication. People generally smoke excessively, drink large amounts of tea, look depressed and sit down together for meals. Other activities include watching television and playing table tennis, which I became pretty good at. Few patients have sufficient concentration to read for long periods. Some go for walks around the grounds if they are allowed to and are up to it. I found refuge in the quiet room. Whenever I had a visitor I would take them in there and we would get some privacy away from the germs and bacteria in the main room. I could play my tapes in there and try and forget about what was happening to me. Time stood still for a moment until a visit ended. As time went on, though, the visits were less help because I was sinking into a deep depression.

I was exhausted by what had happened. I was tired of being ill, worried if I would recover or not and scared that I would be ridiculed if I returned to the outside world. My dad told me on one visit that he thought I was going to be a *cabbage* for the rest of my life. I couldn't feel comforted by what he said as my mood was too low. Now I can see that other people are less fortunate and that helps me keep my balance. Where was I going? What was happening to me? How was I going to explain this to everyone? How was I going to recover? I didn't care much anymore. I had gone through too much to be positive.

Time became the only real healer. It took time to accept the situation and time to adapt to it. I'm not sure how therapeutic psychiatric hospitals are. I mean, all they do is put depressed people together. How are they going to cheer each other up? They just add to the misery. The other patients might have helped me gain a perspective but it was not a positive one. It was still the loonies on the inside and everyone else on the outside. It felt like being in prison when I was innocent. I'd been caught but had not done anything wrong.

They had stolen my free spirit. My soul would have been better off wandering around on an island designated for people experiencing mania. Years later, one of my university professors agreed with me. Once I'd left, he told me that he had experienced similar problems. This didn't surprise me as he was very sharp and quite eccentric. I would be able to reach my manic potential on this island that I imagined myself on. Who knows, I could have come up with moments of inspiration and genius there and even acted upon them? I would have been special and capable of changing the world for the better. And if saving the world was beyond me, then at least I would have maintained my humanity and dignity. My free spirit would have thrived and blossomed.

I planned to try and be positive. I would fight this plague. I was glad that I wasn't normal. Ignorance may be bliss as Socrates once said; perhaps that was why I was so unhappy. I turned to epigrammatic poetry to raise my spirits. I would read them to everyone on the ward even those who were in a trance. They evoked a lot of rhetorical questions and assessed my mood better than I could in reality. I wrote hundreds of them only to throw them away in anger when I was trying to adjust back into society. Could I come back from the abyss? If I could then how could I fit back in, be told what to do by the system and suffer new burdens? I wasn't going to be a modern-day Sisyphus – pushing a stone up a hill all the time only for it to fall back down again wasn't my idea of fun.

I spent my eighteenth birthday in hospital. It was one fucked up occasion. About half a dozen patients were well enough to have some cake with me and we finished one bottle of buck's fizz in under three minutes. There was a celebration at my grandmother's house where my mum and brother were present. My mum and grandmother took several photos of me. My eyes were more dilated than they were when I was E'ing my bollocks off. They were worn out, beaten by all the medication that had gone through my mind and body. I felt nauseous whenever I thought of my mum and Nan's photo albums so I asked them to take those photos out. My mum wrote "Jason's eighteenth birthday" next to it. It was a loving but futile attempt to pretend that everything was normal. I feel that I looked like I'd injected an ounce of ketamine through my forehead with a syringe the size of a baseball bat. People's eighteenth birthdays are meant to be special or fun, not utter humiliation like that. It wasn't anyone's fault though, just how I felt.

I was to spend another three months in Coney Hill. I spent a lot of the time writing poems, playing the ward guitar, chain smoking, watching TV, playing table tennis, speaking to visitors, going for walks and participating in general ward activity. As I regained consciousness, the routine of the ward helped me to focus and the occupational therapy I undertook, along with mixing with patients and staff, helped me to regain a morsel of my self-esteem.

I had lots of visitors. My mum and dad would come near enough every day. My dad would often bring me a Mars bar and say that he loved me. My mum left her job in Wales for as long as was necessary and moved in with my Nan so that she could visit. This really helped me. She would try and be strong when seeing me and cry when she got back to her mum's house. My brother would come a couple of times a week and ride up after work and be positive. I know that it really upset him but never really knew

Bipolar, Recovery and NLP

what to say to compensate for all the suffering he endured because of me. What could I do? I was no Houdini. I couldn't stop him feeling this way.

I noticed that my mum and dad never came at the same time. This must have been planned. They still hated each other at the time and probably blamed each other for my being in there. They knew that any confrontation on their part would upset me. I guess it was also nice to see them separately as that meant that the time I spent with visitors was far greater. I wouldn't have wanted them to come together anyway. I couldn't have handled it.

It really helped when I had a visitor. It broke up the despairing monotony of ward life. I looked forward to seeing Brad the most. He was recovering from injecting speed by going to the gym most days and coming to see me. His presence made me feel that I could cope with returning to society as he was doing exactly the same thing. I remember him visiting me when I was particularly manic. As soon as I saw him I ran into my room and put all the clothes on in my wardrobe. I put on about a dozen tops, four pairs of trousers, half a dozen pairs of socks, two hats, gloves, shoes on my hands and feet and packed my rucksack full of the rest of my belongings. He laughed.

"Jase, what are you doing?"

"I'm getting out of here man. I've had enough of it here."

"Do you fancy a game of table tennis?"

"All right."

I kept trying to smash every point for a winner and Brad laughed throughout the game. He won pretty easily because of this. Afterwards, we went back to my room, stuck on a hardcore tape, sat down and lit up a cigarette.

"What are you doing now?" asked Brad.

"I've decided to stay here for a while."

Brad is in stitches and I have a grimace-like smile because of the high dose of medication that I'm on.

I also looked forward a lot to Tim coming. He was in my original year at school and visited me almost as much as Brad. He saw me at one of my lowest moments. We were sat in the living room one time when my jaw started to twist. I had not been given enough Procyclidine and was unable to speak. I was crying because of the extreme pain. My jaw would wind down, rest for a moment and then start up again. They gave me some Procycladine that worked very quickly.

Years later, Tim told me that after that visit he burst into tears. He couldn't believe what had happened to one of his closest friends. This made me realise what it must have been like for others that had watched me suffering. I was so lost in my own depression and self-pity that I didn't stop to think of the lasting effect it had on my family and friends. My dad never said how it affected him but he was very calm and positive about it all. He understood that I had had a rough time but encouraged me to get on with it. My mind was often in a state of flux so any positive comments I heard would be mixed in with the negative effects of my depression.

A handful of people came to visit me once. Derek Gabb, Nicholas James and Paul Kingsbury, Kerry Tamlyn and Jenny Tomlinson, Helen Cosgrave, Petal and Sam Checkitts. They either came because I asked them them to, because they were concerned or because they were simply curious. People are generally curious about what it is like to be mad but don't want to get too close. I had a card delivered to me sent by Denmark Road High School for girls. That was very moving – dozens of girls had signed it. I knew most of them.

Chris, the dancer from school, and his friends came to visit but were turned away. The staff thought that they were going to give me drugs. Fucking hypocrites. They wanted to see me, not give me drugs. Anyway, the drugs the consultant had given me had fucked me up more than anything else. They had given me amnesia and caused me to have a serious relapse. I had no energy to fight anything. My will was weak, and I was tired, worn-out and ill. My confidence had been shattered and my sense of reality was permanently altered. Nothing would be the same. After a brief recovery period, though, my attitude to life changed. I was tougher and didn't want to take any shit from anyone anymore.

One day, my classical civilisation teacher, Mr. Moss, visited. This was a pleasant surprise, and he told me that he looked forward to me coming back to school when I was back on my feet. He was a wonderful man who gave me the confidence and inspiration to become a writer. He apologised on behalf of my French and English teachers who couldn't come but sent their

Bipolar, Recovery and NLP

love.

I was gutted that my English teacher couldn't make it. I had only known her for a few months but she had been an inspiration to me. I guessed then that she just couldn't handle the drugs thing. I felt that she had let me down as I had heard that she had intended to visit. For a while afterwards, I regarded her as a selfish bitch that talked the talk but didn't walk the walk. Eventually, I forgave her.

I clung anxiously to Coney Hill's recreational activities to try and stop the depression taking over. I somehow had to escape the monotony of the ward. The first activity I tried was football at 8.00am in the morning. This forced me to change my sleeping pattern at the time, which was to hide in bed until at least one in the afternoon. Sometimes, I was pressured into getting up by the staff. At other times, I was prodded but they often gave up after a few attempts. They wouldn't physically force me out of bed but would draw the curtains or steal my sheets. When I was sunk in depression their actions would make no difference and I would sleep without any covers. During the most severe bouts, I lay in bed for 20 hours a day. I would only get up for food, to go to the toilet or if a visitor came in and coaxed me out of bed. Then I would return to bed as soon as they left. However, when I started playing football I had recharged enough to consciously make up my mind to get back into society, and this seemed the appropriate place to start.

We had to do warming up exercises in a group. I found it rather embarrassing as I was a sporty type and knew of better warming up techniques. I felt like I was in a junior school games lesson. Then, to my despair, we were issued with a foam ball. For fuck's sake. Anyone who's played with a sponge football knows that it's impossible to achieve power and fluid passing. There again, the exercise was good so I went a few more times during the weeks that followed. Not many people turned up and the opposition was rather poor but it did my self-confidence some good.

I soon took up another class. Relaxation classes were more popular than the football, probably because everyone was depressed and just wanted to sit there like cabbages. Also, the room was only 20 metres away from the ward whereas the gym was a 10 minute walk.

Bipolar, Recovery and NLP

During relaxation classes, a group of up to 15 people would sit upright in chairs. Soft music was played in the background and the co-ordinator would ask us to close our eyes. She would tell us to make sure that our backs were straight, our feet and knees together, and our palms and elbows resting on our upper legs. Then she would ask us to follow her, breathing in deeply and slowly, and breathing out in the same manner.

The first few times I went I found it refreshing and relaxing. Then I lost interest. I would start to cheat and see if everybody actually did close their eyes. They did and were unaware that I was looking at them. The last time I went, I even fell asleep. I didn't see that as especially relaxing as I could fall asleep back on the ward. What's more, when I was on the ward I could have a cigarette when I wanted to. Fags were a great comfort for putting up with the endless boredom and the periods of anxiety that I so often felt. Most of the patients were heavy smokers and you were permitted to smoke anywhere apart from the lounge, dormitory, kitchen or staff room. That left the main room and outside – if you were allowed to go out for a walk, that is. Some patients were voluntary and could go out if they told the staff where they were going, while those on section had to wait until a member of staff was available.

There were other forms of occupational therapy, but I didn't participate in any apart from pottery, which I went to only once. I was a great fan of sixth and fifth century BC, Attic Black and Red Figure Pottery. I was most impressed by the magnitude of the *François Vase*, and was impressed by the fact that after it had been dropped somebody had managed to put over 1200 pieces back together. All I could think of when in the pottery room was the love scene in *Ghost* where Patrick Swayze and Demi Moore get covered in clay. This love scene made me feel lonely. Five months before I had thought that I was the most attractive man in the universe and the most appealing to all women. Now I was living in a mental hospital in the company of grannies who were knitting and sewing; and despite having seen a dozen or so naked women and received some good blowjobs I had only had sex properly a few times. Maybe this was why I was ill. Maybe I lacked the emotional support that a caring relationship would have given me.

I had one vaguely sexual experience in hospital. I went to have a bath and, passing the unlocked door, saw a girl called Karen lying in it. She was demented and cried out my name so I left the room worried that the staff would come in and put me on a six month section. I didn't want to be trapped for longer because of one incident and I was too shy and considerate to make a move on her.

It took the approval of three professionals to put me on a month's section – the whole process being quite thorough. There was a ward round once a week that was intended to discuss anything on the patient's mind. Unfortunately, these are often overcrowded and full of student doctors whose presence can often intimidate the patients. They are also rushed and the patient will usually come out of one even more stressed unless represented by an advocacy worker. If you're ever in this situation make sure you get one. It's unlikely, however, that you'd be told that you have a right to one if you are in hospital. Apart from the ward round, there is no contact with the consultant who prescribes your medication unless you persistently beg the staff to make an exception.

The nurses keep an eye on you and are sometimes pleasant. However, they're careful not to get too friendly as it's deemed to be unprofessional. In any case, the patients don't usually want to get too close either as they are generally not in the mood to make friends and deep down resent the authoritative figures that wake them up every morning, figures from hell that keep stepping on your toes. Such views are, of course, unfair in a way but commonplace nonetheless. These nurses were genuine people who chose to help others for a living. Still, I will always be a bit sceptical about this. Nobody can deny that the job involves a kind of power trip. This is most resonant when medication time is called. Every patient is given their medication in a particular order and is expected to be grateful. Only the charge nurse is permitted to give out the medication in case any mistakes are made, and sometimes they dish out crushed tablets to the patients. I know some people who've said that it's fine to eat crushed tablets when probed. But if they ever read the little notes accompanied with Lithium or Sodium Valporate tablets, they'd learn that this is not the case.

Why should we be grateful about taking pills anyway? It's a bloody nuisance having to take lithium every night for years, I can tell you. When taking the pills they feel uncomfortable, get caught in the throat, give you a dry mouth, make you wake up to go for a pee and then sometimes you can't remember if you've taken them or not. Because they are so important, however, your lifeline in fact, you get stressed out about it and confused.

Some patients would spend the whole week demanding to speak to the consultant and as soon as they'd finished talking to him or her they would demand another consultation. These psychiatrists were busy enough. Patients would revere them and think that they could cure not only their illness, but their emotional problems too. It was as if the consultant ruled the world. Well, then I guess they have the same power cravings as the nurses, probably even more so. But then doesn't everyone have these tendencies? We all want to be in control of something or someone. Why do so many of us have pets? To have a loyal companion? I don't buy this assumption and I never will.

To help me adjust back into society from hospital I was allowed weekend leave. My first night out I went into town with two of my friends, Kevin and Brad. We went to the pub and got slaughtered. People knew where I had been and greeted me with a simple "Hello Jase" or "All right Jase". We then went on to a nightclub. As I hadn't drunk any alcohol for five months I was legless by the end of the session. My two friends rang my dad's doorbell, propped me up against the door and made a quick getaway. My dad answered the door, stopped me from falling and put me to bed. I spent the rest of the weekend sobering up. As time went on, I would spend more and more time at home. I felt embarrassed as I recalled manic thoughts that I had had in the house. This was very difficult for me as my dad and his girlfriend were both acting as if everything was normal. I'm sure it was extremely difficult for them as well. I mean how were they supposed to act? There were no guidelines for them to follow.

I had started to see a counsellor regularly towards the end of my stay in hospital. He was helping me establish a firm footing with the outside world. I would continue to see him once a week for the next 12 months. He was a polite, perceptive and reasonably intelligent man but was a bit robotic and always gave the impression that he was telling me what I wanted to hear as opposed to the truth.

Bipolar, Recovery and NLP

I would sometimes feel patronised, paranoid, humiliated and belittled. This was hardly surprising considering I was relaying my innermost thoughts to a complete stranger. I don't really feel that he ever got to the bottom of what was wrong with me. No matter what I told him about my past, my family or my mania he would never actually know what it was like to be me. What's more, he didn't really understand me. When I told him that I wasn't going to see him again, he didn't believe me. He still made an appointment for the following week. It was as if, despite his intelligence, he was somehow artificial, too squeaky clean and incapable of true empathy.

Maybe it was the nature of the profession itself, being too regimental, too organised, too out of touch. I know that I left at the right time because I was becoming too self-analytical, too honest and too engrossed in my own psyche. I would leave school when everybody else was having lessons and go and speak to my psychologist about things that I had only just found out about myself. This was part of my weekly routine and it was absurd. I felt different, an outsider.

I would never be able to return to being normal after living in Coney Hill. No matter how secure my recovery was I would always have the knowledge that I had lost my sanity completely and the people sat next to me in class hadn't. They knew what had happened but never uttered a word. They covered everything up by just saying "All right Jase." That was fine with me, as I would have felt uncomfortable talking about it.

One of the last days I spent in hospital I had a long talk with my key worker. His name was Alan and his role was to follow my progress on the ward. He was a nurse that I was allocated to for special attention. He was a very chirpy chap who always tried to reassure me that everything was going to be all right.

I asked him if a diagnosis had finally been reached. At last, he told me it was called "manic depression". He told me not to worry, though, as it may never happen again. I was relieved because I wasn't sure I would be able to cope with another breakdown. I wish that Alan had got his facts straight or been more up front with me at the time and informed me that 95% of sufferers have another relapse – if he had, maybe I would have taken better care of myself in the years ahead.

Bipolar, Recovery and NLP

Chapter 3 – Back to reality…?

Because I only made it back to school a month before the end of the year I ended up dropping down to the lower sixth for a re-run. I also switched from A-level French at school, which wasn't going too well, to politics at Gloscat College on Tuesday evenings in Cheltenham.

In my new year, I had only one real friend, Kev, who'd visited me in Coney Hill a couple of times despite his dad telling him not to. I didn't really question his dad's reasoning – after all, I could understand that, as a parent, he didn't want his son hanging around with a card-carrying loon.

I appreciated the fact that Kev had ignored his old man. Here was someone who was really making an effort to get closer to me. As a result, we became close friends. He accepted my madness and found it intriguing – exciting even. This helped me relax when I was in his company and I even made a joke or two about myself.

At weekends, I'd usually go out with Kev, although sometimes Brad would come along too. We drank a lot of alcohol but steered clear from drugs. Christ, drugs had put me in hospital, made Brad lose the plot and turned Kev paranoid.

Anyway, it was pretty depressing seeing everyone from my old class leave Gloucester for university when I had to stay. I mean, it wasn't as if I'd failed my exams – I'd just been, how do you put it, held back. When I was in hospital I was told that the whole school had prayed for me to get well. This was a comforting feeling as I thought that I was going to be expelled for taking and selling a few drugs. But why?

I'd put loads of effort into extra curricular activities over the years, had been a member of the school chess team from the start and was even about to be school Chess Captain for the second year running just before I got ill. I was also a key member of the 1st XV having scored loads of tries over the years, even in a Schools' Cup Final. Fuck, I should have been made school captain but I ended up in the loony bin.

I'll always remember what it was like to play, win and score a try on Gloucester's infamous rugby ground, Kingsholm. Twenty minutes had gone in the first half of one cup final and we were getting hammered by a tough comprehensive school called

Bipolar, Recovery and NLP

Saintbridge. We were lucky to be only one try down. Hundreds of their pupils had taken the afternoon off school and we got booed when we went out onto the pitch. It seemed to intimidate the whole team as we only had a couple of dozen supporters, if that. Anyway, I was so pissed off with the way that our team was playing that I ripped the ball out of my scrum half's hand and ran forward yelling, like a man possessed. I was so proud of Tommy's that I simply couldn't envisage losing this match and not holding up the trophy. As I ran forward I broke one tackle, then two, then three, then four using my famous hand off every time. When I was eventually tackled, I managed to stay on my feet until reinforcements arrived. I'd run from my own 22 into their 22. We were awarded a scrum and two minutes later we scored our first try. My run had totally changed the impetus of the game – until that moment we were fucked. We ran out deserved 23–11 winners and I scored one of our three tries. After the game, Bilous, one of our toughest players along with me, came up to me for the first time ever and congratulated me on the way I'd played. He mentioned the run and called me a psycho. I knew that he meant it as a sign of respect. The scrum half also mentioned the run I'd made and both of them knew that it had changed the psychology of the game.

I was the only pupil from the school to represent Gloucester at Under-16 level and got into the county squad. I proudly wore my tie at school which was different to everyone else's. I also competed for the school at chess, cross-country – and even on the streets. When anyone from another school, be it state or public, put Tommy's down for being full of pompous geeks, I put them right, sometimes verbally, sometimes physically.

However, one thing that really pissed me off when I left school was that I wasn't in the hall of fame – unlike my black friend, Panji, who played for England at basketball. I was also surprised that I wasn't chosen to play for England Under-18s at chess.

I hadn't really got to know Panji that well at school despite the fact that we'd been mates in the first and second years. As he moved through the years he became increasingly introverted, playing his Walkman all the time. However, Panji was fucking hard. In the first year, he'd even make some of the kids cry when we played "stinger" – a game in which whoever had the tennis ball

Bipolar, Recovery and NLP

threw it as hard as they could at whoever they wanted to. With Panj, you could hear a real sting when the ball made contact.

In our year, Panj and I were the best at that game – the hardest throwers – although he was probably more accurate than me. Maybe that was why we were good mates. He had a lot of willpower and endured a lot of racism at school. He took it all in his stride until he was about 16 then started beating the crap out of everyone who'd taken the piss out of him over the years. It was fucking great. I remember a big group of us about to play football one day when this fat kid called Stuart Finch said: "We're not going to let the nigger play, are we?" Panj went over, decked him and kicked him in the head once, in a clinical fashion. I said: "Nice one Panj, come on, let's pick teams." One thing that always amazed me was that Panj said he could never remember the incident. Well, I did: it was a classic moment of justice, of freedom beating years of oppression. After that, and after he'd beat up the other ringleaders, people finally shut up. Not only did they respect him but they feared him and that gave everyone a buzz whether they admit it or not.

...

The day after my A-level examinations I flew to New York with Kev. We were going on holiday for six weeks and staying with acquaintances of our families. For the first half of the trip we stayed with Bill and Francis Spicer. Bill was the chief of Woodbridge fire station which was about a half an hour drive from the centre of Washington. Basically, my dad had worked as a fire officer for 30 years and had organised several exchanges between families and fire fighters of Woodbridge and Gloucester fire station, so knew Bill quite well. For this trip, he had planned everything: the flights, excursions, who was staying with who, etc.

When he heard that I was keen to go to America he wrote to Bill asking if we could stay with him for a couple of weeks and Bill was happy to oblige. My dad said that he had written instead of phoning because he wanted to give Bill "thinking time", as he put it. I'm always amused when I hear my dad repeat this story, partly because I like the way he tells it, and partly because I appreciated it and I knew that he was pleased that he'd helped me out.

Bipolar, Recovery and NLP

When we finally got there our accommodation was great. We had a huge downstairs apartment with a five-foot square TV, a fridge full of food and refreshments, an outdoor basketball court and a hot tub. They made us feel very welcome, taking us out to restaurants, bars and malls. Kev wasn't really into the tourist stuff so we spent a lot of time drinking and chatting up girls – although we did go to the Whitehouse and even saw the President. That day there were about 50 people queuing up by the entrance. They stopped the traffic and then a convoy emerged. There were four huge black limousines and the president of the time, George Bush Senior, was in the third. The entourage consisted of a dozen police cars and motorbikes.

Everyone was really friendly and loved our accents. We even went on a firemen's training exercise where real buildings were burnt down. We put on all the equipment and went into two different fires. I was positioned near the exit and was told by one of the fireman to put my thumbs up when I wanted to get out. As the fire was lit, the tops of my feet were the first part to heat up. Then I could feel my knees, the palms of my hands and my face stewing. I was in there for about a minute but got out safely. I took my helmet off and wiped the sweat from my forehead. I handed the helmet to Kev – it was his turn next.

His experience was far more dramatic. He said that when he was inside a huge part of the ceiling smashed on the floor right next to him. He couldn't believe that it hadn't hit him. He thought that if it had landed on him, he would have been dead for sure. He was fucking relieved to get out of there.

Bill took Kev and I to our first ever baseball game. It was a minor league team and there were 6000 spectators. It was a much friendlier environment than at a football match in England. One thing that struck me was how Bill and his second son Patrick stood up and put their hand on their hearts as they sang the American national anthem. For as far as I could see everyone was stood up and singing it, and this was only a small domestic match. It showed that the Americans have a great deal of pride in their nation.

Maybe this is one of the reasons why they're so successful economically. Christ, every person we met, car we went in, house we visited, restaurant we ate in, shop we looked in, whatever, was

Bipolar, Recovery and NLP

bigger and better than its English counterpart. Even Big Macs, which came in at just under a dollar, were twice the size of the ones back home.

One great day out with Bill and Francis and their three sons (Billy, Patrick and Billy Junior who were fifteen, nine and six respectively) was when we went to a huge amusement park. There was one roller coaster that went upside down three times and even underwater. Another great afternoon was when Bill, Kev and I had a go on the automatic baseball machines. We took it in turns to go in a cage with a helmet and bat and hit balls at different speeds. It was cool, and so was America. It was a great place to be.

The next family we stayed with lived in the posh fishing town of Annapolis. This, like Woodbridge, is a half-hour drive from central Washington. The mother was an old friend of Kev's mum, and her husband was a former admiral in the American navy. It was like living in Fort Knox. We couldn't stand them. We weren't allowed any alcohol in the house and they said that they wanted us back early each night to sit down and have a formal lunch with them. We wished we were back at Bill's making huge sandwiches from his enormous fridge.

We were also being hounded by their stuck up eight year-old daughter who was trying to follow us everywhere. She was even bossier than her parents were. After a few days of suffering, we met a local lifeguard called Drew and told him about our dilemma. He was a few years older than us and said we could spend the rest of our holiday chilling out with him and his friends.

We'd stay round their houses most nights, get pissed and stoned and have a wicked time. We bought loads of crates of beers, with the fake driving licenses we'd picked up, and drank them at gatherings and parties. One night we went to see an American legend in concert. We were part of Drew and his mates' convoy. There were about 20 of us all together. We bought a shit-load of Bud and other lagers on the way. We got there six hours before the show started and parked the cars up next to each other. We must have had the loudest stereo system there. It was four hundred watts and we blasted out Guns and Roses or chilled out to Bob Marley as the sun shone down on us. Spliffs and beers were being passed around left, right and centre.

It was a beautiful day. The weather was so hot that summer.

Bipolar, Recovery and NLP

Hotter than anything I had experienced before. I remember walking out of a mall with Kev one day and it was so extreme and humid that neither of us wanted to walk to the phone box to ask for a lift. I loved the sun like most people and realised how much I had been deprived of seeing it by living in a country without a sunny climate.

The man in concert, Jimmy Buffet, was a cross between Bob Marley, and Country and Western, and could really play the guitar – although I've never met anyone in England who's heard of him. 15,000 Americans sang to his famous song which started: "Come on, let's get drunk and screw." To get into the concert we all climbed over a 15-foot wall. There was a middle bit that you could rest on and people were pulling their friends over from the other side. There was a lot of fighting after the concert, though, because people were getting squashed crossing a footbridge on their way back to their cars. This dampened the occasion somewhat but I had still had a great day.

When hanging round with our new friends during the day we'd play a lot of street basketball with the local black kids. I became a pretty mean player by the end and could even do a one-handed slam dunk, although I admit that the basket was a foot lower than professional height. At parties people would be taking helium, swimming, fucking and getting wrecked.

One game that was often played was called "asshole". It was a brilliant drinking game. You'd basically play a game like whist and each player would be ranked: there would be a first in command, say a general, then a second in command, a few other ranks and finally the asshole. Each player could tell the players below them what to drink at any time within limits agreed before the start of the game. Positions would alter depending on the outcomes on the next hand. So the asshole could become the general in the following round. The game livened everybody up and people would team up against others and get revenge when they could. Lots of people would throw up and everyone would cheer when somebody had a good swig of beer or downed a big shot. The funniest thing was being able to say "drink up asshole." It was such a humiliating experience but so funny when saying it to somebody else.

Kev and I got really drunk at one party and had some powerful bongs. We ended up having an argument in which we threatened each other and I suggested taking it outside. This guy, who was 6' 5" and 18 stone, declined. The next day, we had an in depth discussion while relaxing at an outdoor private swimming pool. He said that he could have beaten me up when I was asleep. I don't think we would ever have hit each other, though. I mean, I could never imagine hitting Kev – we had been through too much together. He'd become a close friend when Dominic was at university and I owed a lot to him. He'd basically befriended a madman and risked his own sanity and reputation in the process. Not many people would have done that. I also admired his ambition and respected him as a rugby player. I would still have returned to school if he hadn't been there but he seemed to make the transition back easier.

Back to the States. One bloke called Butler, who knew Drew, drove us down to stay with his aunt in a place called Ocean City. It was here that I was to discover the beer bong – a funnel joined to a tube resulting in an accelerated form of drinking. His aunt was an alcoholic so we got on well. She lived in a trailer that looked identical to the other 5000 trailers that surrounded it. Later that night, I split up from Kev and was wandering round pissed out of my mind looking for the trailer until five in the morning. I only found it because a policeman ended up driving me around looking for it. All I knew was that there was a brown Pontiac parked outside and that the trailer was green or blue.

...

On returning from America I worked full-time as a summer holiday 'Play Scheme Leader' for two months. Dominic had got me the job. It was fun and we were responsible, with two other staff, for the safety and entertainment of 40 five to eleven year-olds. I also started back at the video shop that I'd had worked in since September 1993. I would open the shop on Saturday mornings and work Saturdays and Sundays. I was the only person working in the shop and would study when it was quiet. The job helped restore my communication skills with people after my stay in Coney Hill and helped nurse me back to having a structured life. It also gave me a bit of extra money.

I'd spent a week in Manchester on a politics course in the

Bipolar, Recovery and NLP

January before my A-levels and had been shown around by some of Dom's mates from university. I knew I wanted to go there. I helped them shift loads of fake designer clothes by telling all the kids at school. They gave me a fake jacket and took me out for a drink. That was fucking tight considering I must have made them over 500 quid for less than half an hour's work. One of them lived in Manchester and his name was Oliver. He was the biggest drugs dealer I knew. He would buy and then shift 10 kilos of weed and 2,000 E's at a time. I was taken in by his flash Volkswagen GTI, designer clothes and slick personality. Thing is, I knew he was a bit of a wanker at the same time, happy to rip off his mates and all that. Once, he sold me loads of fake designer clothes to sell at school. I knew they were fake but I trusted him and gave him the money before I could work out how much I could reasonably sell them for. I had to rip off another mate to make any kind of profit. In just a few seconds, Oliver had help to ruin a friendship that I had had for several years and which didn't heal until I got back in touch and apologised in January 2002.

I was embarrassed that I had been so gullible. I can't believe I never beat him up. Kev only met him once and swore that he would beat him up if he ever saw him again. I was attracted by Oliver's charm and wealth and thought that if I hung around with him then I'd get rich like him. Instead, I just allowed him to be cheeky. He got his dues though. A couple of years later he bottled somebody outside a nightclub in Swansea and did some time. I wrote him a letter while he was inside saying that I knew what he was going through as I'd been sectioned and I made comparisons between the two then wished him luck. I've seen him several times since and he's never even mentioned it. These days he's a very successful and legitimate businessman. He always had that drive to do something different. I guess we were very similar in that way. As for me, back then, I was clearly living a risky life and I was lucky things hadn't got worse.

One fight, when I was 18, was a close call. It was on the way back from college and was pretty ugly. Kev picked me up with two local crims. They were working on a pure commission basis but we had no intention of paying them. We drove them around for an hour and they stole about eight stereos. One of them became restless and said he wanted some speed. Kev took his friend aside and I refused to pay him. It was dark and he tried to make a grab for the bag that contained the stereos. I pushed him away and he hit me on the side of my eye with a screwdriver. I went into a frenzy like Agave when tearing up her son in Euripides' Bacchae. He could have blinded me, that fucker. That motherfucker. I grabbed him and smashed his head against the car bonnet. He kept falling down but I kept pulling him back up and doing it again. As I smashed his head against the side window he somehow managed to slice me with a Stanley knife across my forehead. I got him in a headlock and punched him in the head about 200 times. He had a broken nose and a lump on his forehead the size of a tennis ball. He wriggled himself free and I kicked him as he ran off. He started to cry, saying to the other two that I was fucking crazy. We ended up keeping the stereos and made some cash, but I nearly lost my eye in the fucking process. I cleaned myself up round Kev's house. His mum and dad were very concerned and helpful. Then Kev's dad took me home and explained to my dad what he'd been told had happened. We told our parents that we'd been trying to prevent some men from stealing Kev's car in the college car park in Cheltenham. My dad said that it was lucky Kevin was with me, otherwise I could have been even more injured. What little he knew about my life, I thought. The irony was that it was Kev's great plan that nearly led to me losing the sight of one eye. My dad's remark made Kev sound like a hero and there is never one when violence is concerned. It's hypocritical to use violence to stop violence – anybody knows that. It takes a braver man to walk away. The guy I beat up didn't come out for three months after the fight, and at the same time his girlfriend started wanting to go out with me. I got off with her once or twice but by the time I came back from America she was being fucked by another thug.

When I got back from America I was to get my A-level results. I'd set my heart on Manchester confident that I would get the grades. When I found out that I'd got in, I was over the moon, all the more so for the fact that my grades hadn't been great – I'd got four C's in English, politics, classical civilisation and general studies. It was a phone call from my classics tutor that had made the difference. He became a character reference and said that my grade C was a great disappointment given the fact that I'd had an "A" in my mock. I've never seen or spoken to him since but sent him a thank you postcard the first week I was there. I stayed in Whitworth Park during my first year. It was situated close to town and on the borders of the infamous Mosside estate. There were 1,500 students in these halls and in the whole of Greater Manchester a total of 50,000 students. This total consisted mainly of students from Manchester University itself, UMIST, and the Metropolitan University which was really a Polytechnic.

Manchester was much bigger than Gloucester. It would be a challenge living there and a whole new experience. I knew living there would broaden my mind and give me a university life to remember. I could go to a new city and forget about being a madman. In a strange way, though, I was somehow proud of it as it made me unique.

Bipolar, Recovery and NLP

Chapter 4 – Mad for it

In September 1994, about 15 months after leaving Coney Hill, I went to live in Manchester to study a BA (Honours) in Classical Studies. In April of that year, I'd visited a friend there with Kev and we'd both fallen in love with the place. On one of the nights we got tanked up and went straight to the Hacienda. Inside, Kev told me that I was a really good dancer. Quite a compliment really: this wasn't one of those cheesy nightclubs in Gloucester. The Hacienda was hardcore – and I fitted in because I'd seen the dark side of life.

My attendance of lectures was poor from the start although, in hindsight, I suppose I was simply fulfilling the fresher's role: students, in particular freshers, try to make themselves look intelligent and try to show that they can get the best possible grades with the minimum amount of effort. It was all part of the game.

Anyway, I was so excited about being in a big city and having a grant and student loan that I didn't really think about studying. This was compounded by the fact that I'd actually intended to read politics at Manchester, rather than classics, and was probably in the wrong state of mind from the start. I also kept postponing my work because I knew I could write good essays and easily catch up when deadlines started to loom.

There was also a lot less discipline at university than there was at school. If you didn't hand in a piece of work most of the tutors failed to chase it up. What's more, I'd already studied a lot of material on the first year's syllabus at A-level and found it boring, so much so that I even tried to make my thoughts known. During the second week, I even went to see my personal tutor and asked her to advise me on writing an essay. Basically, a lecturer had set me an essay but he hadn't discussed the length of it, etc. I wanted to know the difference in quality between a good A-level essay and a good university essay. I wanted to get ahead. I also wanted to know the difference between a good first year and a good second year essay and the difference between an "A" in the second and an "A" in the third year. Then I could set my benchmark and go for it when everyone else had hangovers. Me? I had the answer to hangovers: Lucozade, and lots of it.

Bipolar, Recovery and NLP

I really wanted to tell her about my illness although this urge was more subconscious at the time. You see, I needed to trust somebody first before I could open up to them. She just brushed me off saying that she couldn't write the essay for me and looked shocked to see me taking my studies so seriously.

That same week, I went to the University Counselling Service and spoke to a receptionist and told her of my illness, but there was a long waiting list and I didn't feel comfortable. Instead of having a discussion in private we were in the middle of a room where other people could hear what we were talking about. I never went back there and my university life was markedly worse as a result.

My first few weeks at uni were spent in a drunken haze like most freshers but afterwards, and unlike the others, I failed to settle down. I started drinking more and more. There were the usual distractions at first – selling speed, ecstasy and hash to students, nightclubs, meeting new friends, and women. And then, a few days before Christmas, things took a downward slide and I really started to throw it back. I arrived in Gloucester just in time to see my dad having lunch with his girlfriend and her daughter and boyfriend. That upset me even though I'd told them I was having tea round Dom's. But then the shit really hit the fan. Running upstairs and into my room I noticed that it had been turned into a guestroom. This really sparked me off. Yes, I'd felt guilty removing my brother's stuff from his room, when he was in London, but now it had happened to me.

At that time, my brother lived with my grandmother down the road. Now my dad was doing the same thing to me. As I ran down the stairs he shouted "Jay" but I slammed the door and jumped into the car with Dom. Ten minutes later, at Dom's, I called him on my mobile and said that I wanted to kill him and hung up. He shouldn't have taken my room from me and given me the small room, and put most of my stuff in the loft. I'd planned to catch up on my work during my break. How could I do that without a desk and, above all, with this mental trauma? Wasn't my head already fucked up enough? And now I had to go through this shit. I mean, he didn't even warn me. How did he think I was going to react? Happily? For fuck's sake!

A few nights later, having stayed round my grandmother's and

Bipolar, Recovery and NLP

at Dom's, I saw my dad. He apologised and said he'd give me some money to help me through uni. He would give me £50 a month which amounted to one drinking session and entrance into a club, or 50 litres of cider. I didn't want to talk to him at all so I went out and got pissed.

...

On 23 December, after going out in Cheltenham, I went to one of the local pubs, The Wagon and Horses, with Dom. A girl that I was seeing, Karen, met us there with some of her friends. Around closing time, Dom and I were chatting up some other girls when we got into an argument with a gang of blokes. Or rather, they started an argument with us.

There were two of us and about twelve of them, most in their mid twenties. We were arguing with this one bloke who said we should watch who we were trying to pull. It turns out that one of the girls we'd been talking to had been the girlfriend of one of his friends. He told me that I'd better keep hold of my pint glass. I didn't think anything more of it until, a few minutes later, this huge bloke threw Dom over the fruit machine. Straight afterwards he punched me in the face. I just fucking stood there and instinctively smashed my pint glass in his face. He fell to the ground and I kicked him in the head shouting: "Mosside, motherfucker you're dead."

Meanwhile, Dom had regained his composure and had started to kick him in the head too. This all took place in the middle of the pub. Fifty people must have seen it. We proceeded into the games room. A little crook I knew was congratulating me when five of them picked Dom up and threw him against the light on top of the pool table. As I ran over and decked one of them I cried out. Despite the fact that I'd been drinking for several hours I could feel a throbbing pain on my knuckle. Whenever I raised it the pain was agonising. Anyway, because of this somebody had got me into a headlock and three or four other drunks were trying to punch me in the face. I was hitting the guy who had me in a headlock in the head with a pool ball when he shouted for me to stop. When I stopped they all punched me in the face. In response, I grabbed a pool ball and knocked another one of them out. I then threw one – which, thank God, connected – until Karen screamed for me to stop. She took the pool balls from my hand, but then our assailants started hitting her too.

By this time Dom's dad and some of his local drinking friends had plucked up enough courage to try and stop the fight. The only way we could escape was to hide in the women's toilets and phone the police on my mobile, but it needed recharging. Several peacemakers came between us and the gang, and after a few seconds I realised that the police were on their way and that I could come out.

On leaving, one of the gang shouted: "You're dead" to me. At the same time, Karen asked me if I was "all right", but as she said this somebody punched me straight in the face. I ignored the misplaced punch in the jaw and told her to go home and that I'd call her the next day. A police van was already there and a car was approaching.

I got into Dom's dad's friend's car and, with his wife, he drove me to the hospital. I ended up with several stitches in my knuckle caused by glassing the bloke whose teeth I'd helped remove with my size twelves. I'd been waiting there for a while when, as luck would have it, the guy I glassed came in propped up by two girls and wearing a headband with blood all over it. He sat next to me, apparently not knowing who I was, and as I motioned to punch him, Mark who had given me a lift, suggested that I sit on the other side of the room which I reluctantly did.

The fight had taken place less than 500 yards from where I grew up and where my dad still lived. One of the gang phoned my house the next day and pretended to be the landlord of the Wagon asking to speak to me. My dad knew it was one of them as he had just spoken to the real landlord himself to see what had happened. The event marked another scar on me that grew and grew. It wasn't necessarily the fight itself but what I felt to be the injustices afterwards. I was banned from the pub and they weren't, and I had to watch out that I wasn't on my own around town or I'd be in trouble. Basically, the only fight scene in any movie with as much panache as the one I've just described is when the gangsters in De Niro's *The Bronx Tale* lock the bar door and smash the bikers and their bikes to bits.

...

Bipolar, Recovery and NLP

In my second term at university, in January 1995, I decided to bunk off lectures – I hardly ever made it in with my hangovers anyway – and go to see Dom for a week. Four of us headed off in a brand new Mazda to Pau, at the foot of the Pyrenees in the south of France, where he was spending a year abroad. I went with Todd, a mate of mine from uni, and two of his mates from Chester – Sharif, a complete nutter who drank hard and gambled most of his money on the boat over and Hung, the driver, a short, excitable, possibly crazy nip whose family were apparently triads.

I went skiing for the first time and was a natural. I remember seeing the snow-capped Pyrenees when we were driving across to Pau. It was an amazing sight and a frisson of freedom pulsed through my body as we all sang along to the DJ SS and Seduction lyrics: "Like a bird in the sky, flying so high." It was one of the most amazing sights I had ever seen.

Going up the ski lift and skiing down the mountain, through the clouds, was beautiful. I felt as if I was in a different world and that wasn't even due to the bottle of Archers and spliff I'd had in the cable car on the way up. After successfully negotiating the learner slope Dom led me onto a blue slope. I picked up speed and after I had snowploughed well out of control, began to fall for what seemed like ages. I fell for about a minute. It must have been nearly a mile. I lost my shades that I'd bought that morning and ended up about 20 yards away from falling off a cliff. Fucking hell, and I thought crashing through the line and scoring a try at rugby gave you a rush.

At night, we all hung around the bars, although they were full of pretentious English university students, and got shit-faced. One night when we were drinking flaming vodkas or some other drink, Dom and Sharif got arrested for kicking off dozens of car wing mirrors. I gave up after a couple – I'd done enough of that when I was 14. My record with a couple of assailants was about 30 in a night. We only went skiing twice but I loved it and knew I wanted to do it again sometime. One time, Oliver went with us. That's right; the flash guy from Manchester was now living with Dom in France. It was good to see Dom though and I left feeling human even though I was still just as hooked on alcohol as I had been when I had arrived.

When I returned I found out that Kev, who was also at

79

Bipolar, Recovery and NLP

Manchester and lived only 10 yards away from me in halls, had been beaten up with a baseball bat and had received 50 stitches to his head. Craig, also from Gloucester, had been stabbed in the leg and smashed over the head with a bottle of vodka. They'd been doormen in Manchester for three or four months and with their boss, Terry, had beaten up the wrong doormen. They were unprepared and attacked during a lock-in.

My drug dealing was by now non-existent. I'd refused to pay my dealer some money as some of the speed that he'd laid on was dodgy, but ultimately I couldn't organise anything anyway because I was drinking too heavily. I was sceptical about being ripped off and didn't have the right contacts to get a big deal. Also, I think I'd just grown out of it. So I turned to 8.4% cider instead. I would knock it back with a fellow alcoholic called Roger.

Roger was fucked up but right on the level. He knew what it was like to be on the edge. He used to cut himself all over his body with razor blades and once claimed that it was better to hurt himself than hurt somebody else. I guess there's a certain kind of logic to that, albeit pretty warped. The first night I met him there were a dozen people at a gathering and he didn't utter a word. He was just sat there drinking a couple of bottles of neat vodka until he threw up.

All this drinking wasn't doing my lithium level any good but I tried not to care. I tried to blot it out. I couldn't accept that I needed medication to be normal. I couldn't face up to the fact that I was a loon. Anyway, fuck it. I forgot to take it half the time. It had toughened me up and, as Alan had told me, it probably wouldn't happen again. I assumed that because I was well at that particular time I didn't have to stick to a strict regime with the medication. I was at university enjoying myself, or at least trying to, and I tried to take comfort time and time again from the words of the key worker: "It might never happen again."

I was fucking this medic, Sarah, for about two months. If I hadn't had her as an outlet I'd have probably ended up in prison or something. We had sex every night, usually three times, and it was good, but we always seemed to have the same conversation. The night I met her there was a party at her flat. It turns out that Kev had scared a few lads he was arguing with and armed police had burst into the flat. They were wondering what was going on.

Bipolar, Recovery and NLP

Apparently, somebody from Mosside had threatened the people in the flat and pulled out a gun. This somebody, in fact, was Kev, but the fact is, he had really put the shits up them. Sometimes he was brilliant; he could be so convincing. It changed him when he was attacked. He was more angry, defensive, paranoid and even wanted to kick-off with me.

This was largely my fault because when we were still at school he brought his new girlfriend Karen round and in a drunken stupor I got off with her in front of him. He went to the toilets in the pub and when he returned, saw us snogging. This was a tragic moment as we were very close up to that point. He said that if it were anybody else he would have hit them. I said that he could hit me and I wouldn't retaliate as I felt so bad for what I had done. As misfortune would have it, this Karen was the same girl I'd been with on the night of the brawl in the Wagon.

There were also practical reasons for me not kicking off. Not just that we were good friends but also the fact that he was actually massive. All this was before he became a doorman and then he went really crazy. Fuck! Was this guy, the mate I spent most of my time with, as crazy as I was? What was going on? Our lives were spiralling out of control and, instead off calming each other down, we were both playing on it. It was as if we would rather be feared, than liked, by people.

We would hang around with thugs and proper gangsters although it was always hard to tell the difference. There was no pattern – you don't really know who's really crazy until something happens. That's when the men are sorted out from the boys. Of course, they're all muppets at the end of the day. There are many better things in life than becoming a gangster – being a writer; being an entrepreneur, as Kev always planned to be; or even being a monk as my brother sometimes daydreamed about.

Soon, Craig and Kev were turning into bigger head cases after every shift. As Kev said, this wasn't *Goodfellas*, this wasn't a movie; it was real life. They even made me want to become a doorman.

One night, I had some Italian girls round cooking us dinner. We'd met them in a snowball fight the previous week. Half a dozen of us were pelting everyone who went past with snowballs and nobody tried anything, as they were scared of Kev, Craig and

Bipolar, Recovery and NLP

me. One bit of eyeball and a stare, grunt or "All righteey then" from Craig and anyone would shit themselves. Craig punched a huge hole in my lounge wall one night. It was plasterboard, but he was massive. He was on steroids and built like an ape.

Once, when we went to Leeds, I remember him swinging metal lampposts from side to side. You could see them swaying all down the road when we walked off. This remains to this day the greatest example of brute physical strength that I have ever seen.

Smashing my wall in Manchester pissed me however. It angered me so much that I pretended not to be in my room when they knocked later on. They kept banging and then ran at the door, knocking it off its hinges and taking a big chunk out of the bottom. What kind of animals had they turned in to? Deep down I was pissed off because they'd acted violently towards one of their best mates but really, in my warped drunken haze, I was upset because they'd done something more violent than I had. They'd done something that had rivalled the madness of Jason Pegler, certified nutter from Coney Hill. I didn't want to give up my reputation as the class "A" nutter. I was proud of it. I was one warped motherfucker.

Mind you, I could talk. I had already threatened two of my flat mates and was later to threaten another two. I had smashed several windows with a golf club, smashed every plate and glass left in the lounge, urinated on Kev's flatmate's eggs, and persuaded Hung to menace two of Kev's flatmates with nunchukkas – but Kev never minded. At least, he never said he did. I'd only met Hung twice and I'd persuaded him to be something that could have got him into trouble. This Chinese youngster who, although he was a bit flash like Oliver, essentially had a friendly and passive nature, turned into the devil when I told him to. Everyday, it seemed that I would do something vile or morally corrupt. I reminded myself of Juvenal's description of Rome which was of a place full of "stupidity, ugliness, vice and crime".

The only sane part of my life was giving Sarah a mindless fucking. She was pretty square and one day I think I went too far for her. I had veered away from the drugs apart from the very occasional spliff and the few E's I had taken when Dom came to visit once, but this time it was Roger's birthday. My drinking partner had never taken any drugs apart from speed once and hash now and again so I bought us a couple of trippy E's each, some billy and the regular White Lightning cider. I bought eight litres which didn't prove quite enough. We sat in his room and had some erudite conversations about life, the world, the universe and what song we were going to play next. I was also trying to teach Roger how to dance but the pills were so trippy and full of strictnine that I was stumbling all over the place.

By early evening the following day I was wasted. Roger was sat in the living room trying to drink some more cider that somebody had brought him. I kept telling everyone that I felt very odd and drank vast amounts of water. I must have drunk 20 pints in a little more than an hour. I phoned Sarah and asked her to come over. I said that I was wrecked and was desperate to see her. She came and we went to my flat and had sex. I told her that I was dying. She said that I would be OK, and the fact that she was a medic made me believe it; she was bound to know the score. She led me back to her flat where we had sex again. During it, I felt very hot and breathed very slowly. I thought that I was going to pass out but the sex did feel good; it was the only tonic for my ailment.

A few days later I went to Tenerife with Kev. Before I left I tried to see Sarah but she said that she was busy. She did, however, leave me a nice note on my door saying that she hoped I had a great time, and sent her love. Now that's the sort of open relationship that I want, I thought. Fuck, she must have known that Tenerife was a pulling joint – all my mates certainly did and most of them had never been there. Did she want me to pull other women or stay with her? I analysed the message and showed it to Todd. Was it a nice message or did it have a hidden meaning? After all, she had never said that she didn't want to see me before.

She'd been really upset the previous week because she'd had to take the morning after pill. I'd said I was sorry but didn't really understand how cut up she was about it. I mean, I had said that I was sorry a few times and asked if she was OK, but I didn't offer her any support. I was no shoulder to cry on, just an alcoholic mess. That talented chess junior had transformed into a beer-drinking monster.

The week in Tenerife was really hot and I got a good tan. We stayed next to a brothel. I was really tempted but couldn't afford it.

Bipolar, Recovery and NLP

I thought back to when I was 17 in Amsterdam. I'd fucked this horny model-cum-Chinese prostitute, but her beauty was diminished by the seediness of the occasion, and my paranoia and inexperience. I walked into the Tenerife brothel a few times when drunk but was escorted out by the bouncers after refusing to buy women drinks. Kev and I pulled German and American birds. The night we pulled the German birds Kev threatened me. He said I was chatting up the bird he wanted. I didn't mind because I wanted the one he was talking to.

Our nights consisted of drinking Tequila slammers with Sprite, and lots of lager and cocktails. We had some great chats, good laughs and drank ourselves into oblivion. We would go to some bars and then a club until about six in the morning. We spent all day sunbathing and cooling off with brief swims. My illness was not apparent. I was often depressed but this was probably because of the amount of alcohol that I was drinking. I didn't feel that I was going high or low on a daily basis – Christ, I didn't even know that manic depressives could go high or low on a daily basis at that time in my life. I'd tried to forget the illness by drinking as much alcohol and acting as recklessly as possible. It worked to some degree because I was blotting it out and had made a conscious effort to drink more than anyone else.

I had had the same attitude to drink when I was younger. The problem now was that the stakes were higher. I had met Roger who got drunk every day and had beaten him. Now I was in a futile competition against myself. A slippery slope where all I lived for was alcohol. It got to a stage that nobody wanted to drink with me; I would pressurise everyone I met into getting out of control. I wanted them to be just like me.

...

After the holiday, in April 1995, I returned to Gloucester. I was about to enter a nightclub with my mate Duncan, who was in the marines, when a gang approached us. One of them asked me menacingly if my name was Jason. Wanting to avoid trouble, I said no and that my name was James. He said: "I know it's Jason Pegler" and took a swing at me. I moved out of the way and said I didn't want any trouble. As he took another swing I got him in a headlock and told him that I didn't want any trouble. Dunc was

Bipolar, Recovery and NLP

trying to stop the others from joining in. Some of them were in the same crowd that I had fought in the Wagon four months previously. I let the bloke go and repeated that I didn't want a fight. Then he got hold of a bottle and threw it just missing my head. My patience snapped, I grabbed hold of him and threw him through a car windscreen, dragged him out and punched him repeatedly in the face. Then I saw a policeman approaching and swapped places with him so that it looked like he had thrown me through the windscreen. I was even punched after a second policeman had arrived.

I was arrested for so-called Breach of the Peace and referred to as a "prisoner" by one of the officers. I protested that I shouldn't be called a prisoner as I was the one that had been attacked. He ignored me which enraged me. I was left in the cell for about 20 minutes and then two policemen interviewed me.

I told them that I was attacked and they said that the aggressors had said that I had glassed one of their friends a few months before. I owned up to it but said that I was attacked first that time as well. I said that I was just sticking up for myself. I was actually proud that I wouldn't let other people push me around. The police must have seen some validity in my argument as I persuaded them to give me a lift home. These types of brawls, however, couldn't have been doing my sanity any good.

...

I was released without charge and glad to return to Manchester a few days later. In Manchester, I could get drunk and nobody would notice. I could be my anarchic self and not be interrupted. I could be me. In Gloucester, people just got in the way and they knew about my past – they knew about my mental illness. I thought it made some people want to challenge me to a brawl.

The reality was, that as time went on, I played up to my madness more and more instead of accepting it as a problem and trying to prevent it from happening again. When I was drunk, I was loud, obnoxious and acted like a muppet. I remember once being really pissed after having played snooker with Kev, Todd and a guy called Ronnie. What was meant to be a quiet night turned out to be an ugly one when for no reason, apart from my alcoholism, I threw a huge breeze block through a club window. It was the snooker club that we had just been in. I could see the irritation in all of my friends' faces afterwards. It was one step too far for all of my mates but I didn't give a fuck. I was the crazy one and I didn't give a fuck. I was the crazy motherfucker and I might as well have been born in fucking Compton.

I had gained a reputation for fighting, and playing rugby, in Gloucester which naturally made me a target for thugs. Living in quite an affluent area and being known as the County Chess Champion also made people want to take a pop at me. That was why I hated going back there; it was too violent. The narrow-mindedness didn't really sink in until afterwards. Gloucester was quickly turning into a place that I didn't want to go back to at all. It was absurd. I was becoming just as irrational and narrow-minded in my behaviour – probably even more so – than the thugs in Gloucester who I despised so much.

I spent my first day back in Manchester drinking Stella Artois and waiting for Sarah to return as Kev was working and Roger was still away. She didn't return until the next day and when I helped her carry her stuff in she was more interested in talking with her male friend than me. I asked her what was going on and she told me that she wasn't ready to have a relationship. I left calmly but felt rejected and gutted that I couldn't have a regular shag. I also knew that I had lost the only sense of stability in my sad and chaotic life. This was exaggerated by the fact that I was only taking my lithium sporadically.

A few days later I started fucking this girl called Harriet. She was fat and, although her face was reasonable, I only went anywhere near her because I wanted to sleep with her friend, Meredith. When I first met Meredith she was very obnoxious, conceited and temperamental. She had short bleached blond hair, was about 5' 4", slim and trendy. She looked like a pretty horror doll as she was very good looking but wore way too much make-up. Sometimes, after we'd got together, I felt like I was fucking Darryl Hannah in Blade Runner. I wanted to get into her pants, though, the moment I saw her.

Within a week, I managed that. We started to sleep with each other most nights. Some nights, I would walk into her flat and, when her flatmates said that they thought she was asleep, I would say it doesn't matter. I would walk into her room, half wake her up

Bipolar, Recovery and NLP

then fuck her senseless. She always seemed distant and I soon discovered that she was on Prozac. She was also a drunk like me. Interestingly, we would never speak to each other when any of our friends were around. I also felt that I had to humiliate myself to get her to say something nice to me.

One evening, for example, in front of Meredith and two of her friends, I drank a pint of their piss for 15 quid. It tasted horrible even though it was supposed to be full of vitamins, and I had to wash my teeth hard for the next few days. I can't believe that people used to clean their teeth with piss in the days before dental hygiene. I felt like Egnatius in a Catullus poem. Catullus laughs at him for cleaning his teeth with piss – imagine how he'd have laughed at me for drinking it in the modern age...

Although I wasn't officially crazy at this time, because I wasn't living in a mental hospital, I was certainly crazier than anyone else in my social circle and always would be. I was the loony and I was obsessed with it. I thought the experience of being in Coney Hill would feel like a noose round my neck for the rest of my life. It was something that I had to live with inside of my mind and it caused lots of problems. I had achieved my goal. I acted crazy to protect myself from going crazy. *As I saw it, if I was always crazy I couldn't go crazy again.* I was a manic-depressive with a classic case of denial. It became difficult for me to socialise with people on a normal level, my university work was being neglected and my overdraft was steadily increasing. The sporty fellow was now no longer sporty.

After I'd started to see Meredith I managed to settle my score with Sarah. I couldn't have her so in my jealousy and anger I set about enacting revenge on her through making her friends suffer. I went into my hall's bar, The Grovel, brewed out of my mind. I was with Kev and this guy Tom who tried to give the impression that he was as crazy as me and Kev. Well, that was one hell of an effort, man. Anyway, I went up to three of Sarah's friends who were sat down at a table and punched them all in the face with the help of Kev and Tom who were holding them down. I ran out as the bar manager came in, and was banned from the bar for the rest of the year. I later found out that one of the lads I'd punched left university for good the following week. I guess my beating him up was the last straw.

Bipolar, Recovery and NLP

The next day, Sarah came to my flat and told me how nasty I'd been. I said that she hadn't given me a choice. Who did she think she was, screwing with my head like that? Fucking slut. My head was fucked enough as it was. However, after I listened to her moral argument, I agreed that I'd been out of order and apologised. What had I become? I had turned into a wanker. I was a monster.

This wasn't the life that my parents had expected me to live but parents can never predict how the lives of their offspring turn out. They can only do what they think is appropriate. It's often not enough, though, as we live in an imperfect world. We live in a place of survival of the fittest. There isn't enough sympathy for the madman, the homeless, the third world or humanity in general.

I was having more and more thoughts like this in my drunken state. By now, I was drinking at least four litres of extra strong cider every night – usually White Lightning or Wild n' White. I had also mastered my beer bong, which I was thankful to Butler for.

The physics of the beer bong is as follows. It consists of a funnel and a tube joined together. You pour, say, a can of 8.4% cider into it making sure that your thumb is at the bottom of the tube. You straighten the tube and wait for the bubble to hit the top. Then you put the tube in your mouth and lift up the funnel. The bong creates a vacuum and the liquid rushes into your stomach quicker than anyone can neck a pint. The concoction is lethal. I've even tried it with small bottles of vodka, whisky and the odd can of Special Brew – dangerous but a good party trick.

I frightened some people, excited others, but whatever their view only geeks would forget about the beer bong. Eventually, I got bored with it. For starters, nobody could stick me when I was using it. But it also made me violently sick when I overdid it – the beer would come out in a huge gush of puke. The world record, according to Butler, was somebody in Los Angeles. They apparently drank 40 bottles of Budweiser in two minutes and then their stomach exploded. Now that was a great urban myth. But I didn't believe it.

Once, I had 10 cans of Lowenbrau Pils, which is 6%, in 90 minutes and kept it all down. At one time, I used it every evening but now I was happy to drink my horrible cheap cider. Basically, I didn't have much money and needed to get drunk everyday so cider was the obvious choice. My first year at university had started by going out to three or four clubs a week and had finished with me sleeping with a girl that I never spoke to and becoming one of the best drinkers in Manchester.

I had managed to avoid hospitalisation, though, and, on the surface, even felt strong. My stream of consciousness went as follows: only a strong man drinks strong cider and I could drink more strong cider than anyone else. Now I look at tramps drinking the same shit and go through a mixture of emotions. First, I identify with them because I know what it's like. Second, I feel sorry for them because it's not a good state to be in. Then I think they're weak as they should choose to do something more positive with their lives. I feel relieved, as I'm not like that anymore, although I know that I always have the potential to go back to the drink. A leopard never changes its spots and neither does an alcoholic.

I hoped that I would never get ill again but I was risking my health by drinking heavily, and so far the gamble had paid off. Thing is, because alcohol's a depressant, there was nothing to win except for a short-term removal of inhibitions. Deep down though, I was terrified that it would return and was trying to forget somehow – via alcohol – that it had ever happened at all. As with most people, alcohol was a form of escapism.

Alcohol had taken over my life. On the plus side, it helped me chat up and fuck dozens of women. On one occasion, I had a brief relationship with a woman from Stockport. She was a 33 year old single mum and had a 12 year-old kid. I pulled her in a club called the "Boardwalk", although probably wouldn't have if the booze hadn't made me dance like a maniac. I was dancing so well I would have made James Brown raise his eyebrows. I had lightning quick hands and feet, and was bang in time with the music. I looked like a professional.

One night, at about 2.15am, Kev and I left the club where he was working. We were both smashed and he shouted at some black girl calling her an Afro. This was not like the Jean Rhys that I had pitied in a rare moment of manic lucidity and sensitivity. What was going on in my life? I was now hanging around with a racist. Sure, I used to call my white mates "niggers" but that was a joke. Panji even told me to call him "nigs" when we were at school together. I was not racist though. I was into rap and had a massive poster of Snoop Doggy Dogg holding a gun in my room. I had had a fight with Panji at school when I was 12 and called him a nigger. He had thrown a stone by mistake in my eye and had laughed when he did it. I kicked off although it's something that I regretted almost immediately. Soon after that, we became good mates and my prejudices faded away. I empathised with him. He had it hard enough as it was. Being mixed race, he had enough problems as it was trying to forge an identity for himself in a school full of white kids.

After the Afro taunt, two students starting punching Kev in retaliation. I decked one of them and started to kick him in the head repeatedly. We then ran away from an approaching police van but were soon arrested. A few hours after being locked up I was told that I had a phone call. That was odd as I hadn't told anyone that I was there. It was my solicitor. He told me that the bloke whom I had allegedly assaulted was in hospital. As things turned out, we were released the following morning with no charges. I couldn't walk as my feet hurt from kicking the bloke who had hit me.

The next day, we were on the front page of the main student newspaper, *Mancunion*, and in the same paragraph as the BNP for "a racist attack". You see what newspapers do, distort the truth. Or was it actually true? After all, my friend had called her an Afro. However, we had been hit first even though Kev had made a clumsy comment. We certainly weren't in the National Front. To suggest so was absolutely ludicrous. What did these student journalists know anyway? They were all fucking geeks. They didn't have any balls like us, our gangster friends, or Snoop or the mob in those gangster movies. A part of me, as ashamed as I am to say it, felt some pride in what we'd done. I'd been victorious in battle and had had some publicity. I was turning into a twisted motherfucker. I also wanted to write at that point, but never got round to it. It was something I dreamed of. Anyway, you couldn't know a lot about life if you're always writing about it – you had to go out and live it, I thought. I got Meredith's address in London before I left Manchester for the summer and went back to Gloucester.

...

Bipolar, Recovery and NLP

On my first night back in Gloucester, in the summer of 1995, I got into a fight with an old friend Daniel Roberts. I hadn't seen him for a while as he'd spent the previous two years in prison for burglaries, robberies and assaults. I'd started the fight by grabbing his pint out of his hand and drinking it in one. It was my way of celebrating seeing him and I was even prepared to buy him a drink afterwards. Moments later, I received a weighty punch on the side of my face. Most blokes would have been knocked down by it, but not me. I just fucking stood there.

The punch was from Daniel. He'd been doing a lot of weights in prison. His hands were twice the size they'd been before he went down. By way of response, I punched him to the floor and started kicking him in the face. As Duncan tried to stop me, I strangled him. The bouncer pushed me out of the pub, as I was off balance, and closed the door. I regained my composure and tried to get back in. It was a futile task. Daniel had also been thrown out. Was this how I treated my friends? Were these the sort of people that I should be hanging around with?

The next day I apologised to Dunc and sort of did to Daniel. We were round Peach's house and I remember Daniel swinging Peach's eight year-old brother around and saying: "If I ever had a little brother like yours, Peach, I'd kick fuck out of him everyday so when he's my age he'd be hard as fuck." For God's sake. My life couldn't go on much longer like this without triggering other episodes could it? I declined my friends' offer to go swimming that day as I knew I was crazy enough without hanging around with them. One nudge too far and I might be pushed over the edge again. It wasn't as if I had to prove my madness as everybody knew I had been in Coney Hill. Sometimes, I convinced myself that I was proud that I had a reputation like that but really I knew that I pitied myself. I felt that there was something lacking in me: total sanity.

That summer I drank every night and after a week in Gloucester went to stay with Dom in Hossegor, in the South of France. He was with his girlfriend camping and they lent me a tent. Dom had become pretty good at surfing and, after trying it for a couple of days, I took his advice and bought a Boogie Board and all the extras including a summer wetsuit, fins, some surf magazines, and wax so I could stay on the board when riding a wave. I learnt to boogie board and doing that for several hours every day for six weeks makes you fit no matter how much you drink.

Going to France provided a much-needed break from the grey, rainy climate of Manchester. Hossegor was beautiful, hot and sunny everyday. Temperatures got up to 33 degrees centigrade in the shade. It didn't feel as hot as it had been when I went to Washington though as the humidity was low. The campsite was huge and I stayed there rent free, doing a runner when we eventually left. We'd cook a barbecue every evening and eat chocolatines and French bread for breakfast.

I got my first great sun tan. The only time the three of us would argue was about who was going to do the washing up. We bought some plastic chairs and would often eat with a German couple. The man, Axel, had a long board and all the expensive gear. He went surfing every summer but I don't think he ever caught a decent wave. The beach was topless and there were some bloody sexy women there. Thing is, it was difficult for me to pull as Dom was happy with Paula and everyone else, surprise, surprise, was French. We drank Kronenbourg 1664 every night and cheap French wine called "Grappe" which was 12%.

We bought some metal boules and played most evenings on the sand. One time, in the middle of an argument, Dom threw the boule at me. I was 20 yards away and it went about 30 feet in the air smashing through the plastic chair and just missing my foot. Now that was close. He had a temper like all my friends seemed to. I think part of it was just male hormones, but I had always tended to hang around with charged up people.

Paula left after I'd been there six weeks and Dom only wanted to stay there a few days longer. The two of us flew back from Biarritz. I was never really into it but when Dom and Paula disappeared in their tent I would wander off to a large group of French puff heads nearby who were always happy to share spliffs with me. Most of them would sleep in hammocks and they all had huge bamboo bongs. That was the last time I ever had a spliff except for when I was manic once several years later.

A few days after flying back from Biarritz, I went to Newquay with Kev and rode the biggest wave that I've ever seen. Out of 40

Bipolar, Recovery and NLP

people trying to get out back only two or three managed it. It took me several minutes, mind you, and when I did I had to sit on the crest until the cramp that had locked my leg went away. When I took off, it was one of the most intense and thrilling moments of my life. I rode the wave for what must have been a minute and had to jump off the board when I realised I was heading for the rocks at Fistral beach. I left unhurt and with a feeling of great freedom and exaltation that I had never experienced before.

Kev and Craig were working as security guards at Trevelgue campsite and tried to get me a job, but after a couple of weeks we all left as we ran out of money. I remember fucking a virgin in our poxy little caravan which Craig had broken into. Kev was sleeping on the floor and Craig slept outside. We hung around these Scousers and ate their food, borrowed their car and trashed their caravan. The Gloucester boys were back together again but there was always a sense of violence in the air that made everything so intense. Anyone who came into contact with us was lucky that we didn't knock them out for the sheer hell of it.

We made friends with some South African doormen. At least they were on the level. Kev and I had arranged to get jobs as doormen in a Newquay nightclub and one night, when Craig was working, we went out with the two South Africans to celebrate. We played pool all night in the pub blatantly using everyone else's money on the table. Nobody would dare ask to play as they saw that there were four steamed up lunatics playing doubles who were ready to kick-off at any moment. When we left the club Kev and I walked back and he must have threatened a hundred people. I'd never seen anything like it. He was crazy. He'd go up to a gang of four blokes and demand a fight. First, he'd demand a fight one-on-one and then he'd challenge them all. I was acting as a diplomat, but nobody was up to the challenge of having a brawl with Kev. He had fire in his eyes and something in his belly that night. The memories of the relaxing weeks in Biarritz were fading away as I got back in with the Gloucester boys. Soon, I would return to Manchester, move in with them and seek refuge with an alcoholic by becoming an alcoholic myself.

...

Bipolar, Recovery and NLP

In August 1995, I returned to Manchester to sit two retakes. If I'd passed my philosophy coursework I wouldn't have had to take these exams, but I got no marks. I'd asked my brother to do an essay on Plato on Aristotle. He was a philosophical genius but was so unstable at the time that he ended up copying a big chunk of the essay straight from a book. Years later, I asked him to tell me how he could do something like that. He said: "I was so weak I didn't even know what I was doing... There was a time three years previously when I could have dictated the essay from the top of my head. I'd recently been kicked out of dad's and had to move in with grandma. I'd gone from having a study and planning on being a professor to sleeping on a couch and living with a geriatric old biddy. No one will ever know the psychological impact that having my room taken away from me had. I felt as though someone had ripped the floorboards from underneath me and I was sinking into the abyss." Dad and Claire had their reasons. Claire had done domestic chores for Harvey and I for a couple of years. She had already brought up two daughters. Wasn't it time we stood up on our own two feet? I could understand this. It was just the way things happened – without any consultation.

Back at uni I also felt let down by the department. I was fascinated by philosophy because of my brother's influence. He encouraged me to read Plato and Bertrand Russell when I was 11. By the time of my first class, I already knew about all kinds of philosophy from ethics and aesthetics through to epistemology and metaphysics. Afterwards, the lecturer said that there would be a tutorial the following week for those who were interested. I was really looking forward to it. Just as I had loved debating at school and hanging around with intelligent people, philosophy was also my forte.

In the event, nobody turned up apart from me. I was so angry. I couldn't believe it. In my view, the lecturer had shown a complete lack of responsibility. But maybe I had scared everyone off. Maybe I had been so engrossed in the class that people saw me as pretentious and didn't want to sit in the same room as me. They could have switched locations without telling me, but I wasn't that paranoid and knew I had the right time and place.

I was so pissed off I didn't go to a philosophy lecture until three months later and only then because I had been told to in a

Bipolar, Recovery and NLP

letter that said I must improve my attendance. The philosophy professor had destroyed my dream start at uni. I was like a time bomb waiting to go off and he had pressed the detonator.

I ended up passing the exams and did a week's labouring. Six of us lived in a house in Mosside: Kev, Craig, Roger, Chris, Todd and me. We moved to another flat in November as nobody could be bothered to clean the house. The backyard looked like it had gone through a nuclear melt down. The nearest anyone got to it would be to open the door, eyes closed, and throw the rubbish as far as possible so it wouldn't make you feel anymore sick the next time you opened it. I also didn't pay any rent which helped fund my drinking.

By now, I could drink six litres of 8.4% cider in a night – and each of the 12 pints in one go. I was proud of myself and thought that nobody watching the World Embassy Darts Championships at the Lakeside could do that. The new flat was in Victoria Park and we were burgled five times in six weeks. Everyone's stuff was taken except mine, as my room must have been mistaken for a cupboard (even though it was massive). I had a suspicion that we might get burgled as the area was a bit rough. I mean, we nearly had a fight with a group of Asian lads when moving in and that was in the afternoon. As a precaution, I covered my stereo and everything else that was visible with dark sheets so they couldn't be spotted by someone looking through the key hole.

I eventually moved in with Meredith as I knew I would get thrown out of university if I kept on drinking with Roger. My relationship with Kev had turned into a Jekyll and Hyde scenario. He was frustrated that I didn't want to go out and get drunk and pull. I mean, I was an alcoholic who could drink from the flat and had a regular shag that came round when I said. I didn't need anything else. I was becoming socially inept and couldn't deal with the violent moods of a doorman. He threatened me when we were in the new flat and that was the last straw. Kev told me how he hadn't got the deposit back from the previous landlord. I told him that he should have knocked the fucker out. I told him that he shouldn't have paid so much rent in the first place. I hadn't. Kev's response was to say: "Maybe I should knock you out." I was pissed off and we left the house two minutes later after necking some Stella. I would still occasionally start off drinking the same as Kev. It was a kind of bonding ritual when we went out. By this time, though, I was more prone to necking a bottle of wine in one through a straw.

Just after leaving the house, I saw an Asian bird that I had shagged some weeks before. I told Kev to cross the road as I didn't want to see her. After the girls crossed over, Kev shouted at me. "Who do you think you are telling me what to do? Nobody tells me what to do except my old man. You ever say anything like that again and I'll knock you out."

The drunken threat by Kev made me think where my life was going. My life couldn't go on as it was for much longer without disastrous consequences. I would fail university, certainly go mad again and probably end up in prison for any one of several public disorder offences: vandalism, GBH, ABH or even murder. What could I do?

A few weeks before the threat, I tried to get off with Meredith's flatmate, Lucy. She and Harriet, who lived with Meredith, treated Meredith really badly, took her money and food, and even left her locked out of her own house. I was so fucked up that I had initially gone round to have a go at Lucy. They were having a party which Meredith had not been invited to. The evil cow and me slept on the same bed with our clothes on but we didn't get off with each other. She wouldn't let me, as she put it, "score a hat-trick".

The next morning, I went into Meredith's room and told her what happened the previous night. She said it was OK but I said I couldn't see her anymore because it wouldn't be right. I left kicking bins in the street and crying. It was the first scrap of sensitivity I had shown in a long time – months, possibly even years.

Five minutes after getting back home Meredith was at the door. I couldn't believe it. Was this the same girl who was so cruel to me when we met? Was this the same girl who had dared me to drink a pint of piss and implied that I had a small dick? Yes, it was. I told her it was too late. She left and a few minutes later I got a phone call from another girl that I'd been shagging. I told Roger to say that I wasn't in. He did but told me she'd said she wanted to see me. I'd ignored her previous couple of phone calls and it was the last time that I would get a call.

Bipolar, Recovery and NLP

I called for Meredith a week after she left my doorstep in tears. I'd discovered that she had tried to overdose the night after I had split with her. We'd missed each other and for the first time talked to each other properly. All the bullshit had gone out of the window and it was evident that two incredibly fucked up individuals each needed a shoulder to cry on. She was clever and unique. We spent the next few nights and the New Year in London together. We really got on well and things were really romantic. Although Meredith decided to quit her degree in Art History, we agreed to move in together in Manchester. We moved to Chorlton-cum-Hardy, a friendly neighbourhood where the Bee Gees used to live. My relationship with Meredith improved and became more interesting as time went on.

We moved in with each other in January 1996 and were happy until October of the same year. I particularly liked not having a television for the first few months. It meant we talked to each other more, got to know each other better and used our imaginations. She was very artistic and we had her drawings framed on the walls in each room of the flat. We were both in a bad way when we moved in but gradually got our heads together and were grateful to each other for it. She was the first girl I loved.

My alcoholism had reduced to binge drinking about three to four nights a week. It was a fresh start. I started studying and my grades improved a lot. I actually became interested in my course. I admired the Roman race again and became absorbed in Greek tragedy. I even read Lucan's *Civil War* from start to finish. I liked the gruesome bits that described, in detail, blood splashing when heads were being hacked off. My life was more stable although I still had that violent streak in me especially when I was drunk.

This was evident on the day of my twenty-first birthday. I got drunk with a guy who'd lived with Kev in the first year. His name was Charlie. I drank ten Stellas, while he stopped at eight and met up with his geeky friends. I was furious and hurled an empty pint glass across the bar. It smashed against a bottle of spirits and I didn't look back when I walked out. Meredith had gone straight from work to meet me for a quiet drink but I guess I ruined her night by being shit-faced, moaning and being so fired up. Also, for my twenty-first, mum and dad had made a special effort to come and visit and buy us things for the flat. They bought us a toaster, some crockery, an ironing board, kettle and stuff like that.

In the summer, after comfortably passing my second year, I worked for Ladbrokes for two weeks and at Safeway for six weeks part-time. I didn't like the bookies: it was full of drunks, chain smoking and throwing their money away. They never said thank you, just grunted and were glued to the screens showing horse and dog racing.

The job at Safeway was OK to begin with. I worked 6am to 10am Mondays to Fridays and was responsible for assessing and reordering the stock in the store. It took a few weeks to be trained up and I could use my natural ability at mental arithmetic to count how many cheeses were on each shelf. If there were 13 rows and 13 columns then that would make 169 slabs of mature cheddar.

I also used a computer database and inputted my results. I was doing a job that was important to the store. Then, when my manager was away, the bureaucracy arrived. I was given a machine that would count the products for me. I told one of the senior managers that it was slower than my head and that it was a nuisance, but I was told to keep using it. That was the last straw. I left and never went back to get my P45.

Although I didn't stick the jobs, I had changed and was a human being again. I hadn't seen my friends for months. They no doubt felt I had deserted them. But I'd been brave enough to make a change. By leaving the hectic lifestyle with my mates I'd made a decision and stuck by it. This decision was proving to be beneficial.

In the month before my final year began, I read the entire year's syllabus to get ahead. I wanted to make sure I got a 2:1 and believed I could make a miraculous recovery and get a first. With help from Meredith, who was working as a receptionist in Chorlton, I started the preliminary work for producing and directing a modern film of the ancient Greek Tragedy, *Ajax*, written by Sophocles. It deals with the theme of madness and shows the noble warrior Ajax going mad then killing himself when he returns to sanity because of the humiliation he has felt. This was it, I was dealing with madness in my own way now. Nobody could stop me. I was sorted. I was together. I was going to get a first. I had secured funding from the Hellenistic Society and the Classics Department. Members of staff were giving advice, I had a producer, a cameraman, a place to hire equipment, storyboards written and had advertised, and set a date for, the auditions. My personal tutor was even helping me to choose the actors. Everything was in place.

Bipolar, Recovery and NLP

Chapter 5 – Oh no, not again…

Just when my life seemed to have some meaning and I had at last found an identity that I was content with a catastrophe unfolded before (or rather *through*) my eyes. I was hit by a thunderbolt from Zeus.

In the same way that I'd failed to turn up at the Oxford University entrance exam three years previously, I failed on this occasion to turn up to my own audition. *I was a bit preoccupied… a little bit crazy… a little bit high… really high.* I had gone manic, too manic, once again – although how it all started is still a bit of a haze.

I remember walking through Mosside buying ethnic minority newspapers and thinking how I could save the world through the medium of film. I stayed up all night writing messages in books and on pamphlets that I had collected, also leaving my phone number to let people know who to call when the inevitable nuclear war broke out

News of the war was about to break the following day. At about 4am, I thought I'd call Snoop Doggy Dogg to ask for his help. There was an emergency number on the back of the CD cover of Doggystyle to contact his crew if anything went wrong. I rang the number and it didn't matter that I couldn't speak to anyone as my powers of telepathy had returned. Throughout the night of the 26 October, I was performing sexual rituals that are too disgusting to mention or recall. By 7.30am, I thought that the whole world had turned into the Red Light District in Amsterdam and that Chorlton in Manchester was the centre of world consciousness. I had never been so happy and intrigued in my life, not even during my first manic episode.

Meredith knew something was wrong and went to her boss to ask for time off. Well, I did need somebody to help me prevent nuclear war, didn't I? When she went to see her boss, I started to put my plan into action. The first people I could communicate with on a telepathic level were the homeless. To help get them off the streets and make them my recruits, I would skate round giving them bananas and books which I had left cryptic instructions in. I was so pleased to have saved the world from another nuclear war as a result of conversing with people like Dogg Pound. To confuse

Bipolar, Recovery and NLP

the enemy, I had bluetacked my *Usual Suspects* poster to someone's garage only a hundred yards away from the house. My mind was racing and my critical faculties were gone. I was completely unaware of this at the time. Instead, I was in heaven – the fleeting moments of hell hidden deep in my consciousness, the mania so powerful.

We stayed in during the afternoon and I put my boogie board on my back thinking I could fly anywhere I wanted to in the universe. I was also very proud that I could swim underwater to Australia in five seconds. While these thoughts were coursing through my mind, Meredith decided to take me to my mum's in Powys as she didn't know what to do. I had told her about my manic depression before and she'd said that it didn't bother her. Like Kev I think she thought the idea of it was cool, but she was about to discover first hand the traumas of what she'd let herself in for. She got more than she bargained for.

We went to my mum's by train from Piccadilly station. I was glad we took this route as I discovered time travel on the way which was most satisfying. I knew I had discovered it every time I clicked my fingers ... now ...now ... now ... I sat opposite a really nice old lady who was so senile that she seemed almost as loopy as me. I bought a great magazine on the greatest sportsmen in the world. It was refreshing to discover that I was the best at every sport in the world. Forget the cartoon *Sport Billy*, this was *Sport Jase*.... and this was real...I was real...

We arrived at Leominster and got straight into a taxi. I didn't want to be seen in public as my position in society was too important... It was too crucial. If I was going to fail in bringing about world peace then the world was doomed. I was the only person who had the potential – I was Jesus Christ, God on earth...

It was also my destiny to become the greatest film director on earth... People would come to the cinema and be influenced by my films... Their lives would change as a result and so would those of their friends and any other people who they ever came into contact with... No matter how slight the influence it was everlasting and continual... I could not fail. This was my destiny... My destiny was a destiny that even surpassed that of Aeneas founding Troy. Virgil's *Aeneid* was my favourite book and I was delighted to have surpassed the achievements of the hero...

Bipolar, Recovery and NLP

When we arrived at my mum's Meredith explained that I was behaving strangely and that she was worried. My mum looked worried but that wasn't unusual as she always looked worried. Like most mums.

Mind you, wouldn't you be worried if you were the mother of God? That's a lot of responsibility, a lot of pressure to be under. Of course, I didn't mind them worrying... I knew that they wouldn't understand yet but would in due course although I wasn't sure when... but sometime soon ... sometime real soon, that much was certain ... Meredith soon went to bed as she was exhausted.

I stayed up talking to my mother while telepathically intertextualising programmes on television for everybody else in the world so as to instil world peace. I had slept with, and therefore conquered, my mother without her realising it by playing with her fire tools and holders, and was now king of the world. I was king of the castle, king of the mountains, king of the past, present and future, even king of Old Trafford. I was king of everything and everyone...

Before I went to bed I had to perform rituals. I did this by cleaning myself in the bathroom and rinsing my mouth out with soap and water. Indeed, just as in my first episode I had gone from believing I was dominant, king of all, to submissive, a mere subject, so too now I had suddenly become an abject slave to womankind. My mum and Meredith were the bosses now and to be a good slave I had to suck on a small teddy of Daffy Duck that I had covered in soap. I sucked for several minutes until I was led away by the two goddesses. I was glad I had performed these rituals as I was now guaranteed a life of eternal slavery. I was going to become the next manager of Manchester United. We would win everything and, by playing sexy and exciting football, would be able to influence others and instil world peace... All it needed was for more women to take up the game and we were on our way...

However, that night as I lay in bed with Meredith, I realised for the first time during a manic episode that I was actually manic and that I was ill. I said: "I know I'm ill and I need help." I burst into tears and received comfort in the form of a cuddle. Now there were two people crying and things got worse. The next day a social worker came round and wanted to section me after I'd been reading the Classics and the Hellenistic Society handbook cross-legged and naked under a tree in the garden. It was a cold autumn day and my stepfather had ordered me to get in as my behaviour was extremely odd. I ran away from the social worker thinking she was evil… and most of all terrified that she was the enemy.

I ran into a pub and challenged a traveller at the bar to a competition. The two of us went into the games room and I bet him I could get the white as close to the pocket as possible without potting it. He accepted and I duly did this with the white stopping by the edge of the pocket. He bought me a pint and I drank it in one. On the way out I said that I didn't have any money and couldn't have bought him a pint if I'd lost. He said that was fine and pulled out a knife. "It's OK. I'd have stabbed you in that case, you cunt." As he laughed I laughed too and, thinking he would make a good extra in one of my imaginary movies, left the pub before things got too complicated. I didn't want to get distracted from my mission…

I walked down to the health centre and my stepdad got out of his car. He told me to get in the car and threatened to tell my dad about it and would even punch him if he didn't do anything. He said my mum shouldn't go through all this on her own and that my dad should help shoulder the burden. However, at the time, I didn't really register what he was on about as there were far more interesting manic processes and formulations going on in my mind. When I got back to mum's there was a doctor and ambulance there. They said they were going to take me somewhere for a rest. Well, I was happy with that. I thought I deserved a rest – after all, it's not every day that you find out you're God, is it? I might even meet some people to cast in my film… I lay down in the ambulance as though I was on a luxury yacht cruising around the Caribbean.

About 45 minutes later we arrived at the Mid Wales mental institution, Talgarth. There was a big lounge, even bigger than the one in Coney Hill and certainly more colourful. The first person I saw was a Scottish patient heckling the staff. She turned me on because I thought she had telepathic powers like me. I also thought that she was into bondage. The nursing staff interviewed Meredith and my mum as I was shown around my new film studio… They both cried as they left, and I only realised something was wrong

Bipolar, Recovery and NLP

when I was prevented from leaving by five hospital staff who injected Haliperidol into my arse. (I did not discover until 2002 that I had an allergy to this and it was a lawyer who told me not a doctor.)

I spent over two months in that hospital in the Black Mountains in the middle of nowhere. It seemed like two years, however, because this time the depression hit me harder. In January, at my own request, I was transferred to Withington hospital in Manchester. This was the closest image of hell that I had ever seen. It resembled then, and resembles now as far as I know, something that Michel Foucault would have written about in *Madness and Civilization*: small wards, no colour, staff that treat patients like criminals or retards and certainly not the kind of place for any kind of rehabilitation. Perhaps I'd gone back to Manchester too quickly.

The consultant in Mid Wales wanted to put me on ECT, the horrific treatment Jack Nicholson went through *in One Flew Over The Cuckoo's Nest*. I knew as much about it as anyone else – very little – although being electrocuted didn't strike me as being particularly humane. I was told that it helped to shorten depression quicker than antidepressants on their own but could sometimes lead to short term memory loss and, in some rare cases, permanent memory loss or brain damage.

ECT is increasingly rare these days but the public should still be made aware of it. Perhaps the best medium is film which has the power to really get across how sick and disturbing it can be. *Fight Club*, for example, touched upon it, as has Birdie and Me Myself and Irene. Anyway, me? I declined the treatment as I kept thinking of when Chief put Jack Nicholson to sleep. I couldn't get that image out of my mind.

When I was offered ECT by Dr. Cooper in Mid Wales, I was frightened and humiliated. We discussed the matter in the weekly ward round.

"Is life worth living?" asked Dr.Cooper.

"Don't care."

"You don't care?"

"Don't know."

"Are you more depressed than the last time we met?"

Bipolar, Recovery and NLP

"Yes."

"Do you have suicidal thoughts?"

"Sometimes."

"Do you think you might act upon them?"

"Yes."

"It looks like the antidepressants aren't working as fast as we'd hoped. We talked about the possibility of ECT treatment last time. Would you consider this an option?"

"How quickly does it work?"

"It works with the antidepressants and should double the speed of your recovery."

"What about the side effects? I've heard you can end up brain dead."

"The treatment is a lot better nowadays. There is very little chance of that happening."

"Won't I lose my memory?"

"Short term memory loss is likely, but the chances of long term memory loss are very minimal."

"How minimal?"

"I don't know how much exactly."

"I heard it was one in fifty."

"No, I would think it would be less than that."

"The thought terrifies me."

"It's a scary thought but it has benefited thousands of patients. I'll give you some time to think it over. You can ask one of the nurses to contact me and we could start the treatment. Is there anything else you wish to discuss?"

"Don't know."

"Well, Jason (shaking hands), I hope you feel better soon."

"Thanks."

I felt like a python was slowly crushing me. All my will to live was being drained out of me. Nevertheless, I resisted taking the ECT treatment. There are a maximum of eight sessions over a period of four weeks and the anaesthetic stops you feeling any physical pain. Techniques have improved over recent years and my previous consultant and current psychologist both said that they would opt for ECT if they were given the option during the lowest ebb of an episode of bipolar effective disorder (technical term for manic depression). Well, I guess they know their stuff but they can see it from a more rational perspective than me. I've seen people straight after they've come out of the ECT treatment room and it's made me cry.

Andy, who taught me to play *Imagine* and *Jealous Guy* on the guitar in Mid Wales, was one of these. He kept repeating conversations that we had already had before. He had forgotten everyone's name on the ward and he was only middle-aged. It was soul-destroying to see such a talented man humiliated. He'd lost all his confidence and had turned into a fumbling wreck; this was a man who'd played solo guitar in front of 2000 people.

Most people who have ECT experience short-term memory loss and a few experience long-term memory loss forever. In 2001, the mental health charity, Mind, reported that there are 1300 "shock treatments" carried out each week in the United Kingdom. Two thirds of those who've received it would not choose to have it again, 40% of respondents reported permanent loss of past memories, 36% have difficulty concentrating, while three quarters of the total sample said they were not given any information about side effects.

Well, there you have it. Whether or not a patient should take ECT needs to be very carefully thought out. You have to look at cases individually and in-depth. You can't implement such powerful, arguably inhuman treatment, however scientific it is supposed to be, without looking at the state of mind of an individual person extremely carefully. Otherwise, you risk fucking up their life for good. I know if I was a doctor I wouldn't want the responsibility of someone's death on my shoulders whether during the treatment or afterwards through suicide. How would you explain it to their family? How would you explain it to their parents?

On the other hand, it would be naïve and defeatist to hold science back and most doctors believe that, when used with antidepressants, ECT halves the time of depression of a sufferer who only uses the antidepressants. In many cases, they believe it prevents suicide and is the most preferential form of treatment for somebody who is a suicide candidate. All I can say is that science is surprisingly ignorant when it comes to mental illness. There is no cure for it – only a series of attempts to try and stabilise patients as best as is possible. Manic depression is like the flu: it can come

Bipolar, Recovery and NLP

and go at any time – and it's hard to say why.

The same is true of the schizophrenic. One schizo in Mid Wales had the greatest mind I have ever come across – the wit of Paul Merton, the critical accuracy of Germaine Greer and the fascination of Shakespeare all rolled into one. His name is Magnus Robertson, and we wrote poetry together. He was totally paranoid and believed that spirits were following him around the hospital and invading his psyche. He was born in 1953 and was 45 when I was in hospital with him. He was always in and out of hospitals and, the last time I heard, lived in Neath with his mother. On 7 January, 1997, he gave me a poetry book. The note read:

For Jason, with warm and deep regards, never to be forgotten, Love Magnus. "When shall we three, meet again ...?

Whether he was referring to me, him and the book as a separate entity I can't remember, but this man's poetry was amazing. He even put my brother's intellect to shame and made me feel privileged to have met him. He wrote poetry in a luminous pen on his bedroom wall and we would hand our poems to everyone on the ward to try and cheer them all up, even the staff. As creative people, we also needed reassurance that our poetry was good and writing it was a great form of therapy for both of us.

I also kept in touch with a 60 year-old man I was in hospital with who lives near my mum. His name is Alan Greenwood. He has manic depression and, at his last count, had 18 hospitalisations to his name. He is unable to work, chain smokes roll ups, watches TV until the early hours of the morning and his flat is a health hazard. It's disgusting. Seeing the toilet would make you want to throw up. It's as close to the one in *Trainspotting* as I've ever seen. He's tried to kill himself several times and I believe seriously meant it. Thing is, he's too clumsy and too much of a mess to do it properly. He wanders around the pubs in the small, local community asking people to buy him drinks and is generally regarded, by people like my stepdad, as a pain in the arse. Despite all this, if you start talking with him, it's clear that he has a brilliant mind. His use of language is advanced and so is his critical thought and he has a powerful imagination. I've read short stories that he's written and they're fascinating. Rather subliminal, perverse and a little fucked up, but ingenious in parts. Alan, however, does not take care of himself. He may have manic

Bipolar, Recovery and NLP

depression worse than I do but even if he hasn't, I'm not going to live like that – I'm not going to give up and bow down for anyone.

The longest I've ever stayed awake for is eight days during my second episode. I was just about to start work labouring at a building site in Manchester when Mark Doran, a friend, persuaded me to go to see the doctor instead. It was the right move as I was manic, already two hours late and so confused that I probably wouldn't have made it to the building site anyway. In any case, I could use my magical powers to lift bricks so why go to the site? Christ, I was so fucking magical that the magic worked itself through me rather than at my will. I didn't even need to consciously imagine it. How about that for magic? That would make me win the battle to be the slave for any mistress.

Sexual perversion and fantasy often takes over when I go manic. I'm not sure if this is common with other manic-depressives or whether it's peculiar to me. Too embarrassed to ask, I suppose... Something I'll discuss with my psychologist when she's ready. I keep mentioning it but she changes the conversation. Maybe she's conscious of avoiding transference, who knows? Maybe I've been and always will be a pervert. Don't think I've got the potential to become a rapist or a paedophile, but who knows? What is it in a man's psyche that constitutes this kind of behaviour? Show me the most revealing anthropological study so I can stop it happening to me and to others in the future. I know I could be a murderer if I was pushed to the end of my tether. I've been fortunate not to kill several people in fights I've had. That's why I stopped drinking. That's why I tried to change my life but still the mania came back and catapulted me into oblivion.

More research needs to be done on mental institutions, and more money given to them because they're pretty awful places. They're over-disciplined, regimented even, consist of too many untrained and uncaring staff, have too much bureaucracy and severely lack rehabilitation activities, humanity and any kind of release from depression, for example, comedy. Why can't they play comedy videos everyday, bring in clowns, entertainers and comedians? That's what my grandma always suggested and she'd been saying it for 60 years. It's because people don't generally give a shit about something unless it happens to them or somebody they are close to.

Bipolar, Recovery and NLP

Mid Wales hospital had a TV area with several armchairs, a large dining area, a free pool table, a quiet room and a punch bag outside. The pool and punch bag were good forms of therapy and allowed me to escape from the other activities. However, the hospital was still militaristic in its make-up. Every mealtime, a patient would have to lay out all the cutlery or nobody would get served. The staff would order people around as if they were naughty children. I was only given my room after my father complained that I couldn't sleep because of snoring in the dormitory.

One patient wouldn't speak to me because she thought I was the devil. This was one of the few times I laughed when I was in that institution. I nearly got assaulted by one of the patients. She insulted me and called me stupid so I said: "At least I don't look like a whore." She picked up her mug of coffee and I dared her to smash it over my face. She looked like she was going to until she burst out crying and fled the room. When she returned, a few minutes later, I apologised to her after having been advised to show some humanity by one of the other patients. She was a middle-aged lawyer who had retired to become a writer and was normally quite pleasant. She said that she had never felt like doing anything violent like that in her life and that everything was getting on top of her.

I knew I had gone too far but there was a part of me that didn't give a fuck anymore. I was so depressed it was as though I had given up. I had gone through so much shit that my will was too weak, or so I thought. In fact, I was clinically depressed and the only way out of it is to wait. Time is the only healer. Drugs and environment can only do so much to lift you out of deep depression. When you experience it you feel that you're to blame for feeling like you do but that's not true. It's just something you have   to   endure.

I went back to Manchester to be with Meredith. My mum said it was too soon and that I wasn't ready. She said that I could only depress her, the mood I was in, and she was probably right. Thing is, I wanted desperately to get my life back on track and was even happy to accept the fact that Meredith now worked in the week so I would only really get to see her at the weekend.

Although I was severely depressed there was still some fight left in me. I was driven to Withington hospital, in Manchester, by a member of staff from Talgarth. I was handed over at 9pm. Being "handed over" was a term used by nurses when they changed shifts. It made me feel more like an unwanted dog than a human being.

The place was dark and barren. The ward was tiny compared to what I now look back on as the luxury of Mid Wales hospital. Why were they going to demolish Mid Wales when it was clearly a much more favourable environment than where I had ended up? Why had they demolished Coney Hill when it was paradise compared to the hell I was now faced with? How was I going to cope with this? I was depressed enough as it was. Now I had to face this fucking shit. I didn't know if I was up to it.

My first intention was to try and be positive as I still believed that I was a positive person. The first patient that I said hello to shouted at me to "fuck off". And that was after the staff had been so cold on my arrival. They had written my name up on the board in a green highlighter pen as though I was some kind of prisoner or, at the very best, some kind of experiment. Everybody was drawn up on a kind of ward diagram so that an eye could be kept on them from the office. They could be watched and controlled if anything got out of hand.

I was placed in a ward with four beds despite having pleaded for my own room before my arrival. At least there were only four people in the room, though. Sleeping was bound to be easier than in Talgarth and I prayed that there would be no fat old man snoring. While a new member of staff showed me around the ward, in a hurried manner, I noticed that the only form of activity was a four-foot pool table which was stuffed in the corner of the corridor. There was no room to play properly. A large woman said hello to me in a Manchester accent. I could tell that she was depressed and that it was a real effort on her part. I felt a spark of humanity reaching my soul when she asked if I had a cigarette. The spark soon faded, although she told me her name. It was Cecilia.

The handover was completed. I was subdued, felt very uncomfortable, and even frightened, as I was led along the corridor to my room. There was a teenager a bit younger than me already asleep. I liked his trainers. There was no bedding on my sheets and

Bipolar, Recovery and NLP

a window that wouldn't close next to my bed. The covering around my bed was like that in a hospital except that people could see in if they wanted to. I had no privacy. I heard the echoes of the member of staff who had dropped me off. He had told me to make the best of it and that I was over the worst. It was 10 minutes ago that he said this but it seemed so long. In fact, it seemed like years.

The nurse left me in the room and told me to leave any valuables I had in the office as the wardrobe doors were broken. The state of the people in there made me worry that all my clothes would be stolen and that I'd be walking around naked by the morning. When the nurse walked out an old man came over to me. He looked about 80. He said: "Give me a cigarette." I said that I only had a couple. "Give me a fucking cigarette." I gave him one and tried to leave the room immediately. As I walked out I heard him say: "I fought the Korean War for you and you won't even give me a cigarette. You fucking ungrateful little bastard, you'd better watch it. I'm going to fucking get you. You'd better watch your back."

I was distraught. This man was living opposite me – what could I do? If I hit him I'd be put on a six months' section, but I was so weak that I didn't feel I could win a fight with him anyway. I was also sure that if I told the staff they wouldn't give a shit and it would probably aggravate the situation. But I didn't like not standing up for myself as it made me feel a coward. As I left the room he said: "I want a cup of fucking tea when you get back and all. Make sure it's got two sugars." I left and went to the toilet almost in tears.

I walked along the corridor to the corner of the ward and lit a cigarette. Just as I was walking to another corner of the ward which the member of staff had not pointed out to me Cecilia told me that I couldn't smoke over there. It was one of the rules of the ward. The member of staff that had showed me around had not told me that. I sat down even more anguished, looking at her, the television and the floor. "Where are you from?" she asked. "I've got manic depression and I've come from Wales." I said.

She nodded her head and took a huge drag on a cigarette. I noticed that her hands were covered in cigarette stains and she looked like she hadn't exercised since birth. She looked liked she ate hundreds of donuts every day and had been wearing the same clothes for weeks. Was this my only form of rational contact? There again, speaking to a woman who was so fat and ugly made me question my prejudices. I was prejudiced against her because of her appearance, just as people were prejudiced against the mentally ill in society.

I guess other people feel the same way about extremely fat people as they do about the mentally ill. They're both in the minority and are therefore persecuted by the masses. These prejudices are typical of the foundations of racism in our society and need to be stamped out. Britain is now a multicultural society and people need to understand different cultures to function in an orderly fashion. It's an embarrassment to the nation that the British National Party has had so much support in places like Oldham and Bradford. We're in the new millennium. I mean, what the fuck is wrong with people? Are they fucking ignorant or what? The more different cultures mix and blend, the more educated and happier everybody should be. It's as simple as that. It doesn't take a moralist or a puritan to work this out – it's just common sense.

I had to get out of the shit-hole I was in. I knew I was ill but Withington hospital would make me worse. It couldn't be good for anybody staying in there. Time passed extra slowly in my new environment.

One of the staff approached guarding a sandwich trolley. "Only one sandwich each." she said to the black man who had told me to fuck off. "There's tea as well", said my new friend as she pointed to a huge teapot. The teapot looked almost as big as her in proportion. It must have had enough for 30 cups of tea in it. I drank the lukewarm tea in a few seconds and ate some egg sandwiches without chewing them properly.

Soon, I went to bed wearing a T-shirt, jumper and a pair of socks as I was freezing. The old man was talking to himself, cussing and swearing about being hard done by in life. I thought that he was some kind of schizophrenic. He was clearly not well and had an aggression problem. After trying not to hear him talk gibberish for two hours, I asked him if he wouldn't mind being quiet. He went mad and said: "Who do you think you are asking me to be quiet? You've only just got here and you think you own the fucking place. Where's my fucking tea anyway? I fought the fucking war for little brats like you, and this is how you treat me.

Bipolar, Recovery and NLP

You ought to be ashamed of yourself. I've killed people before, you know, in combat with my bayonet and I'm not scared of anyone." I said: "Look, I only asked you to be quiet, forget it."

"I'm going to fucking sort you out," he said walking over to my bed. I went to get out of my bed and he stopped me standing up by putting his hand firmly on my knee. "Don't think you're better than me you little prick." I'm 6' 4" and bulky but this mad, old, evil bastard was really scaring me. I was really weak and I left the room asking him to "just leave me alone". When I arrived in the ward I was confronted with a dirty, perverted, podgy man. He smelt awful and had yellow stained fingers from smoking too many roll ups. He tried to pinch Celia's arse so she attacked him, punching him and slapping him repeatedly. He cried for her to stop. Then he walked away hastily with his pyjama bottoms falling down and his own bare arse showing. She kicked him in the back and called him "a fucking pervert". She sounded quite scary with her Scottish accent, and looked it too, with her booming voice and eyes raging. "Don't come back in here tonight or I'll beat you up, you fucking pervert. He's a fucking pervert. Stay away from him", she advised me.

For five minutes, we sat there in silence smoking cigarettes. She had given me one of hers. The dirty man walked back in asking me for a cigarette and she chased him down the corridor. "He's a fucking pervert, a fucking pervert. A pervert." she repeated. One of the night staff came in and asked what the disturbance was. "He's a fucking pervert. He's a filthy old man. And he's ugly", she cursed. The member of staff walked off looking cross that a retard had had the audacity to disturb her. She was no detective, I thought. Why wasn't she doing her job, I thought, instead of reading the bloody tabloids? "You should all be in bed. Be quiet. And go to bed soon", she snarled.

I've often wandered around at night in hospital and discovered staff, who I've presumed should have been awake, sleeping. I used to feel a great antagonism towards mental health nurses as they held power over me unlike anyone else had ever done when I had been an adult. I used to think they thought the patients were unworthy beings. They were in charge and had nobody to boss them around. I was paranoid that the staff who didn't speak much thought that the patients on the ward weren't really people anyway and didn't warrant any special care or attention. The difficult thing about being mentally ill is that it's such a lonely experience. I also feared that the general staff consensus was that the patients were crazy and needed to sleep as they would be less of a nuisance then; that's the best remedy – sleep. They don't want to talk to anybody about their problems. Even if they did they would be incapable of being rational as they are mentally ill.

Meanwhile, back in the cesspit known as Withington, a girl aged about 15 popped out of the women's quarters into the lounge carrying a book and smoking a cigarette. It was now 12.30pm. "What are you doing?" I asked. "I'm writing a poem", she said. "I'd like to read it sometime", I replied. "Have you got a piece of paper?" She tore off a piece of paper. "Goodnight", butted in Celia. "And stay away from that old man in there – he's a fucking pervert", she said. "Goodnight", I replied. I wrote a rhyming poem in a couple of minutes. It was not very memorable and one of the thousands I'd lost or thrown away while being in, or coming out of, hospitals. At that time, though, it helped. "Can I read your poem?" I asked. "Sure", she said. "There's more in the back." I started reading through them and they weren't bad. "Can I look at your tapes?" she asked. "Yeah", I said.

We sat in silence. I read her poems as she smoked a cigarette, playing one of my hardcore dance tapes in the background. I said I liked the poems, and when she went to bed I went back to my sleeping quarters. The old man opposite was now asleep and I curled up in the chill of the night trying to forget everything that had happened to me – all the shit I was going through, had been through, and which was yet to come. That night was one of the lowest ebbs of my life. I knew I was going to have to get out of there if I was going to survive, going to save any self respect. I was losing dignity and the will to live fast. When my eyes were closed, I could still see the light of the moon through the flimsy curtains. My thighs felt as if they were covered in ice and my feet had terrible cramp. I was too depressed to do anything about it except to curl up even more. After a while, I got up and put my jeans and another jumper on but I was still freezing and the window wouldn't shut. A tear dripped down my eye as I said: "Fuck." As I curled back up in my sheets I started to cry. My only comfort was that Meredith would be there the next day. In the darkness that clouded over me I tried to imagine her as the light at the end of the tunnel.

Straight after finishing work Meredith would come to see me. At least there was something reliable in my life – something that had a little meaning. There was a sense of purpose and together we made a good team. We had come together under extraordinary circumstances but had grown to care for each other. It was a peculiar way to fall in love. We were devoted to each other and I was monogamous in a relationship for the first time in my life. We were thankful to each other for sorting each other's heads out and neither of us seemed to be able to function properly without the other.

She had inspired me, or certainly made it easier for me, to write my first screenplay in the summer of 1995 entitled: *A Can of Madness*. (Sound familiar?) It was about my first manic episode, although I had changed the names of the characters to avoid offending the people closest to me. Putting my own thoughts and behaviour through somebody else also acted as a form of therapy. It was the first thing of any real substance that I had written. I had written short stories about various fights that I had had and endless poems – my favourite of which were a collection on the theme of ecstasy entitled *E*. The collection describes taking ecstasy and its effect on my psyche and the chemical generation that I am part of.

When morning arrived, I noticed that my tapes had been stolen from the ward. They meant a lot to me and the staff showed no sympathy. They merely repeated hospital policy. "Any valuables that you have should be kept in your room." I told them that I had no lock for my cupboard and they said that they would "try and get a lock for me when it was not too busy". Well, in a hospital, especially this one, that was likely to mean never. Staff just forgot things like that – I knew from experience. My expectations of getting back the tapes were low and no member of staff ever came back to me on their possible whereabouts. I made several futile attempts to get somebody to look for them but nobody did.

There was no justice in there. Just a head fuck. You were just fobbed off all the time and if you persisted they just belittled you by saying there were more important things to attend to. They'd make you wait for ages. It seemed deliberate. After I gave up looking for my tapes, I gave my money to the staff and they put it in the safe. When convenient, I would have to ask permission to get access to it. Then I would have to sign and the member of staff would record how much money was left. Sometimes it was like Fort Knox trying to get in the staff room and then they would loathe you pestering them to get money out to buy cigarettes or sweets.

On the night I arrived, there was an act of gross misconduct by a member of staff. The cunt wouldn't let me take my lithium, I mean, he took it off me. I told him I needed it and that it was my lifeline but he said it was hospital policy that patients couldn't have any drugs on them. I told him that I understood that but said that I had not been given my lithium at medication time because my name was not on the meds board and they agreed I could take my own that evening. That fucking cocksucker. I spent a night without lithium because of him and he was supposed to be looking after me. The other staff told me that I would have to wait until the morning. I felt so pathetic: I couldn't even hold onto my pills. What a loser I was turning out to be.

The food in the hospital was appalling. There was a canteen along the corridor although usually the staff members that served the food were rude and impatient. It was another one of the demanding chores that an NHS mental nurse had to deal with. It was an example of them doing menial tasks instead of being able to concentrate on nursing. A typical comment you would hear was: "If you don't like it, then that's too bad. I'm sure someone else will have it." The only thing I can remember liking was sponge pudding with custard. The taste made me feel, for the merest part of a second, OK; like I felt when I was writing a poem. Time stood still for just a few fractions of a second. These moments were becoming fewer and fewer though, as I was starting to go deeper and deeper into depression when I arrived back in Manchester.

When Meredith arrived on my second afternoon there she looked exhausted. She hadn't eaten and her hair was dyed auburn brown. It didn't suit her and her clothes weren't as clean as they used to be. She was wearing too much make-up to try and cover up how physically and mentally exhausted she was. She'd lost that spark and she looked shattered. She didn't stay for long. She had to find the landlord because the heating in the flat wasn't working. Several months later, she told me that she used to cry herself to sleep because she was so cold. I hate that when people tell you things months after they happen. Why can't people be up front with each other? It would save a lot of pain in the long run. I mean, the more direct people are with each other the less their emotions are fucked around with.

Meredith was pleased that I was back. She'd wanted me to transfer to Withington Hospital for weeks but I hadn't been well enough. Now she thought I was better. It was a good job that I hadn't moved to Withington before as it was so nightmarish. I had no option but to discharge myself and did so the following day. I also cancelled an appointment I had arranged with a university friend the following day. It was with the guy I used to get drunk with, Roger. I didn't want him to see me in such a shit-pit. When I telephoned him and he didn't suggest an alternative time or place to meet I said: "C'ya" and put the phone down with regret. None of my friends had come to see me in Wales or in Withington, only Meredith and my family.

Going back to my flat was almost as big an ordeal as going to Withington. I went back to the place where I had discovered that the whole world would be in an orgy together, the place where Chorlton-cum-Hardy was the head of world consciousness. This was the place where I had to restore my sanity. What the fuck was going on? What the fucking hell was happening? Things went from worse to even worse. It was January 1997 and the depression took over. I began to sleep more and more. My only activity was watching cable TV late at night and the occasional shag with Meredith. I would sleep up to 16 hours at a time and at random times of the day. When Meredith got back from work, the flat was a mess and I was either in bed or had just got out of it. She came back for lunch every day and woke me up making me a sandwich, or we would share a salad.

She became more and more messy and more stressed every time I saw her. Back then, though, I didn't really notice or care; I just wanted to sleep. She asked her boss for a week's holiday. He had been very reasonable in the previous few months and she had told him about my illness but this time he said no.

A couple of weeks later we went to the travel agents looking

Bipolar, Recovery and NLP

for the dream holiday. We chose a week in Benidorm as opposed to a week in Bulgaria skiing as her ski kit didn't arrive from her mother's in time. She bunked off work and we went to Heathrow. I had had 10 cans of Stella by the time we boarded the plane and literally filled two of them with piss as we were taking off. My animal mentality had returned and became a metaphor for denying my illness. Something had to give sooner or later.

This was not a romantic start and was similar to how things were when we first started seeing each other. We spent three nights getting pissed up in a tacky bar where a woman would extract bottles of wine and candles from her fanny. We didn't see any of the sights. I was drinking incessantly. I would drink at least 15 pints of strong lager in one, and each one through two thin straws as they didn't have the thicker straws that I had become accustomed to back in Manchester. I had to have a witness for each one. We were hung over in the day and only managed to spend a couple of hours on the beach.

On the fourth night it was Meredith's birthday. We went out for a nice Chinese meal and then I started drinking more than usual. We befriended two Scottish heroin addicts and somehow got separated. Meredith had stormed out because we had had an argument. I was too pissed to remember what it was about. She was probably jealous of me gawping at the girl who did the magic tricks. I left one club and made my way to another. As I ran up the stairs to the exit I slipped on something and went flying. As my jaw hit the floor, I must have passed out straight away.

The time was 7.50am. The place was Alicante Hospital. The reason I was there was because I had broken my jaw. This symbolised a moment in my life when things had to change. I started writing my first novel. It started off being a positive book about an alcoholic with a mental illness who was trying to lift himself out of depression while recovering from a broken jaw in a Spanish hospital. He had a girlfriend who loved him but then he would fantasise about being a paedophile. After writing a couple of pages about the latter, I ceased writing and wondered what the fuck I was on about. The depression had really got a hold of me this time. I'd lost my own identity for real and I wondered if I would ever be able to get it back.

The night before, I had threatened to jump off a walkway onto

Bipolar, Recovery and NLP

the beach. I also remember threatening to jump off the balcony of our apartment on our first night there. It was on the eighth floor. Meredith didn't need that shit. I didn't know if I really gave a fuck about anything or if it was a cry for help, a cry for somebody to lift me out of my depression.

The fact that I had broken my jaw turned out to be a blessing in disguise. It knocked some sense into me. It forced me to put my life into perspective before any serious suicide attempt took control of my mind. Meredith went home at the end of the week and I stayed an extra week for an operation that proved to be successful. The hospital and staff were very professional and I even learnt some Spanish. I couldn't open my mouth for six weeks, though. At least this stopped me getting pissed. I wasn't stupid enough to drink through straws and breathe through my nose. I wouldn't be able to puke up my own vomit and could swallow it and die. Jimi Hendrix and Sid Vicious would have been proud of me if I'd done that, but I wasn't that stupid. I wasn't as stupid anymore.

Before I'd gone on holiday Dr. Cooper had put me on Sulpiride. The pills seemed to start working soon after the metal was released from my mouth. Six weeks free from drinking had sobered me up and lifted my mood as well. I could now face life again, but first I had to face coming to terms with madness. I had experienced two manic episodes. It was no one-off and it was likely I was going to have others. There was still hope though, as Dr. Cooper told me, as I had not been maintained on Lithium and for 90% of people who have the illness it controls their mood swings. This could prevent an episode. My girlfriend had stood by me and I was determined to go back to university later in the year and finish my degree.

It was only April so I decided to get a job. I knew it would give me some much-needed confidence and I could also pay off my £1,200 overdraft. I joined several temping agencies and got a job through one of them as a security guard at Manchester airport, preventing protestors from sabotaging building work.

I met someone at a bus stop on my first morning to work. He later proved to be one of my best friends. Tom Robertson understood what it was like to be a bit crazy and his positive attitude and constant encouragement to, from and during work sanitised me and helped me deal with the biggest dilemma of the illness. Relying on Tom for spiritual and philosophical support enabled me to come to terms with going mad. The transition back into society became more bearable. My conversations with him also cleared the path in my relationship with Meredith which had been very rocky up until that point.

We worked 12-hour shifts, from either seven in the morning to seven in the evening or vice versa, seven days in a row. In between changing shifts we would alternate between three and four days off. I worked from the start of April until the beginning of June. Life was looking up. Meredith got a promotion – which included a good pay rise – to a marketing position at work, and even set up a website for her boss's company. I bought her a new outfit to celebrate. It was a professional looking designer aqua blue jacket and skirt. We had the occasional row and she would sometimes shout at me. I never raised my voice, though, and if I felt really frustrated I would call my old school friend, Panji.

He played basketball for Manchester Giants. He deserved it as he had practised so hard before and after school from the age of 14 onwards. Panji liked to party and was usually available if I wanted to get out of the house. He was finishing a degree in Mechanical Engineering at Salford University and was disillusioned with basketball. He would come and pick me up and we would go for a few pints and talk about what we were doing and wonder what other people we used to go to school with were doing. We would go to the sports bar, Cheerleaders, and other bars in Deansgate, or cruise around student hangouts.

The Panji I knew had always been a very quiet and determined individual. He drank too much but managed to lead an extremely active life. I admired him for that and liked listening to stories about what he and his team-mates got up to when they went out at night. I remember drinking polish vodka with him on his birthday. Panji introduced me to the best player on the team. His name was Mark Robinson. The guy just blanked me. I couldn't believe it. If that was what a bit of fame did to him then fuck him, man. If I ever had a bit of fame, which I always wanted, I wouldn't treat anyone like that.

When it was time to come out, I felt as if I was one of those 12 year-old boys being hit on the backside – the most painful place apart from the nuts and face – by one of Panji's flying tennis balls. Meredith wanted to go back to London and leave me, knowing that I had to stay in Manchester for another year and finish my degree. She said that she wanted "her mummy". We had been living together for eighteen months and she had enjoyed the first six. My illness had taken its toll and she had no fight left in her. Having discussed things in detail and cried throughout I thought it best to grant her wish. I made the most painful phone call that I had ever made. I rang up the landlord, an amicable man called Joe, and gave him a month's notice. The following month I have never cried so much in my life. I was a pitiful wreck whose heart had been broken. I didn't know that it was possible for a man to feel so weak. She was crying almost as much as me but it was she who had deserted me just when things were turning round. She had given up. Run out of steam. She'd run out of the juice, man.

We stayed together for the next few months with me spending most of it in London with her parents. We did the things that normal people do. We visited art galleries, went out and socialised and even did some of the tourist things like visiting Madame Tussauds and going on a Big Bus London bus tour.

Bipolar, Recovery and NLP

Chapter 6 – Back to life (the second transition)

In September 1997, I moved into some quiet university halls on the outskirts of Chorlton. This was just the kind of environment I wanted to be in to focus on my final year, and the exact opposite of what I'd wanted in my first year. Within a few weeks of starting the first year a group of us had wanted to leave halls and get our own flat. Thing is, the halls wouldn't give us our money back until they rented our rooms and since they couldn't guarantee this we all stayed put.

My new digs were near a huge green, with the local pub bordering a canal. The flat was very smart and a cleaner came round once a week. The cleaner even did the washing up which was pretty essential with six blokes living in a flat. It was a multicultural flat. My male flatmates were from India, Portugal, France, Malaysia and Ireland. It was a new home and a place where I could concentrate on my work. There was a little green outside the kitchen window and I could see people going to get their mail from my bedroom window. I would play football whenever I saw people kicking around – it was always a nice break from studying.

I made a conscious effort not to tell people of my illness. Ironically, of course, I always ended up letting the cat out of the bag. I was embarrassed by it and didn't want to be asked too many demanding questions in case my head exploded. Basically, I felt that I could never be my real self, especially when meeting people. People would ask me what I wanted to do when I graduated and I told them that I wanted to be a writer. They would ask if I had written anything or ask me what I was going to write about. I would tell them that I had written and would continue to write about drama. Eventually I would write comedy. They would try and make me be more specific. I would tell them that I wrote empirical texts and conclude their interrogations with profound remarks stating that I had had an interesting or crazy life that was too complicated and too personal to explain to somebody that I had just met. I couldn't open up to complete strangers. I didn't want them to judge me for what I had become: a retard. I was somebody who passed in and out of madness and who was unable to control when he did. Just as Oscar Wilde had been persecuted for being gay, I didn't want to be maltreated for being mentally ill. I knew I had a problem and writing about it would be the most cathartic way of dealing with it.

On 5 October, 1997, it was my Nan's eightieth birthday party. I bought her a picture of Van Gogh's *Café Terrace on the Place Du Forum*. It was one of two hundred canvasses he painted in 1888 and this man, like me, was a mad genius. I stayed with Meredith in the luxury suite at the hotel where my mum worked as the receptionist. We had some champagne the night before the party and pretended that things were OK. For that night things actually were ok although, as a whole, our relationship was resting on thin ice. At the party, Meredith looked stunning, mature and sophisticated, as she always did if she made an effort.

The party itself was a bizarre affair. There were about 20 people there of whom I only knew half a dozen or so. So this was the rest of my living family tree? They appeared so small-minded, simple and content, living in the past. These, then, were the roots whence I had sprung. They were not, however, the side of my family that had given me my mental illness, as this was the sane side, my mum's side – the *caring* side. My dad's side was the one with the mental problem. They were the crazy ones. In fact, it's widely accepted that if a family has manic depression in their genes there is a 27% chance of a member catching it. Well, I always knew I was special.

I remember closely watching Meredith interact at my Nan's party. It was to be the last time that we would see each other for a year. We were to grow apart and lead lives in different directions from then on. How can somebody you have spent so much time with, and been so close to, suddenly disappear out of your life like that? Thing is, it happens everyday to thousands of people all over the country.

Meredith and I tried our utmost to remain amicable towards each other and stay friends, but it proved to be impossible. The human condition rarely allows people to be friends once they have been lovers. It is too weak. Love is either painful or a delight, and ex-lovers are unable to remain friends, in most cases, as the emotions that run through them are too strong and lead to jealousy, resentment and anger.

I guess the ending of my relationship took a course similar to

Bipolar, Recovery and NLP

that of many others. It slowly fizzled out. She had visited my new digs the week before the party, which was my first weekend there. Some of my flatmates remarked how good-looking she was and I was proud to show her off, but that was the last time she came. She asked if she could come up the week after the party, but the truth is I didn't want her there. I couldn't forgive her for leaving and although I still wanted her in some ways, I wanted a new life. Above all, I suppose, I wanted to see if I could cope without her. I told her that she couldn't come up that weekend and she pretended not to be upset. If she had pleaded, on the other hand, pleaded like I did to her to stay with me I would have let her. But she would never do that. She would never resort to begging like I had. She was too good, too strong for that. She was too well-brought up. She couldn't humiliate herself as I had done. She had given enough up already, looking after an invalid.

Meanwhile, I had asked another girl out to the cinema and she had accepted. This could be the start of something new, I thought. It could be the start of a new relationship where things could be right from the start. If it didn't work out long-term then at least I might get some sex during the week. In the event, nothing materialised with the girl I went to the cinema with – I think I scared her a bit. I mean, she started shaking when I put my arm round her in the cinema. Anyway, I didn't give a fuck really. It really helped me stop thinking about Meredith – as to my great annoyance and frustration I was thinking about her nearly all the time. It's hard when someone is such a part of your life and then you become separated, especially when it isn't your decision.

...

Over the next few weeks, we were both coming up with excuses and the phone calls to each other became less and less frequent and more and more detached. We fell out on the phone in January 1997 after I asked her if she had a boyfriend and she said: "It's none of your business." I told her that I had had a girlfriend since and she told me that she did have a boyfriend and hung up. Her response was to write me a nasty letter blaming me for her troubled life. It was so melodramatic it would have been more appropriate in a Shakespearean comedy. I think of the ass in *A*

Bipolar, Recovery and NLP

Midsummer Night's Dream when he gets his oats. His lover doesn't know what's going on just like Meredith. She had blamed everything on my illness and now hated me – it was crystal clear, the evidence was right there in front of me. I didn't need that shit. So that was it. That was fucking it. We were finished. Fucking finished, for good. I burnt her letter and put that episode of my life behind me as best as I could and started my final year at university for the second time.

In halls, I had become an avid student for the first time since I was 17 and drank heavily only once or twice a week. The main reason for the reduction in alcohol consumption was my love of tae kwon do. The instructor, about my age, was a charismatic African and his sense of humour and positivism, combined with my own fascination, was enough to get me hooked. It restored me into the physical world and did a lot for my self-confidence. It also helped control my aggression which had been a problem since I started drinking when I was 14.

I showed my screenplay to two of my lecturers who admired me for having the stature to put my experiences onto the printed page. I remember the head of department, after I had told him that most of my script was autobiographical, saying: "I hope your life really wasn't like that." I brushed his remark off with a deep sigh and some extra tae kwon do training.

My personal tutor was encouraged by the way I could accept criticism of my work in an unpretentious manner. My marks improved from medium to high 2:1s, to low firsts and eventually to high firsts. I made applications for postgraduate study in writing, theatre and film. I entered my screenplay into the Manchester University Film Competition. To my bewilderment, they claimed that they never received my entry. I went to the University Film Society and discovered that the students there had the home number of Danny Boyle, the director of *Trainspotting*. He had been the patron of the Film Society for two years and they had been too scared to phone him even once. They refused to give me his number as he was making some film in Bali (*The Beach*) and my creative mind was left wandering around again. My final year studies were keeping me more than occupied thanks to all the essays that needed to be submitted for coursework.

Whenever sane, I found it difficult to avoid playing on the fact that I was a loony, especially when people got to know me better. It was my way of saying: "If you fuck with me, I'm gonna fuck you up." I still had that Snoop Doggy Dogg mentality in me and although I was white, I was, in the words of Ice Cube: "The wrong nigger to fuck with." The halls consisted mostly of foreign students which was both refreshing and annoying. All in all, it helped me to socialise on a superficial level. This was good for two reasons: one, I didn't feel so much of an outcast, and two, I could revert back to my studies without too much distraction.

On New Year's Eve, I had my best fuck for a long time. She was a 33 year-old Irish stunner. She was extremely slim, blonde, pretty, looked sophisticated and laughed a lot. I had gone out on the piss with my Irish flatmate, Mark, and his brother, and at the beginning of the evening had said, in a Larry Fishburne (*King of New York*) manner, that: "I'm gonna go down town, find me a girl and get my nob polished." It worked.

We latched on to three Irish women prowling outside a public house in central Manchester. One of them was really good looking, the other two were not. That was OK as I didn't have a great deal of competition that night. In fact, I didn't seem to very often. I set about putting my plan into action. I ignored the good-looking one but made enough innuendo and gave her just enough attention to keep her interested. I kept cool, so I could reel her in when I wanted.

When the New Year approached, she called for us to join her friends who were dancing. I knew she was up for it and New Year's Eve led to a snog, a good fuck and an interesting couple of months. It was unfortunate, though, that she turned out to be a bitch. And I don't mean a bitch. I mean a fucking ho. You know, a prick tease and all that kind of shit. First, things went great. Lust is natural. After I'd fucked her, she remarked how relaxed a person I was. I spent the next few days and nights drinking with her and her friends and then fucking her in their hotel room. After five days of horny fucking, with her mates spending a lot of time out of the room leaving us to it, she went back to Dublin but invited me over whenever I wanted.

Half term was coming up and I had worked hard so I decided to go and stay with her the following week. When I arrived in Dublin, she kept me waiting in a pub for two hours as she was with

Bipolar, Recovery and NLP

her mum having her nails manicured. I mean, what kind of shit was that? I didn't make an issue out of it, though, as I desperately needed to empty my bollocks. They felt like fucking watermelons man. I mean, I didn't have elephantitis of the nuts or anything, but I had nowhere to stay and I wanted to fuck some pussy and have my balls sucked.

We eventually got back to her flat after getting rid of her mate and I realised what a spoilt bitch she was. Daddy had bought her a brand new pad in a trendy suburb of Dublin. She was manageress at a travel agent's and went to work during the day. I read and answered exam questions on the great Roman orator Cicero and went to University College Dublin to check out their film studies department. I had an in-depth conversation with one of their lecturers and he convinced me that I should apply. I fucked Debbie and came over her nine times during one episode of Grandstand. I was quite proud of that achievement and it was nice to watch a bit of Football Focus while I was doing it. There was a lot of shagging during the week but the relationship had nothing else to it. It consisted of her insulting me, apologising, cooking a nice meal, me watching her get drunk and trying not to drink much myself. Hardly the cultural side of Dublin. I met her sister who was even more vacuous than her. There was not a jot of intellectual capacity to them, only a belief that their daddy was better than everybody else's because his BMW had cost £80,000. They were totally fucked up and unlikeable, but when you think through your dick, you think through your dick ...

I left Dublin and spoke to Debbie (yes, she has a name although it clearly isn't an aristocratic one) a few times in the weeks that followed. She had arranged to fly over for Valentine's weekend. I mean, talk about being a hypocrite – what's a tart like that doing flying over for Valentine's weekend? What the fuck? What the fuck was going on? By this time, I was studying harder and getting closer to having a six-pack by taking tae kwon do more and more seriously. I met her at the airport and we stayed at the Copthorne Hotel next to Old Trafford football ground. She was paying. I could get used to this, I thought. It wasn't long, though, before I was made to look stupid. We were only into our second drink at the bar and she was chatting up the barman. He was only about 18. What the fuck was going on? If any bloke gave me shit

Bipolar, Recovery and NLP

I'd kick fuck out of them, but when a woman gave me shit I kept quiet and became paralysed. Better to do that than lose my temper, I thought.

I reluctantly took Debbie's bags up to the hotel room as she flirted with the barman. I remember asking her if she'd had any abortions. She admitted that she'd had two and said that it was none of my business when I asked her how she had felt. It seemed that any attempt I made to get closer to her rebounded off a wall that had already been strategically set in place. We eventually got to the hotel room and I remember the sex wasn't as good as it had been the last time. I had bought her a Valentine's card, as I thought girls always liked that kind of thing even if they said they didn't, some aromatherapy oils and handcuffs to try to add a bit of kinkiness to the proceedings. She replied that she didn't want a card, as she guzzled the chocolate that accompanied it, and said that if she put me in handcuffs she would leave me tied to the bed and fuck off to the bar. I was sick of her cruel humour and knew that there was a good chance that she meant what she said. It would be something that Debbie could tell her friend who would be arriving on a later flight with her boyfriend from Dublin. The weekend was a frustrating one.

We went to a nightclub but they wouldn't let me in, apparently because my shoes weren't smart enough. I had to go all the way back to my flat in a taxi to get some smart shoes because the stupid cow I was with insisted that she didn't want to go anywhere else. The last time I saw her was at the airport and when she guessed that I had had a shit weekend, she said: "Don't worry I've only been messing wid ya." I had shown my sensitive and jealous side and she was not interested in it. She just wanted to have a good laugh by humiliating me. My head was fucked enough already without being trampled on by a callous bitch like that. That was the last time we saw each other. I rang her a few times after that due to lust and confusion; I was grateful that she never called me back.

Tae kwon do became more and more an inspiration and a way to channel my aggression. It helped relieve the tiresome hours spent studying and acted as an escape from anything that was bothering me. By Easter 1998, I was training everyday, sparring privately with my teacher and doing advanced yoga classes. I was

Bipolar, Recovery and NLP

as fit as a fiddle and agile as an anteater's tongue. I had a few close friends and my self-confidence had returned. I hadn't missed a lecture at university and had handed all my work in on time, usually ahead of schedule. I was a scholar most of the time and managed to channel my aggression effectively for the first time in my life.

I was totally absorbed in tae kwon do and other martial arts such as jujitsu, judo, ninjitsu, karate and kung fu. When things became too stressful, I would go for a few games of pool or snooker and have the occasional drinking binge. I was so proud of my figure that I would limit my drinking for the first time ever and burn off the fat the next morning or afternoon if I ever had a hangover. The return to the physical world helped my health and work. I was also conscious of complying with my medication everyday and for once my lithium levels were normal. Every couple of weeks I might forget, in which case I'd take an extra dose. Sometimes, though, I simply didn't need to.

I had a few loose relationships with women. I slept with this Austrian bird and would kick her out because she kept me awake. The most unforgettable was a pissed-up venture with a girl who lived next door and who was studying Russian. She wanted to go out, but once I'd sobered up I didn't want to go out with her. After a meaningless one-night stand we never spoke to each other again apart from when I would say the occasional: "All right." She was too embarrassed because I was a "good catch", as she put it, and although I felt guilty about being picky I had my standards. I knew I was prejudiced but I just couldn't help it. I had another fling with a girl I met on the internet. I sent her a picture of my cock in the post and after a five-hour telephone conversation decided to stay with her for a weekend in Scunthorpe without even knowing what she looked like. It was a pleasant surprise as she was very pretty. She was 20 and had a two year-old kid. We didn't see each other again as the situation was too bad. She must have thought that I was some kind of psychopath ... If she only knew ... Ha, ha, ha.

I also met a woman through an advert in the Manchester Evening News. I travelled to Crewe to meet her. Again, this was a blind date. She was thirty-eight and had four kids. What was it with me and single mums? Maybe I didn't want kids of my own as I was told that my illness was a genetic condition and I didn't want my kids to go through what I had gone through. I thought that I could bring up somebody else's kids. Yes, that was it. And if we split up it wouldn't matter. It wouldn't matter if I lost custody as they weren't really mine and it would save me money too. Think of all the money I could save on nappies and shit like that, or schooling and food.

I watched *Golden Eye* at the cinema with the blond, single mum and she was good-looking for her age. We made out in her car as she didn't want me to meet her kids yet. She said she'd call me a few days later. After a while she didn't so I called and asked to see her. She said that she didn't want to see me again as she thought I wanted something that was too serious. Fuck, I was only being a gentleman. I didn't give a fuck about this wrinkled slut bag. I mean, treat a woman nicely and she wants you to treat her like a slut; treat her like a slut and she wants you to treat her better. I never understood women. What the fuck went on in their heads? You think you know what they're thinking and everything's OK and then they always surprise you. They fuck up men's heads, man. Well, that's the attraction I suppose. We're all masochists at heart. Just like we all need loving once in a while.

Soon after I last saw Meredith in October 1997, I started to write to sexy advertisements in naughty magazines. It helped me get over her. Thinking of women as sex objects instead of lovers made me more rational. Most of the ads I responded to were time-wasting women who were prostitutes in disguise. Others wanted naked photos of an erect penis so I obliged after borrowing my Portuguese flatmate's camera and taking photos of myself. I had some good responses, the most amusing of which was seeing a woman I had formed a no-strings relationship with in Escort magazine. "I didn't realise that you had become a celebrity", I said.

The Sunday Sport proved to be the most successful. It led to some interesting encounters which turned me into more and more of a misogynist. Things were really starting to take off when I stumbled into another relationship with an Irish girl. This one was very pretty, tall, brunette, 24, lived in halls and, what's more, had bigger tits than the Irish slut from Dublin. Basically, my flatmate Mark had told me that one of the best looking girls on campus

Bipolar, Recovery and NLP

fancied me but that he couldn't tell me who.

I guessed which girl it was and made my move. Her name was Katherine O'Donnell. I saw her bored out of her mind with a bunch of fuck-wits in the bar on campus and decided to teach her how to play pool. We had some swift pints and went back to my flat. I had five pints of Caffreys in five swigs in twenty minutes as I was pissed off for leaving Scunthorpe a night earlier than expected. We went to my room and downstairs to pinch a bottle of my Portuguese flatmate's wine. She started snogging me and so began two weeks of almost constant, hard-core sex. She gave me all the compliments under the sun; told me that she had fancied me for ages, that she had never met anyone like me, that I was the best fuck she had ever had, that she was falling in love with me, that she loved being in my arms and loved spending time with me, and that I was the most intelligent person she'd ever met. I'd never met a girl that was so infatuated with me so quickly.

The only problem was that she had a boyfriend. He was a big fucker and had never lost a fight. That wasn't too much of a problem, though, as he lived in Belfast and I knew I was a crazier fucker than him – and a better man. Christ, I had to be with all the compliments she was giving me. I was also at my physical peak and felt confident that I could knock out four clones of her boyfriend at the same time, *and* on my own. Nobody could fuck with me, I was invincible. I was a fucking mean machine. We debated at length whether she should go back to Belfast or not for Easter, and eventually she did go back and stay with her friends. She couldn't stay with her family as her dad wasn't speaking to her because he disapproved of her going out with a Protestant. I was pleased with this situation in one respect as it made my position of keeping her a little stronger. Mind you, if her dad refused to speak to her because she had a boyfriend with a different religion, wouldn't he be prejudiced against a manic-depressive as well? I tried not to think about that.

Anyway, when she went away, I concentrated on studying as my finals were looming and I didn't want to underachieve. She was going to see her boyfriend but she convinced me that I was the special one. Things weren't going to change – they were going to stay the same. After all, our relationship wasn't just one of lust. She had been going out with her boyfriend for three years and I was the only other person she had slept with in that time. She didn't want to upset him but she intended to stay in Manchester and get a job as a teacher when she qualified for her PGCE in June 1997. I was planning to do an MA in Screenwriting at Manchester University at the time, which could have included a writer from Granada Studios as mentor, so I saw the possibility of a long-term relationship with her. Things were going to plan. I was coming of age and my life had cemented after all the crumbling in the past. I was not going to end up writing for some shitty magazine like Concrete World; I was destined for the top. Soon, I would be on top of the world.

Katherine came back from Northern Ireland a week later and we went out and got drunk the evening she got back. We ended up fucking in the woods in the dark and it took us a couple of hours to find our way home. Our short cut didn't work and there was also a slight problem – we discovered, in the morning, that the condom had split. As she wasn't on the pill, I had to take her down the clinic so that she could take the morning after pill. Afterwards, she was throwing up in a bad way and said that she didn't want me to see her being sick. Then I discovered that she needed time to think as she was not sure if she wanted to carry on seeing me. What the fuck was going on here? Yet another woman fucking with my head? Oh no, not again. I even lent her my screenplay as I thought that would convince her that I was a great writer and to try and impress upon her that she was privileged to find me.

I turned to Mark for support. I had told him about my manic depression after a game of snooker one evening. He was easy to talk to. He had told me that he had warned Katherine not to get involved with me because he cared about me as a friend and didn't want to see her fuck my head up. I found out then that he had told her about my manic depression before even I did. Fuck me, he thought he was such a fucking counsellor that he could control my relationship before it had even started. What the fuck was going on? I felt like kicking his teeth in but he was so easy to talk to that it would have been unjust.

His problem was that he told everyone everything. He was the sort of mate who would fuck your bird behind your back and then, if you found out, blame it on her and try to return to the friendship you had had before with him. I found out that he did this a year later to one of his best friends. And what's more, he did it to one of his Irish mates.

The night in the woods was the last time I fucked Katherine. We spent the next morning getting her the morning after pill at the clinic and she dumped me soon after that. We fell out soon enough at a party. She was pissed out of her mind flirting with a few of the blokes there. Another tart – why couldn't I find a decent bird? Couldn't I find one that wasn't a slut? That's all I wanted. My mum would always tell me that I was too desperate and that girls can tell that. "It scares them away", she would say. "When you least expect it, that's when you'll find one. When you don't go looking for it." She was right. It took me a long time to figure that out. When you frown, you use 60 muscles; when you smile, you only use 16. I guess girls can sense that.

Our break-up now seems quite comical. I was fed up with her flirting at the party and when she sat on Mark's lap and started flirting with him it was the last straw. My pulse was beating pretty hard and in my sober state I poured a glass of tap water and threw it in her face without uttering a word. I left the flat immediately and returned to mine, satisfied with the morsel of retribution I had won, although I was angry that I had been made such a fool of. My ego had taken a knock and I couldn't handle it. At least everyone else now knew that she was a tart. More importantly, they knew that I wouldn't let anyone fuck with me.

My anger turned to Mark. This was the wanker who I had been pouring my heart out to half an hour before. I had only left my studies to go to the party and try to win Katherine back. Her friend had phoned the flat and he had told me that she was round there. I thought he was my best friend apart from Tom. Then I realised he was everyone's best friend – at least he pretended to be. He was not a genuine person; one of those fake people in life who are always out to impress others. Their own life is so shit that they project themselves onto other people. Mark was a loser. I mean, he was 30 and was in his first year at the Polytechnic studying an Engineering degree. He didn't have the required A-level grades like most people I knew so had taken a foundation year instead. His best job had been as a security guard. Once he told me: "Once a security guard, always a security guard – I hoped that wasn't going to be me." When he had moved to London aged 18 his parents had paid for his single ticket from Ireland and didn't want him to come back. They wanted to get rid of him because he was such a fucking pain in the arse. At many different times of my life, I would have kicked the living shit out of him and cracked his skull open. The fucking Irish tosser.

As I went to sleep that night, I wondered what the reaction at the party would have been. I was woken up at two in the morning. It was Katherine on the phone. She started hurling shit at me like women do when they're angry, and once I told her a few truths she forced me to apologise. It was the only way I was going to get any sleep. So that was it: another head buried in the sand and another girl waiting for her fucking prom. I went back to sit-ups, and counted to myself: 1, 2, 3 and 4 kicks, side kicks, flying kicks, punches, all low, middle and high. I went back to blasting out House of Pain on my stereo and making my six-pack even more defined. Soon, there didn't seem to be an ounce of fat on my body. I was ready for battle, ready for my finals – already two years overdue (as my dad would always remind me) because of my fucking illness. I mean, what the fuck did he know? He told me not to go back to university, as he didn't think I could do it anyway. He told me to get a job. He didn't think I had the strength of character to go through all the shit and see it through. Well I did, so fuck him. Fuck him, man. I did have the strength of character and it was nearly over. Then I could get on with different shit.

As my memories of Meredith, Debbie and Katherine became more of a blur and my finals approached, I reflected on university life and what I was going to do after it had finished. Since January 1998, I had spent time in chat rooms having cyber sex and trying to invite myself to stay with rich women all over the world. I wanted to be a gigolo. Unfortunately, I couldn't scan my photo properly and that put an end to that. I was charming enough on the net and had to make do with cyber sex. I was ripped off by several escort agencies, spending a few hundred quid in total to sign on, and not getting any work. Then I noticed an ad wanting someone to become a live-in slave with Mistress Debbie in Leeds. She wanted help writing for a magazine which one of her Mistress friends edited. I wrote her an abject letter and took some raunchy photos. She sent me a printed response saying that I was one of her possibles. I hoped that she would invite me for an interview or even a day's trial. This didn't seem an odd thing to do at the time as the classical literature I was reading was far more liberal towards sex than the puritanical attitude in Britain and the world in general. I guess I allowed fantasy to clash with reality. Or maybe I was just being a pervert. My mind was also a bit racy but this was to be expected with the pressure of the exams.

Sometimes I would feel a bit high, but whenever I did I would try to relax. I also had recurring migraines which were signs of stress. The fantasy was also a pleasant break from everything. My tae kwon do lessons had stopped and, although I did wrestling, boxing and jujitsu with some of my friends, I was often training on my own. My teacher didn't want to fight me in combat as he feared for his safety because I was "too much of a psycho". I wrote again to the Mistress in more detail and the next reply was hand written in greater length. This excited me and I wondered what might happen ...

By now, I had begun my finals. The first paper was "Cicero and the year 63BC". In my view, he is the greatest man who has ever lived. He was a complete all rounder, brilliant orator, lawyer, politician, public relations expert, consul, philosopher and humanist. His poetry and historical works are criticised throughout history and it was unfortunate for him that Mark Antony arranged for his disposal, exhibiting his head and writing hands in the Forum. Then there was "Ancient literary criticism". This was a look at the origins of deconstructing texts, beginning with Homer, Plato and Aristotle and discussing the effect they had had on subsequent writers such as Longinus. The lecturer, Professor Michael Haslam, had spent 20 years teaching in California and was the head of the classics department. He made the course easy to understand from the start. I had already studied Greek comedy in the first semester with Professor Bain, who was an expert on writing about Black Magic and Necromancy in the ancient world. Aristophanes' comedy was the most memorable text. It parodied Socrates and his sophistry in an entertaining and ironic manner. That left only two exams to go.

I was mentally drained but also excited when the penultimate exam approached. The course was "National identity and the Roman past". It was a disappointment throughout because the lecturer never made clear what she was trying to accomplish. The course had no real structure and was too general a topic. In the exam, I made some grandiose comments almost trying to correct the whole course.

The final exam was "Latin love poetry". I wrote two essays on Catullus and one on Ovid. The essay about Ovid went too far. I was making literary allusions, quoting the text and saying that he was taking over the world. Shit like that. I got pissed immediately after the exam and passed out early in the evening.

The little boy whose teacher, when he was six, told his parents he was far more intelligent than anyone else in his class and was definitely university material, could finish what had always been expected of him and get on with his life. It was time for a change, a new beginning, and a new chapter.

Bipolar, Recovery and NLP

Chapter 7 – End of uni, third time loony

After another drinking session the following day, I travelled to the Lake District to meet up with my Gran and brother for a few days. Now, if there are two people you shouldn't be with when you're going manic it's these two. Their characters and peculiar relationship made it difficult for my mind to rest. Nevertheless, spending time with them was "exhilarating" to say the least – my Gran with her senile dementia and my brother, a walking literary encyclopaedia.

They were both eccentric – a couple of poles short of a scaffold – and enjoyable to be with at times, but spending too much time with them could easily make me manic. However, I felt stronger now that I was about to graduate and felt I owed it to them to spend some time with them both, despite their incessant bickering. I hoped, in short, I would have a good time. I knew we would drift into our own little worlds and look back nostalgically to a time when life was better and people were kinder. I longed to see the countryside that they had so often talked about when I was growing up.

I went to the Lakes that year on a positive note. They travelled there together several times a year but this was the first occasion that I had taken up their invitation. We stayed in a lovely country house and saw some wonderful scenery. We also had some crazy conversations that didn't seem so crazy at that time. For the first time for many years, five minutes of conversation with them both at the same time didn't give me a migraine. It was remarkable. We talked for hours about history, politics, nature and I really enjoyed listening to my Gran's stories. Because she was so happy, I even think she told me a couple that I hadn't heard before.

The day I got back to Manchester, after my little break, the halls were really quiet as most people had left. I couldn't get to sleep and stayed up watching TV until six in the morning, thinking how I was going to take over the world. I went to my room and masturbated on and off until nine in the morning. I also reorganised my room while rubbing Vaseline all over my body. After all, it was time to prepare for an important rugby match (not that I had arranged to play one for years) and ready myself for appearing in the Guinness book of records for being the most

137

Bipolar, Recovery and NLP

intelligent person in the world: Jesus Christ (in fact, why Christ when you can be God?)

I went down to the kitchen when I heard Mark had got up and started talking gibberish to him. He knew that I wasn't well; in particular because I was quite convinced the chess pieces I was playing with were flying saucers. He asked for my mum's number. He phoned her and said that he would take me to the doctor's. That's good, I thought. I wouldn't mind fucking the doctor. Mark told me to get ready and have a wash and shower and kept calling me to get out. Otherwise, I would have been in there washing myself all day. We walked to the doctor's. I was acting like a complete lunatic, dodging traffic, leapfrogging over bins and other objects and greeting people I had never met. Fortunately, I didn't hurt myself. Steadfast and determined, Mark led me to the doctor's.

"Jase, stay on the road, you're gonna hurt yourself. I don't want you to get run over. I'm glad you decided to come. You did the right thing, you know. Come on, stop messing around, you're gonna be late for your appointment."

"Did you like playing rugby?"

"No, I was too much of a wimp. They put me on the wing. I was pretty fast when I got the ball if I could catch the goddamn thing."

"Lets get a rugby ball and have a match."

"We'll do that another time. Let's get to the doctor's now and get you sorted. At least your mum knows, that's the main thing. I told her I'd look after you so come on, Jay, if you can't get over here for me do it for your mum. All right. That's a good lad. We'll be there in a minute."

Jason chicken runs in front of a car and smiles at the driver. The owner beeps his horn.

"For Christ's sake, Jase, that was close. Stay close to me. That's it. From now on, you're staying close to me."

"I'm immortal anyway. Cars can't hurt me. But thanks mate."

"Yeah, whatever."

When we arrived at the surgery, Mark convinced me to open up. One jumbled sentence of thinking that the whole world was a brothel and Dr. Black put me in a safe house for a few days. I can't remember if they gave me anything to calm me down – if they did, it wasn't enough. It was too late. I was out of my fucking tree. In the safe house there were two other people having a breakdown and a member of staff. One woman had taken a Lithium overdose. I fucked her when she was asleep by putting different coloured pencils outside her door. This could not have been done without my magic powers.

The other woman was 79 and told me that she had a 15 year-old boyfriend. *That's OK, I didn't mind a wrinkled pussy and her walking stick turned me on anyway.* The member of staff showed me to my room and I went to work… I immediately started performing my manic rituals… First, I licked up all the dirt on the floor. This took over an hour and was quite dangerous as I was constantly chewing blue tack with drawing pins in my mouth. The next stage was to undress and tie all the bed sheets and spare blankets around my cock. This made it ache like a chest would ache if it had to do a 24 hour dumbbell session. When you're manic you can absorb more pain than when in a sober state, so I carried on making links ...

I turned the bed on its side along with the wardrobe and chest of drawers. I thought that my room was bugged so I was turning myself into a huge speaker to detect the bug and keep the thoughts of God away from Satan. The staff member knocked on my door and, when he persuaded me that it was OK for him to come in, lost his temper. He asked me what I was doing and told me to get dressed in the bathroom. I went to the bathroom to get dressed while he started to return the room back to normal. He told me to calm down and suggested I get a drink from the kitchen as my psychologist Kath Porceddu would soon be arriving to see me. That was a nice surprise. I had been seeing her for about six months now and hadn't fucked her yet. Hers was another pussy that was soon to be decoded. Things seem so much easier when you're manic as your imagination seems to become your reality. You don't actually have to do anything to believe that you have accomplished it.

Kath arrived and in due course she told me that I would be transferred to Withington Hospital the next morning, as soon as a bed became available. To start off with, I hadn't wanted to go there but now I was so high I saw it as my duty to make my presence felt and restore happiness on earth. It was time to stop human suffering and make everyone immortal. I was in a celebratory mood. She had undergone seven years' study and training before she had her own practice, far more than the counsellor I had seen when I left Coney Hill, and it showed. She was perceptive, intelligent, logical, understanding and sympathetic. She also knew I was God but kept it to herself. That was very important and a nice touch, I thought. When she had left, I relaxed in my new surroundings and performed the usual manic acts: I fantasised about worshipping the women that I saw, and watched England lose 2-1 to Romania in the World Cup (but was terribly confused as I thought I was controlling the game... so why didn't England win?)

I filled the sink with water and drank as much as I could in one gulp counting numbers in my head. After all, numbers always had significance and made the world go round: they determined how much money people had in their bank; they determined geographical distances ... when people would see each other ... I spent two hours in the bathroom. Most of the time I was doing a handstand and cycling. This was the first time I had ever been able to do a handstand unassisted. Well, as the saying goes, leave the best things to last, and by God, I did.

I allowed the Spice Girls to come down through the air vent and shower with me. Geri was first and then they all joined in. This was far more powerful than Eminem thinking about impregnating them a few years later, although I do think he's a great rapper. I had actually fucked all of them while doing a prolonged handstand and smiling inanely. That was the ultimate hard-core fuck. As a result of my actions, I was soon going to be a TV celebrity, perhaps the best way to get my message across and start saving the world.

After my five orgasms, one for each of the girls, I finished off my salute to myself by moving the metal lockers with my feet and kicking them close together so there were no gaps. This took an amazing amount of balance and strength and was something that nobody in their right mind would attempt as the whole bathroom floor was soaking from the shower that had been running for ages. I pushed one of the lockers too hard and it crashed making an enormous racket. It just missed my feet and would have severely fucked me up if it had landed on me.

Bipolar, Recovery and NLP

I was pleased with the way the ceremony had gone but then heard the same staff member from before yelling for me to come out. I got out and he asked me what the mess was. I didn't say anything. He asked me if I was OK and, when I nodded, he told me to go to bed. I knew he had to clear up as it was a servant of God's duty to do such things, and I went to bed. Not surprisingly, I was wide-awake for the rest of the night.

The first thing I remember about my second stay at Withington was gluing pictures of black women to my bedroom wall. To enact world peace I had to be seen in public with a black woman to reduce racism, reminiscent of the film *Bulworth*. I was telling all this to my black friend Andy, who was visiting me at the time. However, although he was laughing and seemed at ease with me, this was the last time he would visit. That was OK, even though we were close friends. The main thing was that I'd sent him on a mission to train as a junior school teacher: he had to stop little kids playing with action men and teach them how to roll spliffs instead; then they could get into Bob Marley and everything would be all right.

The following days and weeks will always be a blur. My mum and dad came to visit a couple of times but I have no recollection of this. Mark told them where I was and up they came. It was good of them to come together, put their differences aside, and support me. They realised they had made mistakes in the past and had come to see their son who was ill. Did they feel guilty? Did they want forgiveness? Well, any Christian would forgive them. Sometimes I did and sometimes I was still angry – about the past and all the arguments, and how it had altered my psyche and arguably led to my illness. As time passed, though, I forgave because I couldn't be sure that my condition was down to them anyway. The most frustrating thing was that I'd never be able to turn the clocks back and find out what would have happened to my health if I'd had parents that got on. That said, I realised that I was fortunate that I had the love of my parents, friends and family as some of the patients didn't have any visitors. Some families simply give up on members of their family who have a mental illness; they can't carry the extra burden. Thank God I've never felt that isolated. Even if I get upset or angry with them, I know that when push comes to shove, they'll be there to support me. That helps keep the morale up, especially during episodes or at times when I'm too introspective.

After a couple of weeks, the high subsided. In its place, depression had set in so I called my Grandmother for help. She told me to hang on in there and told me about when she had walked out of a mental hospital with her head held high. She was never ashamed and never gave a rat's arse what anyone else thought about anything. I also rang my Nan whose advice was limited as she wasn't the sharpest knife in the drawer. She advised me to eat what I could – fruit if possible – and to drink plenty of water as that's what it said in a programme on television. What the fuck? Still, I was so low that to hear the voice of anyone who cared was a comfort.

I remember Tom and his girlfriend, Perry, coming to visit me. He was my best friend left in Manchester; Panji had retired from professional basketball and had got a job in Southampton as a mechanical engineering contractor. Tom and Perry were really positive people and, after talking with them, I realised that this episode had been a lot quicker than the other ones. There were also justifiable reasons for relapsing. My lithium level had been recorded as too low in March. It was only 0.3 and it needed to be between 0.5 and 0.8. This was due to occasional binge drinking and sometimes forgetting to take it. My level was normal when I was in hospital but being too low over previous months could have triggered a manic episode. Basically, the need to manage my illness more effectively faded as the depression got worse.

My mum and dad came up for my graduation and both told me how proud they were of what I'd achieved, especially after what I'd been through. I was given a 2:2 first of all, but this was later upgraded to a 2:1 because a letter from my head consultant, Dr.Thomas, confirmed that I was as high as a kite when I sat my last two examinations.

Graduation day was far better than staying in hospital for the day but a huge anti-climax. I hate looking at the photos now because it's obvious, if you look closely, that my eyes are bigger than normal. They're pumped full of drugs, man. What kind of a fucking sick celebration is that? Perverse? Fucked up? Unfortunate? Just like my eighteenth...

Everyone else gets to celebrate their graduation properly. I was a walking zombie and nervous wreck during mine and drank orange juice at the social gathering afterwards when everyone else was getting pissed. All I could say to people was that I had had a breakdown. Yes, I had had them before, and I was appealing for a higher grade because I wasn't well when I sat my examinations. No wonder I haven't seen any of them since. Who would want to invite a maniac to a reunion? There again, it was probably the last time they would meet anyway. I mean, I was out of control. I was in and out of my mind from day to day.

There are different stress causing factors for each episode and one contributory factor for my third must have been the nature of my dissertation. It was an exploration of madness in Greek tragedy. Starting with Foucault's *Madness and Civilisation*, I attempted to define the madman and describe his plight across the ages. I made allusions to certain plays, notably Sophocles' Ajax, and Euripides's Bacchae and Heracles, and found prejudices throughout. You didn't have to be a rocket scientist to work out that madness was the ultimate humiliation enacted by the gods upon humans. Such punishment was dealt out as a result of *hubris* and usually resulted in suicide. It was fucking intense. Imagine a mother and daughter parading around with a lion's head, after they had ripped it limb from limb when mad, only to realise that it was in fact the head of their son or even brother. Discussing the treatment of mad people in ancient and modern times was too much for me to cope with at that period in my life. I wasn't prepared for it. I was unable to eat the apple and spit out the pips. I had choked on my own vomit. I had wallowed in my own shit. I would have been better off doing a dissertation on the more stable Cicero. I could have been more creative and maybe even recreated my own Ciceronian speech. I had come top of the class for doing that before.

Writing about madness when it was too close to me had done me more harm than good. Let's take a simple analogy: reading about snooker can make you more of a snooker player if you study where to hit the cue ball for different shots and alter your stance. It will certainly make you think about snooker more. The same is true with madness. Read about it and you are more influenced by what you read. If you're susceptible to it you could end up more anxious, with higher blood pressure, and forget to manage yourself properly. Before you know it you're back in the bin and your opponent has potted the black. You're three frames to nil down and not paying attention. You don't even know if you're up for another game. You're too depressed ... and your opponent is Ronnie O' Sullivan and he's on top of his game. He's already got the confidence as he's world champion and he's showing no mercy. You're one game from being whitewashed and he's just got a 147. In a nutshell, you're fucked.

Withington was still a shit-hole. A 20 year-old girl who had two kids and was getting a divorce from a husband who knocked her about had a crush on me. I had to get out of there, man. A 30 year-old I had a crush on had already left. Once, she actually came back to visit and gave me a cuddle, but after I called her at home and asked her out she declined because she was in love with somebody. I never called or saw her again.

One of the characters in hospital was a massive black bloke. A manic like me, he was a black belt in tae kwon do and had joined the army when he was 17. When I was high, I kept thinking he was 10 years old and even thought he looked like the black guy who had kicked me in the head when I was 14 before another bloke had smashed my nose and a gang had kicked the shit out of me. I would tell him this a lot when I was high and it was the only time that he ever looked serious.

The place was so bad and my mum felt so sorry for me that she dragged me out of there after three or four weeks. I recuperated by staying in all day and watching MTV. My mum would go to work in the afternoons and as I could sleep in till 3pm, sometimes I wouldn't see her until 6.30. I'd spend the rest of the afternoon with my Alsatian dog, Ben, by the fire.

One night, though, Michael gave up the pretence of being the perfect stepdad and I did not forgive him until February 2002 when my mum told me that he was sorry. He came home pissed one Saturday night and threatened to leave my mum if I didn't move out straight away. I couldn't believe it. All those pints he bought me at Christmas and attempts at bonding were just an act. I felt betrayed. The Thursday after the ultimatum, with my pride getting the better of me, I moved back to Manchester in a terrible state. If I'd had time to think I would never have moved back there. I would have spent a few months recovering in Wales and then probably joined the rat race and moved to London. Meet Jason Pegler, star of the rugby team and chess captain. I could have any job I wanted.

Bipolar, Recovery and NLP

Chapter 8 – Gina

I went to stay with my dad for a few days which I hadn't done in three years. He opened up to me for the first time since I was 17 and assured me that he loved me – despite the fact that he hadn't invited me to his marriage to Claire a few months earlier, which continued to play with my mind. Above all, though, I felt under great pressure – from society, my parents and most of all myself – to perform and get a job.

On my last evening in Manchester I'd spent the night with a pretty Bajan Mancunian called Gina. In the morning, my dad had picked me up: he was really good at that kind of thing: being practical; the painter and decorator putting up shelves, etc. In fact, he was so good that he could have had his own TV series. He knew both trades through and through.

Anyway, Gina and I stayed in touch and she invited me to stay with her for a week, or at least until I found my own flat. She was also a manic-depressive but seemed to be able to handle it much better than me. She was 29, 5' 9", slim, large breasts and had a kind nature. Not as intelligent as Meredith but more motherly and easier to talk to. We forged quite a close relationship.

I moved into a house just round the corner from her and we had sex all the time. We lived in a Black and Asian neighbourhood called Whalley Range, next to Mosside. Her brother, MC Buzbee, was famous on the local scene. He was with a bloke called Justin Robertson in a group called Lionrock and wrote some wicked lyrics. I saw him sing live and he was a brilliant performer. He was also a brilliant dancer. He was unlucky not to have made it big. His best friend as a teenager was Jason Orange from Take That. Gina sang on a couple of his albums and there used to be breakdancers on stage. They had danced in front of 5,000 people at some special events. They were a talented musical family. Her mum was lead singer for the African group, Abasinde, and the first time I saw her she was singing solo onstage at the Leeds carnival in front of 15,000 people.

Gina had a 2:1 in Fashion from Liverpool Polytechnic. That was a pretty good effort considering she came from the ghetto. As we saw more and more of each other, however, race became an

Bipolar, Recovery and NLP

issue. I would meet her friends who were polite and then, behind my back, call me a 'honkie'. Most of them were Jamaican. Jejune ones at that. She kept on saying she wanted to be just friends. Two or three times a week I would cry because of this.

The episode I had suffered was still taking its toll. Most of her friends were unemployed and had schizophrenia. This became irritating when I eventually got myself back together. Within a month of returning to Manchester I had found work with temping agencies. My first job was as a mailman within UMIST (University of Manchester Institute of Science & Technology) and it was bizarre. All these students saw me probably thinking that I was uneducated and I already had the degree they were striving for.

Next came a few temporary, but full-time, data inputting jobs. Then, in December 1998, I started at Barclays Bank as a Workflow Processing Operative. I was to work there for six months. Almost everyone there had a degree but couldn't find anything better. I applied for graduate jobs and scored outstanding marks at an HSBC test day that I had been invited to. I went for a final interview in Sheffield and missed out as I had no computer experience and wasn't prepared to become IT-obsessed until I got the job. That was my first big interview and I'd blown it. I remained positive, though, as I had forced my way out of depression by going to work.

I saw my psychologist regularly in order to prevent further relapses and, although I was embarrassed at earning a meagre amount, at least felt my dignity returning. I took my Lithium regularly and stopped drinking entirely. I played squash every week, sometimes twice, with Tom. One of my flatmates was a social worker and he would counsel me if I was stressed out as he knew about manic depression. The other was a boring dip-shit with a PhD in Microbiology. He would only say "all right". Getting a conversation out of him was like chatting to a stiff. There was no response no matter how hard you tried. I became more and more ambitious and saw no quick promotion so got a slightly better job at Barclaycall as a "Sales and Service Advisor". I was proud of myself as I'd passed a telephone interview and two further interviews. I had also started to write again. I started a second screenplay about my second episode and my first children's story

147

Bipolar, Recovery and NLP

about a little bear that Gina, to my great surprise, had bought me for my birthday.

My brother kept advising me to go to London, as did Dominic who had now won a few financial journalism awards. I knew I was destined for greater things and didn't like my new job. What's more, Gina was annoying me. She was argumentative and our relationship was up and down. We were either both very happy, or one of us craved for attention. I felt like a used yo-yo that couldn't find anybody good enough to do some decent tricks on it.

Gina and I went to Paris and Tunisia together. We went up the Eiffel Tower at night and it was a truly beautiful setting, but as I stood there I knew that something was missing in my heart. In Tunisia we went riding on the camels and smoked nicotine-free tobacco through the huge water bongs. We watched and tried belly dancing and made friends with two local journalists. One of them tried chatting Gina up behind my back and to my frustration I never had the opportunity to knock him out because I never saw him again.

Gina also flirted with two different blokes at two different clubs. I had to push the first one off the dance floor to make him understand he was flirting with my woman. I was so pissed off with the way that she looked at the second one that I went up to the sexiest bird on the dance floor and started dancing right in her face. That was enough for Gina to stop and kick-off with me. Man, I didn't want a relationship like that. Her main problem, apart from jealousy, was that she was unable to rid herself of the fear of going out with a white man.

Part of her attraction to these men on holiday was due to my physical condition. I was impotent. For the first time in my life, apart from a few drunken one-night stands, I couldn't get it up. I had a problem with my libido because of the Sulpiride. Although at least it stopped another episode: in February 1998, I felt high and it brought me down. Gina was very understanding and after a few months my libido was functioning as normal again. Manic depression had taken hold of her and she would put on and lose weight in an unnatural manner. It was the pills. They helped us but symbolised that we were not well. Every night we took the Lithium together frustrated that we weren't normal anymore. The illness made us limited in the activities we could do. I had little or

Bipolar, Recovery and NLP

no energy after work and never wanted to go out. I couldn't face going to the pub or anything; I didn't want to see other people having a good time. It's difficult to join in when you're sober but eventually I realised I didn't want to associate with a bunch of beer drinking twats anyway.

Her brother moved in with her in March 1999 and this became a great stress on me, her and our relationship. He made her flat messy and sponged off her. Her priorities were mixed up. She would lend other people money and then ask me to lend her some. I saw that as irresponsible and hated it. I mean, half the people she lent money to never intended to give it her back anyway. She was easy going with people, which was a nice quality. But sometimes she was too easy going and that made it easy for people to take advantage of her.

Like her best friend Debbie, who had spent the first half of 1999 in hospital with schizophrenia, Gina was not diagnosed until her mid-twenties. This shows how mental illness can turn anyone's life upside down. Debbie had had a good job at the BBC in London as a make-up artist until she got sick; she then spent four years struggling through a part-time college course in fashion textiles but managed to make troop winning carnival costumes with Gina. They won the Mosside carnival designs three years in a row and were very talented but lacked the health, and therefore drive, to do anything about it. I often thought of a maxim from Robert De Niro's *A Bronx Tale* when I thought of how their lives were going: "The saddest thing in the world is wasted talent."

However, the saddest thing for me regarding Gina was that she had an angry streak in her that she couldn't control. Her aggressive tendencies erupted once when she'd tied me up. She was reluctant to do so but I kept insisting. She tied my hands tightly behind my back and also my ankles together and sat on top of me. "Do as I tell you. Do as I fucking tell you or I'll hit you", she shouted as she slapped and punched me in the face. I started crying straight away and she untied me looking confused. Her problems stemmed from her stepdad, Burt. He was a motherfucker. Sometimes I pitied him because he was schizophrenic. Other times I wanted to kill him. Once, he touched Gina up when I was seeing her and I only let it go because he was living with her mum and any damage I did to him would be taken out on her. He used to beat the shit out of her.

149

Bipolar, Recovery and NLP

It made me really angry. I couldn't help them as much as I wanted to.

Burt spent three months in prison in 1998 for attacking a woman in Aldi. They'd had an argument about who was first in the queue and he'd gone ballistic. He dragged her into the street and kicked the fuck out of her. He was also a dodgy and lazy bastard. I remember him telling me about a security job he had had. He told me that he used to sleep most of the time and that people would pay him to steal bricks and timber from the place he was supposed to be guarding. I wanted to take Gina out of the ghetto but I never had the strength. In the words of *Naughty by Nature*: "For those of you who've never been to the ghetto, stay the fuck out of the ghetto."

Sean nearly got a gun to kill Burt but Gina persuaded him not to. Sean had two mixed race children who were two and four and Gina used to baby sit them. Gina would scare me by saying during sex with her that she wanted a baby. She wasn't on the pill and I used to pull out of her. She had an abortion with a previous boyfriend and I made sure I didn't get her up the duff as I knew she would want to have a child with me. Looking back, I was a complete muppet not to have had Gina on the pill. My life would have been well fucked up. The offspring would have had a good chance of being manic-depressives and would also be confused as to whether they were black or white. They would also be confused about which culture they should identify with and what role models they should adopt. I would have had to buy them the Public Image Limited song, *Rise*, where John Lydon sings: "I could be wrong, I could be right. I could be black, I could be white".

I wanted Gina's parents to show some kind of commitment for our "future together". Really though, I just wanted some kind of financial reassurance if everything fucked up. When I met her dad, who was going back to live in Barbados and was selling his house, I tried to persuade him to give Gina some money so I didn't have to spend my savings to move us both to London. Why should I have to pay the bill? I'd be fucked if we split up. There'd be no way she could pay me back. She couldn't get a job and if she did she couldn't control her spending. He was no help and neither was her mum. I knew then that there was no way I was going to move in with her. I just didn't have the balls to come out and say it.

I had admitted to my psychologist that I was overly vigilant, obsessive even, with money but it was one of the things that gave me stability. Knowing that I had a bit of money in the bank made it worth drinking water when I saw everyone else drinking a pint. It made it worth settling for Supersaver food instead of the more expensive brands. I was behind others in my career as I had been ill and this was a way of catching up with them financially. I wasn't prepared to sacrifice myself when there could be so many problems in the move to London. Receiving benefit could take a long time. Living in London was far more expensive. Getting free bus passes in London might not be easy.

One night we had a horrible argument because Gina was jealous that I had looked at another girl. It had really upset her because it was on the same day that I met her dad, but at least it gave me the perfect reason for eventually splitting up with her (although I had to repeat it a thousand times as she was so upset). We were lying in bed going to sleep. I had work the next morning. She started punching me really hard all over my body. This happened a few times and each time I calmly pleaded with her to stop and tried going back to sleep. It was nearly midnight and, when I thought she had calmed down, she started kicking and punching the shit out of me. I grabbed her and pushed her up against the sliding wardrobe. One hand was on her throat and my other punched the glass of the wardrobe. I told her that what had happened was the last straw and we were finished. I told her how I had witnessed domestic violence when I was younger and I was not going to lower myself to that level for her or any other woman.

I would move to London without Gina. I felt bad the way I left her, but all along I had doubts about moving in with her. The last time I moved in with a girl she had fucked off and left me. Gina was too dependent on me. *I wanted an equal relationship where my woman had a career. I didn't want to be supporting a kid on a shitty job in a shitty part of Brixton for the rest of life and spending my spare time visiting a manic-depressive wife in hospital or being in hospital myself.*

The more I encouraged Gina about her fashion career, the more disillusioned she got. She had won several competitions with her designs and, a few years earlier, had even been featured in the

Bipolar, Recovery and NLP

Manchester Evening News as the most promising new fashion designer in Manchester. She had a magical quality but I couldn't seem to bring it out in her and I knew that she would be happier with a black man. I only hope that she finds one and she is treated well by him. She helped me out, man. She was a good friend to me when I needed one and I don't know what I would have done without her.

...

I moved to London in July 1999 and enrolled on a Fast Track Postgraduate Journalism course. It was a start and I moved in with Dom until I found myself some shared accommodation. Gina and I were still going out but I was starting to be attracted to other girls. The girls in London looked smarter. They looked like they had more class. I couldn't believe I was being so shallow. They looked more together and career-minded but still wouldn't have the sensitivity or talent of Gina. And we had been through a lot together. Gina still planned to move to London but get her own flat. I didn't think she'd go it alone as she had a lot of friends in Manchester.

Gina was the sort of person who attracted others. She was jovial, kind, friendly and a motherly figure. She was a caring person and we would often hide from people when they called at her house so we could be on our own. I couldn't believe she was prepared to move to London and leave everything just so she could be in the same city as me. I didn't think things were going to work out between us but I could never tell her that. I didn't want to upset her as I cared about her too much. She was like a sister in a way. She was my best friend. How can you upset your best friend? I felt a coward for the way I behaved but I was a sensitive person. We had both gone through enough pain already. Why should we suffer more when I could prevent the suffering? Couldn't we pretend that everything was all right? Couldn't we get ourselves sorted and bounce back at the same time? Couldn't we show these cockneys a thing or two? Show them how charming and tough the people up north really were? Couldn't we be an example of bridging the North/South divide? I was back to my roots in the south and sufficiently psyched by Dom and my brother to cope with any obstacle that stood in the way. I remember when I told my mum that I was moving to London she started crying. That was pathetic. What kind of a fucking response was that? I love my mum but that was a weak response. Hadn't I proved I could make a new start? Hadn't I proved already that I could battle through adversity? She loved me so much that she worried I would get ill if I left the medical back-up and familiar surroundings in Manchester.

The night I told Gina I was going to cancel our deposit and move to London on my own she was devastated. I had never seen anyone so upset in my life. She begged me to change my mind and said she would do anything. I said I was sorry. We didn't have enough money but I wanted out of the relationship. To this day, I don't know what all the real reasons were and that's why I was never able to explain to her why when she asked. I guess I had a Ferris Bueller philosophy within me: "Life moves pretty fast. If you don't stop and look around once in a while, you could miss it." As much as I cared for Gina or loved her or whatever it was, I thought the grass might be greener somewhere else and I wanted to search for it. I wanted a happier life, a change and a relationship without arguments. I wanted to relax and live and behave how I wanted with my future, but I was too scared to let go of her. I was not man enough to let her go and get on with her life.

I found a flat in Vauxhall right next to college. The landlord was called Felix Dilke and he lived there too. He was a really affable and polite intellectual with an aristocratic background. Mind you, he was a little bit odd and a little bit crazy. In fact, he reminded me of my brother. He had graduated from Cambridge University in mathematics and worked as an IT consultant. He was erudite and pleased to chat with me about anything that I wished to discuss. He proved the ideal flatmate for the transition from Manchester to London. He didn't drink either which was a real bonus.

I spoke to Gina at length most nights on the phone. We would have romantic chats and say we missed each other, and we did. She came down a few times and soon became jealous of Felix (she would understandably have been jealous of anyone given the circumstances). He often used the Internet which would annoy us if we were trying to get through. My enthusiasm for the relationship was waning and it was a great relief when Gina said she would stay in Manchester. My course was 17 weeks and we could plan what happened after that.

London was exciting and Gina seemed slow in comparison. People in London worked long hours and socialised a lot whereas she would skip college and sleep during the afternoons to avoid getting stressed. If Gina had been well with fewer problems, I sometimes thought we could have been happy, but there was always an "if". And there was the race thing. When it really boiled down to it my family turned out to be a bit racist which really pissed me off. At that time (though he has changed now) my brother didn't want me to marry a black girl. My dad thought I had "enough problems without having mixed race children". My mum thought "it was not fair for two of us to be together when we both had the same illness as it would be too painful". But this was what brought us together. We would lie to people saying we met in the pub. After all, how many couples meet in a mental hospital? More than would admit to it that's for sure. We learned from each other how to cope with being mad and anxious from day to day, from minute to minute and second to second. Sometimes it was too intense.

One day I acted on my impulses and became a bastard who stopped being monogamous. I deserved having my foot shot like that kid who Joe Pesci's character Tommy shot and eventually killed in *Goodfellas*. Just as Gina didn't deserve being cheated on, the waiter didn't deserve the fate that Tommy dished out for him. I'd talked to girls without saying I had a girlfriend before but that was all until I got some work experience at a top shelf fetish magazine The Forum. I arranged for myself to interview a dominatrix in Brighton. When I arrived, she was dressed in her rubber gear holding a crop and it made me feel pretty horny. To avoid a good thrashing I told her to put some clothes on and bought her a pint of Kronenbourg. I was so nervous that I had one too.

It was the first time I'd touched alcohol since I'd finished my finals in June 1998. The drought had lasted until September 1999 and then the monsoon arrived. We got pissed and went out for a meal. The publication was tight and would only pay for my rail fare. When we got back, I made advances and she was horny. She invited me into her torture room and although I wanted to go I stayed in the lounge and kissed her neck. I eventually gave the interview the next morning after spending the night with her and, after one more interview with the owner of a fetish shop, discovered that I was fired for being unprofessional. This happened in the most theatrical manner. The deputy editor, who turned out to be a complete bitch, screamed at me in the office in front of everyone and told me never to go back there. Then she stormed out. I couldn't understand it. I knew journalists who fucked their clients when the opportunity arose and they got away with it. What the fuck was going on? It wasn't the best start to a career, I suppose. I think I pissed her off because she wanted me for herself. Or maybe I had usurped her authority; whatever, I didn't really give a fuck.

Sometimes there's so much office politics around it's confusing as to what the fuck is going on. I had more work experience the following week at a health magazine called ZM. It proved to be more successful. I refrained from jumping in at the deep-end here and had my first articles published – three short pieces of copy totalling about 500 words that I wrote the first morning I was there. Then I filled up the magazine with things like 100 different ways of describing having sex. This was tabloid journalism but I soon moved onto a more interesting magazine. Every Friday for the next few months, I worked for *Total Film* magazine. The features editor said that I could be the journalist he'd been looking for after he'd liked a few film reviews I did. However, it turned sour when he saw my proposed double spread on the film *Scum* as too much of a sociological study when all his readers really wanted was to read a witty review.

The journalism course was shit although I did make a good friend out of the class, and that was the only positive thing that could be taken from it really. It taught me about copyright and libel and put me off journalism as a 9-5 career forever. I was glad that I would never have to go through it again. Law, current affairs, newspaper journalism and shorthand could send anyone to sleep, especially when taught by the NCTJ and at Lambeth college. Shit teaching and shit organisation. There was good food in the bed and breakfast place opposite, though, and for the first time in my life I became overweight.

I kept making excuses not to see Gina as I preferred going out on the pull. Between September and December 1999 I slept with over a dozen women – making love to one – and that was not Gina. They were from all over the place. There was a good looking, 30 year-old blond tart from Belfast who I pulled at the Plug in Brixton. We saw each other once after which proved to be less fun. There were two birds from Turkey who I happened to pull in the same night. I was going to go home with one but she didn't wait for me to collect my jacket so I took her friend back to my house instead. I gave her my number in the morning and she asked me if it was for her or her friend. I mean, fucking hell. I felt sorry for her so said it was for her. She never called me but I didn't mind as she was just another notch on the bedpost.

In my life I'd fucked well over 50 women. I was back to being a womaniser again and finding it easier every time I went out. One time, I ended up with a French girl who I brought back from a party in the West End. She was a good looker. There was another girl from Dublin who I pulled in the Swan in Stockwell. She ran a pub in Leicester Square. We only met twice, though. She said that I was too young. I didn't really care. I only wanted to get laid. There was also a one-night stand with a girl from Holland who I met in the Dog Star in Brixton. Not to forget the Austrian whore who I met at the same venue. There was a South African rowing champion who was built like a bloke. That was a one-night stand. There was a slim black girl from Kenya whose dad, a psychologist in San Francisco, specialised in looking after Vietnam War veterans. Later, I got off with her Portuguese friend. There was the Scottish dominatrix who I forged an arrangement with and three women I chatted up on trains. One was a pretty blonde from Manchester who lived in Swiss Cottage, a middle-aged businesswoman from Blackburn and an IT Consultant from Cheshire. There was also a hooker, a Brazilian and an American on holiday at Christmas and numerous others.

All in all, things were getting pretty hectic. Binge drinking made me lose my inhibitions and led to more sex. Gina became more distant as I became more deceitful. She didn't know what was going on and I didn't have the strength to tell her. In November I went up to Manchester for five days and took Gina to the doctor's. She was getting high – talking more quickly than usual and extremely excited and passionate. Sounds OK, but if you've seen mania before and if you've had it, it's easier to recognise. *The GP was a bitch. Gina was reluctant to increase her medication as it made her put on weight and she didn't want to get depressed. The doctor threatened to try and place her on a section if she "refused to take the prescribed medication".*

All Gina needed was a bit of coaxing to go on it, a few well chosen words, and a bit of sympathy and she would have done what we advised. She was nowhere near the hospitalisation stage. Look how bad our society is. There was no sympathy, or understanding, just an abuse of power. I bit my tongue to stop myself strangling the bitch to death. Who the fuck did she think she was? That was no way to treat a human being. If a neighbour saw you treating a dog like that they'd call the RSPCA. She was out of order and was a fucking disgrace to the medical profession and the rest of us.

I knew of several incidents where doctors had been unsympathetic and unprofessional. The most obvious one was when Doctor Copestake in Powys told me to stop taking Lithium because there was no sign of any in my blood. (The bloody idiot also told me to stop taking it as I probably didn't need it anymore – he knew my medical history and he told me this!) He should have told me to increase the dosage and cut down on the booze. Then I would have listened to him. I just needed somebody official to confide in but he didn't have the time. The fact that I phoned him from a phone box in Manchester and told him how scared I was of having a relapse didn't change this man's mind. He just didn't give a shit when it came down to it. I'd lost faith in the medical system but was begging this "lovely man", as my mum called him, to take an interest in my life and make me responsible for my own health. Instead of telling me how important it was for me to take my medication he saw me as a lost cause and gave up on me. If I was a doctor I'd never do that to a patient. Thanks to Dr. Copestake I stopped taking Lithium and was in hospital within eight months. I had previously been well for three years.

People are reluctant to criticise the centre point of our communities. That would be a disgrace. Well, I don't mind. Doctors may be overworked, their departments underfunded and they may have too much paperwork and too many patients to see, but some of them have spent so much time studying that they can only act with people on a superficial level. Somebody who is mentally ill needs more than that. They need a doctor who is good at people management, and there aren't many around.

The stigma doesn't help. Doctors work their arses off and see lots of mentally ill patients blagging off the DSS. Well, fuck me it could happen to anyone just as it happened to me. Any one of us could get manic depression just like that and we'd be fucked. The illness takes over your life. If it wants to it destroys you for good. It moves in and out of you at will and there's no escape. It's like clinging onto a ship in a storm. No matter how hard you hold on, if the storm is too strong, you go overboard. You'd just better hope there's something to hold onto and the storm stops before you drown. Doctors are usually middle class people from stable backgrounds so it can sometimes be difficult for them to empathise with lower class and unemployed nutters. It ain't easy ...

Gina took the medication and insisted that we went to church with Debbie on the Sunday. I hadn't travelled 200 miles to go to fucking church but went as I felt guilty about being a bastard. Sean's friend Mark came as well. Within five minutes of the Mosside service it was clear that they were Evangelists. My worst suspicions were confirmed when I noticed that in their magazine they asked for massive donations from their members to build huge buildings for worshipping their gods. Mark and I left while Gina refused to leave. I had a deep conversation with him and he said I needed to be with her through this religious phase. For whatever reason, I agreed and we went back to pick her up. My fears worsened as she described the service as a "bloody amazing" experience.

I tried to get her to leave but the head of the service started to preach shit at me. "You're not a believer are you?" "Whatever you believe is up to you", I replied. "You're not a believer are you ... and you're going to hell ...you're going to hell." As I walked off, I heard him talking to Gina telling her not to have sex with me before marriage. So that's why she was reluctant to have sex with me when I was there. That was the last straw.

I jumped onto the first car I saw outside the church, balanced myself on the windscreen and smashed it to the fuck with one perfectly timed kick. I jumped off the car saying something to the effect of: "He's a fucking con man not a Christian – that will fucking show him." I sprinted off and got into a taxi. Gina went back and told the preacher what had happened. I couldn't believe it. She shouldn't have done that. She had her priorities mixed up. Her loyalties should have been with me. What the fuck? Our relationship was becoming a farce.

Thirty minutes later she arrived home and I had already packed. I got a later train as we made up for a couple of hours. Every time I spoke to Gina after that, that fucking Mark seemed to be there. He became an interfering prick although at least he was a good shoulder for Gina to cry on in the weeks that followed. Mind you, he'd just been in the bin too, was 32 and had never had a proper job. He was also a protestor when I had been a security guard at the airport. His girlfriend had dumped him because he was "a loser", as she put it. Instead of providing for her, he wrote poems, was obsessed with green issues, and ran off to Ireland to work as a part time shipbuilder. He'd promised to decorate his girlfriend's flat for two years and never paid any rent. She was sick of his broken promises. He wasn't a reliable man, not like my dad. If my dad was going to do some decorating then he'd do it. There was no tiptoeing around with him and as I got older I respected him more and more. I had met so many people in my life that had promised things and never delivered them. Waiting for others to get their shit together usually wasted a lot of time.

Come to think of it, Mark's best friend, Gina's brother, was 30 and had never had a job either. Furthermore, he did not have a flat, could not support his two kids and could not even sort out his mum's fucking boyfriend. Gina was surrounded by people who were worse than she was. I had promised to make things up and spend Christmas with her at my mum's when I received a very tempting offer.

Felix invited to pay for me to go on a 10 day holiday to Miami over Christmas. That was the most generous offer I'd ever had. The only condition was that I was to drive him around a bit to see his business partner. I sought advice from people at college, Dom and my new friend Mark, my parents and my brother. They thought I should go. Even my mum didn't mind and this would be my first Christmas without her. I was drawn between upsetting Gina and doing what I wanted to. My dad's advice was the most telling: "Don't let anyone hold you back, you're too young", he said. "What about Gina?" I asked. "You've already told me it's going to end sooner or later so what's the problem?" Gina was really upset and said she hated Felix because of what he'd done. I knew she didn't really hate him – his generosity had just speeded up the inevitable, that was all (I realised afterwards, in fact, that he had saved me a lot of pain.) When she was saying how upset she was and I was apologising to her, Mark, who I didn't even know was round her flat at the time, grabbed the phone. He wouldn't let me speak to her and hung up when I got angry. That motherfucker. If I ever see him again I'll bite his fucking nose off. Interfering motherfucker. Can't get his own life sorted so he'll fuck up somebody else's. In the event, Gina and I talked soon afterwards and arranged to spend New Year together.

Bipolar, Recovery and NLP

Chapter 9 – A ray of sunshine

On 16 December we had an end of term party at the Circle Bar where Dom lived; that night, however, something happened that would change the course of my life – for the foreseeable future, at least. Hopefully, it will change my life forever. After a shed load of Stella and a few shots of Absinthe, a group of us headed off for Leicester Square and ended up in a cheesy nightclub called Equinox. By that point, I'd sobered up a bit and made for the dance floor which was covered in foam. All my college buddies were buzzing around a girl who didn't like me anymore because she'd taken me out a month before but I had ended up in bed with someone else instead. I went round the dance floor on my own. As the music blared out and the lights spun round and round, the alcohol cleared my system and I entered a dream world. I looked at a couple of girls and they smiled at me, pointing to their friend.

I turned to where they were pointing and was faced with this gorgeous little figure; she was majestic looking with longish dark hair, and probably not English. She was beautiful and had the prettiest smile I had ever seen. Her face was covered with her hair as she nodded her head up and down and gently shook it from side to side in time with the music. It was poetic. Time stood still for a moment. Time stood still for a few moments longer. It stood still for longer than ever before.

Funnily enough, I didn't feel the usual "will I get anywhere here?" as I was transfixed by her wonderful smile and small graceful movements. Her knees and feet were rocking and her hands were swaying around in perfect rhythm. She wore a warm blue/greyish jumper and black trousers. She looked good enough to eat. I just wanted to pick her up and cuddle her right there and then. We made eye contact a few times and eventually – I didn't like rejection, especially from such a cute girl – I made my move.

We smiled as we danced next to one another. I was trying to use all my charm and I craved that it would pay off. I consciously made an effort not to touch her yet. I didn't want to spoil the beautiful, Stoical scene. I wanted to tease her a little. I wanted to make her think that I was a bit special – make her think that I was as special as I thought she was. I wanted her to believe that I was

Bipolar, Recovery and NLP

capable of satisfying her needs and making her happy. This dancing went on for a few songs and I felt like a winner. I felt like life had a meaning, like love was the greatest thing.

It was a fresh attraction, but would this one turn out to be one of the great ones? Was she the great one? Time stood still for what seemed like an eternity. I moved my left hand (now, it seems like it took forever) and placed it gently on her waist. When she gave a smile I noticed even more how beautiful she was and strengthened my grip a little. Her eyes were the most beautiful things I'd ever seen. They were like two brown gems, which was great, because all I'd wanted all my life, as Van Morrison once sang, was a "brown-eyed girl". These gems were like a type of stone that nobody had ever seen before. And they were for my eyes only. I didn't want to let her go so after a few more intimacies, which included rubbing my hand on her waist, I plucked up the courage to put my other hand on her waist. She smiled again. I was in paradise. It was like the whole world had been lifted off my shoulders. I felt like Christian must have when he was accepted into heaven; like Sisyphus pushing his rock over the hill, or Tantalus having a drink. We danced and teased and smiled and cuddled, glad to have found someone that made us feel good. She was quite short and that was nice and that also very fitting as my Nan had always told me that a tall man should have a short girlfriend. Like her and my granddad.

Women admire a man who can show this sensitive side rather than all that macho shit and the baggage that accompanies it. If you don't believe me, ask them. Fortunately for me, I've got both but sometimes it can get me into trouble as I don't use them at the right time. I can be so sensitive and then, suddenly, a paroxysm of suppressed violence. That can be quite upsetting for a woman (you know how sentimental they are). On the other hand, they don't want a wimp so get down the fucking gym and pump some iron – cause if some wanker tries to rape your girlfriend, they don't want the coppers to sort it out (or do they?) – they want you to go and get some revenge (or do they want you to cuddle them?) They want you to protect them as well. You have to be able to adapt to the circumstances. Just as in Ovid's *Ars Amatoria,* The Art Of Love, which is his guide to pulling, you have to be on the ball or you'll lose that ho to another bro.

Bipolar, Recovery and NLP

The more you think you know a woman the more frustrating trying to figure them out gets.

Back in Equinox, things were going well. I was reading the signs as well as I used to read those flash cards my mum would wave in front of me when I was two years old. That must have aided my hyper intelligence, although a lot of it probably came from my genes too. The beautiful girl with the beautiful brown eyes was having a good time. There was a connection between us that was strengthening. We became more intimate and my pulse started increasing as I thought what it would be like to kiss the girl with the wonderful smile. I took my time and after some squeezes on the waist and lots of hugging kissed her on the right cheek. At first, she smiled. Then she responded by closing her eyes and putting her lips together.

We kissed for the first time. It was great. All the anxiety in my life turned to ecstasy from the moment we started kissing. We hugged and I stroked her back and her hair. I made sure I kept my hands moving as I wanted to arouse her and also made sure I didn't scare her as she was a great catch. I never knew how innocent she would turn out to be. I would never have guessed that this was not the sort of girl who slept around or not the kind of girl who kissed a lot of boys on the dance floor. I hoped that she was special but had had such a torrid time with women that I didn't really know. Did she really mean it when she kissed me or was I just another snog? The kiss lasted for several minutes and it was controlled. Not one of those really sloppy ones. It was the most natural thing in the world. I was scared to end it as I didn't want that feeling to go away – ever.

You never know when or where you're going to meet the love of your life. I mean, Tom had pulled in a supermarket once. Imagine that. Even in Equinox which was notorious as a pulling joint and where there were plenty of fish in the sea there could be a magical one. One that was better than the rest. The problem was that I had so many defence mechanisms to avoid getting hurt that I would find it very difficult to trust a woman again. I didn't want to get hurt by another bitch.

I stopped the kiss and smiled at her. She maintained that perfect smile and her eyes were even more beautiful. I knew she wasn't English. Perhaps she was from the Mediterranean. It was romantic thinking about it. We danced closely and it was comforting to see her friends smiling at us. It was a relief and a surprise to see that I seemed welcome in their circle. There were half a dozen of them and I was sure as I glanced round that I had made the right choice. Now, I didn't want to blow it, I wanted to progress.

We kissed and danced and turned around for another 10 minutes or so when I decided it was now or never. I invited her for a drink and led her off the dance floor holding her hand. She didn't say anything but seemed happy to accompany me. I asked her if she wanted a drink and she looked confused. I kissed her again more passionately and shouted in her ear so she could hear over the bass. She spoke for the first time: "Que." I paused for a moment. She didn't speak in English. No wonder she was so pretty, I thought. I'm not letting this one get away. "What is your name?" .... I couldn't hear her, so asked again: "What is your name?"... "Sonia", she said in a beautiful Mediterranean accent. "Where are you from?" "I am from ... in ... of Spain." Fuck me, I had pulled a Spanish bird. No wonder she was so beautiful. I'd never seen a girl so naturally pretty.

We kissed romantically and I led her to the bar and bought us two cokes. Time to freshen up and get to know her better, I thought. I asked her if she wanted to come home with me. She didn't want to do that. I asked her one more time and told her that I was a nice guy, that I really liked her, just wanted to get to know her and have some coffee. She still said no, but seemed to be interested in talking some more and having coffee. I repeated that I was a nice guy and that she was safe with me and after a few minutes of persuasion and romantic kissing, we made for the door.

I'd passed the next hurdle. She had allowed me back to her house for coffee. I managed to get my jacket quickly from the coat supervisor and I saw some of my college colleagues on the way out. Some of them smiled. We made a quick exit, careful not to get bogged down in idle chat and settled to getting ripped off by a Leicester Square taxi driver. I didn't care how much it was going to cost – I was in there, man, with a really sexy bird. We arrived back at her home in High Street Kensington and she made me some coffee.

The night was getting better. We were alone in the lounge and now I was sober I felt even more attracted to her. That's a rarity – as most guys know girls usually look worse sober than they do when you've had a few drinks. We talked a little about where we were from and what we did. She was from Burgos, which was a small city in the north of Spain, and had worked as a receptionist in a hotel in South Kensington since September. I told her that I'd dabbled with journalism and about my fascination with writing. The lounge became a place to explore each other's bodies as she told me that we couldn't go in the bedroom because she shared it with three other girls. That gave us a chance to experiment with the small space available in the lounge and she bought a quilt and pillows out from her room. I even managed to make some curtains out of a blanket.

We caressed and hugged each other and had an extremely romantic time. I had never been so gentle with a woman. It was if we were in tune with each other on a metaphysical level as well as a physical one. She was divine and I was privileged to be with her. I would never forget this night and it was the best possible start in forging anything more lasting should the opportunity arise. Of course, there were a lot of obstacles in the way as there always are in life but on that night we were locked as one and happy not to go looking for the key to loneliness.

I left at about seven in the morning and went to college after only an hour's sleep. I had a great night and, once I got her number, told her that I'd give her a ring. She thought I was referring to the ring on her finger and took it off giving it to me. That was the cutest thing I'd ever seen and I kissed her and told her to put the ring back on, explaining that I would phone her later in the day.

Hardly anyone was at college, just three girls and me. Everyone else was too hung over from the night before. I told the birds there that I'd been with this beautiful Spanish girl, intimating that she was prettier than they were which she was. As I left, I saw one of my classmates who I played football with and told him I'd pulled a Spanish bird. "I love Spanish birds", he said. This would turn out to be the response of all my friends. I met Sonia Fernandez Bascones on Thursday evening and persuaded her to come South of the river and meet me at Stockwell tube.

She was radiating innate beauty. We went for a pint and I

thought it was cute that she drank pints and not halves. We had Guinness. After two pints and pleasantries that actually interested me, I realised that she was more intelligent, intriguing and adventurous than I had ever hoped for. She had two degrees in Economics and had spent the previous year in Denver, USA as an au pair. She'd even won a cruise for two around Europe, live on Spanish TV. This didn't make me jealous as she had taken her younger brother.

Sonia also had an older brother who was married. It seemed as if an entire new world was opening before me and that there was now light at the end of the tunnel, as if I could hear the song *Tender* by Blur in my ears whenever I was with her or thought about her. I was so happy that I took her out to my favourite Indian restaurant and paid for us. For those who knew me, this was a great feat "cause I was tighter than a gnat's chuff" when it came to money (have to be if you never know if you're going to be well enough to have a lasting career, if your life is so disordered that you can't create any order out of it). Meeting her, I was careful not to tell her anything about my illness. Not even when she played me *Lithium* by Nirvana. In fact, I was really worried about telling her of my depression.

I had come to terms with the mania. Although it grabs you by the bollocks and swings you round in all sorts of directions, it is an enlightening, although admittedly horrible, experience. I would no longer pretend to my friends that it was a magical experience, one to cherish or one that merited solitude on a desert island. It wouldn't help prevent a nuclear war if manic geniuses were allowed to go without medication, they'd just become more of a mess. They couldn't save the world, they only thought they could.

As I got older, I was becoming more scientific in my way of thinking. I had to if I wanted to avoid another relapse. I wasn't sure if I could go through it again: the depression. Fuck me, the depression man. There's no way to describe it except that I wouldn't wish it on my worst enemy, and believe me I've had lots of enemies (I've still got a few, come to think of it). I had managed to come to terms with rejoining society. And although, after each episode, I felt a lot further behind everyone else as regards my social standing and my career prospects, I trained hard and caught up as best as I could. I may have been lapped but, as in Olympic

Bipolar, Recovery and NLP

track cycling, I could gain extra points on the sprinting laps and get double if I was placed on the last lap. I was the toughest competitor on the track and there's no way I was going to give up.

I've including one of my raps that I have written and performed to show how I feel sometimes. Events in my life have meant I've had to change and evolve as a person, and that is something that can happen to anyone.

I'm MC Jase you'd better watch yourself
I'm MC Jase and I'm full of stealth
This is MC Jase
You'd better watch your health
Cause I'm feeling hyper and I'm fucking crazy
Listening to this rap gonna make you hazy
Lying in bed at 1.30
I'm only 25 but I feel like 30
Can't go to sleep 'cause my head's too strong
Been through too much shit for far too long
I don't give a fuck if you think I'm wrong
It's no fucking use for me to have a bong
Just messes with my head and spaces me out
There's no point in that I have no doubt
Fucking with a bitch is no good for me
Glad I have a girlfriend that looks after me
Cause I'm trippin all the time
Can't even earn a dime
'Cause my head's fucked up since I was 17
I went really manic you know what I mean
I was in the bin for 6 fucking months
Being controlled by a bunch of cunts
No one gives a shit unless it happens to you
Not even any members of ya nigga crew
So next time your gonna pull the trigga
Think of what I say and grow bigger
... Causing more shit's just part of a cycle at the end of the day
...
You gotta get out ... Get the fuck out ...
And shout. Shout what it's all about ...
Before you're another dead nigger or in the penitentiary
For fuck sake's homies, it's the twenty-first century.

167

Bipolar, Recovery and NLP

I'd battled through suicidal periods in my life when each time I thought I couldn't. Oh, I was soon to find out that my life had been so different to that of this innocent and beautiful Spanish girl.

After going to the restaurant with Sonia, we went back to my house and Felix introduced himself in his formal, friendly and welcoming manner. After a few minutes, Sonia and I went to my room and had a great evening. We spent a cosy night together inside. I was getting more and more into her as the minutes went by but was terrified of getting into a relationship that I feared could eventually crumble. The only girl I had moved in with had left me, which was a shock and had made me feel bitter towards women. Also, I didn't want a jealous type like Gina again. I was also aware that whenever I finished a relationship I was prone to dive into another one. I thought I could eradicate all the bad from the previous one and just take the good into the new one. Therefore, I could make the new one work.

The next day Sonia didn't have to go to work until three o'clock so we went to Clapham Junction. She looked so cute dressed in black trousers and a pink cardigan and brown leather jacket. I was going to be sad not to see her for the next couple of weeks but I was so excited about checking out Florida. I got some friendly looking Christmas cards from a charity shop and wrote one out to Sonia. I wasn't sure how she felt about that but she smiled and we went into Battersea theatre for a coffee. We were in there talking, kissing and cuddling for a couple of hours. I wondered what it would be like to know her better and to become a part of her life. I knew I'd want to see her again when I came back from Miami, and I promised to send her a postcard.

That night, Felix had left a note saying that he had felt stressed out and was sleeping round his sister's. He said that he would recover by the next day and looked forward to the holiday. He was like that. He'd work really hard as an IT consultant and hammer away at the computer for most of the evening. After a few weeks he would burn out, sometimes take a day off, recharge and then return to normal. He's a bit of a geek really and rather posh but was always well mannered. He's got a kind heart and is one of the most genuine people that I've ever met. He's been good to me and sometimes I almost see him as another big brother. He happily

Bipolar, Recovery and NLP

shares his intellectual opinions and massive knowledge of literature. We became good friends. I helped him calm him down when he had been overdoing it. He's extremely intelligent, and a technological genius. He tried setting up his own business with a friend in 2000 but this didn't work out. However, he persevered and then forged a different partnership with another friend and now works from home. They're setting up a business in Atlanta, Georgia. His great-grandfather was a prominent Victorian politician by the name of Sir Charles Dilke.

We were both really looking forward to going to Miami. I sat by the window as we took off and flicked through a guide to Florida, which my brother had lent me. He hated lending out his books; it was as if I was taking part of his soul from him. He had lost faith in people and preferred objects instead. Harvey is four years older than me and when I was nine I thought he was so cool hanging around in a skinhead gang and listening to Two Tone. He's basically a genius and is probably the most eccentric person most people would ever meet; anybody can see that. One time, in the late nineties, he was featured in the Daily Star for being an eccentric with the most peculiar looking car in the world, covered in pictures of thinkers, royalty and philosophical quotes. He has such a vivid imagination and sometimes voices his inner thoughts through his teddy bears (a few years later I would pick up on this habit myself, although take it up a step or two).

I used to worry, as did my mum and dad, that he was a schizophrenic but the more I observed him the more I realised that he was OK. He's just in his own little world, unique. He's visited psychiatrists but he probably knows more about psychiatry than all of them put together. My first consultant saw him and said: "You're always slightly manic." When my brother asked what that meant in practical terms, the doctor said: "That means that you will be generally happier than most other people." My brother smiled and thanked him for the interesting conversation.

For my brother, everything is often a game as he doesn't believe in the real world. He believes in the metaphysical world, a world of parallel universes. For example, it doesn't matter that I'm writing a memoir as somebody else is writing it at the same time in another solar system. He's a walking encyclopaedia of quotations and literary facts and can make any intellectual I've ever met feel stupid when he is on form. Sometimes he can be so engaged in philosophical thought that he is unable to do the simplest things – he can't find his way around familiar routes, loses things constantly – but I suppose everyone's got their faults. Even my brother.

On a social and intellectual level Harvey's got an answer to everything. It's futile arguing with him unless you like arguing because he will never give in. He will outwit you, convince you that his argument is right, or otherwise will go off in tangents so that you lose sight of what he was talking about in the first place. He lives, as he admits, "to be deliberately provocative". His goal is to stand aside from the norm and become as educated as is humanly possible. For him, "only in the imagination is one truly free". He can be a good example of how to live your life when in a positive mood. I mean, sometimes he can really inspire me – more than anyone else in the world.

From the summer of the millennium year he had a Scottish girlfriend. She really mellowed him out. She gave his life structure, meaning, and purpose and got him to trust people again. She gave him life again in the real world and I will always be grateful to her for that. Her name was Angela. As time went on, the relationship became a real rollercoaster. But that's another story.

...

Felix and I arrived at the airport close to midnight and took a taxi to our hotel in South Miami. The state is less than 100 years old but seemed far more high-tech than London. Felix went to sleep and I checked out the bar in the impressive hotel. Everyone looked like models. They all looked chilled out apart from the ones who had done too much coke. Even the 75 year-old man sat in the corner, and smoking the biggest cigar I've ever seen, was surrounded by a gaggle of top-notch totty. People were singing karaoke and there was a rapport amongst the locals that I hadn't witnessed in England. The camp barman was really friendly and answered my questions about the places where I might like to hang out during my stay.

Although there were two of us on holiday we had two very different holidays. I would hang out with Felix during the day: we

Bipolar, Recovery and NLP

would go shopping, to restaurants, visit the Everglades, watch Miami Heat play basketball, go to South Beach, sunbathe and meet his business partner Richard. On Christmas Day, we went jet-skiing. I was a natural like I was at skiing. I could get into this jet-skiing. Hell, I might even move out to Miami and buy one. Then I could go jet-skiing every day.

Each night, Felix would go to sleep by midnight and I would hit the town. I made friends with a couple of up and coming actors, one of whom showed me he'd worked with De Niro and Al Pacino. I drank heavily, mostly Budweiser and Jaegermeister. I drove around pissed out of my mind in the flash sports car Felix had hired. I went to nightclubs, strip clubs, toured for hookers, pulled a hooker and a Brazilian babe. I had some coke and stayed up until six in the morning most nights. Felix would sunbathe in the morning and by late morning I would be sobering up by the swimming pool drinking Sprite. We would then drive off to Denies, Dunkin' Donuts and other joints for breakfast.

One evening, I got lost trying to pick up Felix and hit 130mph on the way back. I was buzzing. On the way, I pulled up at a bar and the locals insisted on getting me pissed. One of them let me follow his car back to the hotel. His name was Eddie Bauer. He was from Austria and his brother had won a few downhill races. He was also a black belt in tae kwon do and in several other martial arts so we connected with that macho lark and also on a spiritual level.

I went back to the bar with Felix on Christmas Day and we went jet-skiing. It was my first time and hitting 65mph on the water was an adrenaline rush. It made me want to come out to Miami again and have some fun. We went to a Christmas party that night with the locals from a bar in Hollywood, and my drinking heights reached the old levels. After umpteen bottles of Budweiser we went to a bar to celebrate Christmas, and getting a witness for each one, I drank 12 pints of Guinness in one, and two cocktails. Every drink was downed through a thick straw. One American woman I showed looked unimpressed and calmly said that she had never seen anyone drink like that. This sent alarm bells ringing in my ears but I loved the sound of them and just walked off and carried on dancing to the hip-hop.

The night I had the coke I could have had my head blown off.

Bipolar, Recovery and NLP

This bloke had just got out of prison, for selling the rock, and I was asking him what his five favourite rap movies were. I was a writer and was certified as crazy back home so I had the right to ask these questions. The old man with the cigar was there. His name was Joe and he bought the hotel that Felix and I were staying in for his son as a birthday present. He asked me to give a friend of his from New York a lift back to the hotel at 8am, and I got away just in time.

At 7.30am on Christmas morning I was driving through a small suburb of Miami called Hollywood. I was hung over and had been awake all night. I stopped off to get some coffee. I really needed some as I'd been falling asleep at the wheel on several occasions. The cafe didn't open till eight so I walked onto the beach. The sun was rising and it was the most beautiful landscape that I had ever seen. It was like a wonderful painting, so surreal but yet so full of life. I thought of my life up until that moment and decided it was time to take a chance. Time to move out to Miami, write and work, and hit the real Hollywood later on. I looked out over the ocean and felt stronger than I had ever felt before. I felt a *novus homo* (new man), as Cicero would have felt when he first gained entrance to the senate. He had risen above his own class and I would do the same.

When I'd had a few coffees, and still in ecstasy from the sunrise, I got talking to the only other customer in the bar. I couldn't believe it. He had manic depression. Fate had brought us together. He was a local and asked me my name, saying that he would remember it if I spelled out my surname for him. "P…E…G…L…E…R." My destiny would soon come to fruition. On Boxing Day, Eddie drove Felix and me around and gave us a comprehensive tour of Miami. He knew its history inside out. He took photographs of us outside Madonna's, and Stephen Spielberg's houses, among others. Shit, I didn't have my screenplays on me. I told Eddie that I was going to move out to Miami for good and he said I could stay with him until I got settled. I could work for him cash in hand for $200 a day, expenses paid, helping him to organise concerts in the US and Australia. Well, fuck me that was a good offer. Might never get an opportunity like this again. I would have enough spare time and be inspired enough to write.

Bipolar, Recovery and NLP

Thing is, with all the glamour, Miami could be a dodgy place. It was the sort of place you needed to keep your wits about you otherwise you were fucked. The incident with the hooker exemplified this. I saw this big fat mamma on the street tarted up and she started chatting me up. A guy I walked out of the club with had pointed me in her direction. I gave her $20 and within 15 seconds she'd blagged 50 out of me because I was so pissed up. We went behind a tree right next to the main road and she wouldn't let me touch her up much. She told me to lean against the tree and went straight for my trousers unzipping them. She sucked me off for about a minute with a condom over my cock and it was droopy. I mean, I needed a bit of a warm up – I was fucked. She suddenly walked off. I told her it was getting hard. She walked off saying she had work to do. I called her a fucking bitch and asked for my money back.

Within a few seconds she was back on the main road with three or four of her colleagues. I kept calling her a fucking whore, telling her I wanted my money back. I would never hit a woman so I just walked off in a rage. I saw the guy who had advised me to go over there and he had no sympathy at all. As he saw it, I had asked him for hookers and he had told me where they were. The rest of it was my fault.

People in Miami are also very cliquey. They are vain, sometimes shallow, and money (even more so than in most other places) equals reputation and status. Going into one small club someone offered to get me in for $50. I said it was OK. I really wanted to get into the club next door. I tried to get in the small club in a bad mood and the camp doorman refused to let me in saying that I was rude. I couldn't believe it. I walked back 10 minutes later and asked more politely and he let me in with a smile.

After a few drinks and some funky dancing, I left the club and asked him if he knew of anywhere else as I couldn't get in the club that Madonna had performed in the night before. He walked me over to the other club (I thought he was going to hold my hand), past a queue of 100 people and told the door men of the hip-hop night that I was his friend, "Jason", from England and could they do him a favour and let me in straight away, waiving the entrance fee. He told me to have a good time and I walked in. I couldn't

173

believe it. Shows how far you can get with good manners. I felt that I had unwittingly kissed a gay man's arse and although that bothered me for a few moments I soon forgot about it when I got inside.

All the women had breast implants and model-like figures. They had expensive make-up and wore designer clothes. One woman was eyeing me up a lot and asked me to wait just a minute. She was with some dodgy-looking black guys at the corner of the bar. After a few minutes, I tapped her on the shoulder and her immediate response was: "I'm not going to speak to you anymore." I mean, what the fuck, I hadn't even spoken to her yet. I bowled off and thought how she had missed out. She had missed the opportunity to meet the great Jason Pegler. Within two weeks, I had become as vain as the locals. Well, you need to be vain if you hang out in America, especially in Palm Springs, where I was planning on working with Eddie. I also planned to do some business with a friend of my brother's who was now a good friend of mine, Sean. He was from California and lived in London. His parents lived in the Bahamas and were planning to build a holiday resort and wanted me to keep an eye on it.

I had let my hair down and would prepare for my NCTJ examinations in the first week of February 2000. One more adventure, however, when leaving Miami was pulling an American broad at the airport. She had gone to the same school as basketball legend Michael Jordan and was state manager of a leading cosmetics company. She was on the same flight and we talked and had a few drinks. Felix left for his relatives' farm straight from Gatwick and the horny slut I'd got off with on the plane realised she'd arrived in England a day early. She came back to my house and we fucked a few times despite the heating not working. She left the next day.

I had to break it up with Gina as I'd felt closer to Sonia even though I'd only known her one night. I'd told my psychologist the week before of the inevitably of the relationship with Gina ending, and she'd told me to come clean. She'd advised me not to go to Miami as I hadn't driven for several years. That, combined with other stressors such as exams looming for my journalism course and the recurrence of the binge drinking, could make me ill. Well, I'd only met her a couple of times and I'd put all my faith in a

Bipolar, Recovery and NLP

psychologist in Manchester only to get ill again. What was the use? I was worrying too much about getting ill all the time, becoming a hypochondriac. I wanted some fun. I'd been in a relationship with a possessive woman and not gone on holiday as everyone else had when they'd finished their degree. I'd been in the bin. The last time I'd been abroad I'd broken my jaw. I needed to let my skinhead grow and have a good time. And the holiday was free. For fuck's sake, nobody in their right mind would turn that down, certainly not a manic-depressive who was feeling better than usual.

The American girl had answered the phone before she left and it was Gina. She was really upset and became suspicious. I was still too afraid to upset her so said that it was just a friend. Gina was coming to London for the New Year and I said I'd phone her later. I told her I didn't think it was a good idea that we spent the New Year together and told her that it was over. She was devastated and I felt like the cruellest man on earth. She said that she was coming to London to see me and I said I'd meet her but that she couldn't stay with me. She turned up at my house when I'd asked her to call me first. I let her in and she begged to stay with me, saying that she would do anything. It was horrible to see someone I had been so close to and cared so much about, as if she was my sister rather than ex-lover, looking so distraught and weak.

She wanted to stay with me just one more time and hug. I kept telling her that it was over and tried to get her out of the flat. I couldn't push her out without hurting her as she was so strong. I managed to persuade her to go out for a pint and ran away to get back into my flat. She forced her way in. I would say she was pathetic, but I was the pathetic one for being a two-timing motherfucker and a gutless turd. Still, after all the racism I had suffered, being taken for granted and constantly being dumped by her for the first five months we went out, my behaviour had its own internal logic.

Gina was so upset that I'd tried to stop her getting in the flat and must have known that I'd been unfaithful, as I wouldn't answer her whenever she quizzed me on it, and she eventually left. When she did, she was calling me every name under the sun and we were both crying on the street. I felt relief and a great sense of remorse. How could I have fucked up someone's head like that?

Bipolar, Recovery and NLP

Her head was already fucked up enough as it was and she had manic depression, after all. But so did I. As selfish as it was, I had to look after myself or I was going to relapse and go through the shit mill again. And next time, I might get minced too fine. I might be minced so fine that my identity is lost forever. I might even end my life once and for all during a bout of depression.

I was longing to see Sonia. The events in Miami had been extremely stressful and I needed a girl I liked to save me from my recklessness. She received the postcard I had sent her the same day I phoned. It was a comfort to hear her voice. And it sounded even sexier but still kind. It was the sexiest voice I had ever heard. I was exhausted and slept for the next 24 hours. Sonia invited me out to spend the New Year with her and her friends, but I didn't want to get too close too soon and, anyway, I was planning to move to Miami.

My brother urged me to spend the millennium New Year with him and Sean. They were going to a champagne reception overlooking the firework display across the Thames. Instead, I spent it with Dom's mate, Doug, at the Circle Bar in Stockwell, pissed out of my mind. I was in the pub from ten at night until five in the morning, drinking Stella. Next day, I phoned Sonia and we resumed our intriguing relationship. She looked stunning as usual, like a wonderful oil painting with that endearing smile. I wanted get to know her better and to go to Miami. Why not have the best of both worlds, I thought? She could even come with me if she wanted an open relationship. I didn't mind. I was a writer. I was willing to experience anything. I'd been well for 16 months so why not live it up.

I hadn't really wanted to celebrate the New Year. Whatever I did, it wouldn't have lived up to my holiday in Miami. The New Year had always been an anticlimax for me. I'd spent several with Dom pissed up, or drugged up, with us both slagging off the world in existential, fatalistic or nihilistic terms. *Why did people always get so worked up about the New Year? Nothing ever changed. The resolutions were always forgotten within a week and shit life resumed soon afterwards. People went back to work, even more in debt, with no holidays to look forward to for a while and with accentuated drink and drug problems.*

The millennium just escalated those problems. Fuck this new

Bipolar, Recovery and NLP

beginning shit. Anyway, it wasn't even the millennium until the following year. That's what the Australians thought anyway. What a waste of money all those fireworks were. Why didn't they give the money to the homeless, or to the third world? They could cancel third world debt. They could use it to help people to help themselves. Educate the underprivileged, the disadvantaged ... Yes the uneducated, the backward people, the freaks, gay groups, mentally ill, organisations like Mind and the World Health Organisation. If I went out and joined the party and pretended that everything was OK I would be accepting that I was happy with the way that everything was going on. I would therefore not have the strength of character to fucking change anything. There was also a huge gulf between ideology and reality. I knew that very few artists ever got to change people's perceptions and be remembered for doing so. I didn't want to give in. I never wanted to become one of the herd, one of the cattle, one of those muppets that conformed to what society wanted. Work from nine to five, later if it was worth it, go to expensive restaurants and drink to relieve stress in the short term. Constantly postpone problems and forget about the state of society rather than facing it, dealing with it and trying to speak out against what really matters: justice, humanity, redemption, civil rights, understanding people, making the world a happy place for everyone, giving people a fair go. Especially the mentally ill – that's how I could help so that's what I did.

Thing is, how could I change anything when I couldn't even remember if I took my pills or not, half the time? Not that I wasn't responsible or conscientious, I just couldn't remember the physical act. Sometimes, I could see myself taking pills during a night the previous week. I could imagine myself looking at them, pushing them out of the packets and even putting them in my hand, but not placing them in my mouth and the physical act of swallowing them. I guess my subconscious just blanked that part of it out as it refused to admit that there was, in fact, everything wrong with me. It was only society that told me I was wrong; I was really OK.

Above all, the task is so mundane: putting pills in your mouth. It seems futile because you don't feel an immediate effect; in fact, any effect is hard to identify and, also, what's the point in taking them if you'll probably only get ill again, anyway? The Lithium might not be working, and if it does work the doctors don't even

Bipolar, Recovery and NLP

know why. Mental illness is too complicated a phenomenon for the medical profession to understand. Even if the brightest psychiatrists and psychologists work together they won't have a fucking clue how to control it. They can monitor its behaviour on individuals as biologists dissect frogs and learn things from that, but that's all. Even new psychological theories have their limits. It depends on how strong the individual is, how much effort they can put into it and, sometimes, on sheer luck. Some people have manic depression a lot more severely than others so it will always be difficult to quantify how well proactive therapy is working.

As I started revising for my exams I managed to cut down on the drink and saw Sonia more and more frequently. We got on really well and she helped calm me down. I'd always got nervous before exams as I'd never really done as well as I thought I ought to. Think it just stresses some people out too much, gets their pulse racing. I'd quit shorthand by Christmas and revised thoroughly for the others. They were all over in early February and, before looking for a job, I took some wallpaper down for Felix. This seemed a good distraction from reality. My exam results were very disappointing but I knew I didn't really need them to get a job in journalism. I could talk the talk and walk the walk. I set myself up with an interview at Shares magazine and they offered me some work experience with a good chance of gaining employment if I impressed them. That sounded good as I could get the perks that come with financial journalism. There would be private functions, free drinks and meals, and the like. I liked the idea of being spoilt a bit.

I also did some voluntary work with homeless people in day centres at Victoria and suddenly realised that I had found my vocation. I could help people at grass roots level and actually see people getting better. Journalism was too indirect a way of influencing people, and I couldn't write what I wanted to. Things weren't right with my head. I'd spent all this time setting myself up for a career in journalism and then eventually realised that I'd never really wanted to do it anyway. It was too cutthroat, and most journalists seemed to be rather nosy.

I had an interview as a receptionist at one of the homeless centres. I'd spent a few mornings there serving coffee, doing the dishes, collecting ashtrays and wiping tables. It was a drop-in centre that cooked fried breakfasts (meals were only a few pence), and provided somewhere for people to socialise with others for an hour or two. It must have been good for them as they would spend so much time on their own sleeping or begging outside tube stations. On my first day there, I remember chatting to a posh woman whose husband was an ambassador for somewhere or other. She pointed to one of the clients and told me that he had manic depression. She then started to tell me what a terrible illness it was and that she would hate to be left alone with him as the illness made his behaviour unpredictable. I just stood there flabbergasted. I was going into this career intending to keep my illness a secret. I didn't know if I could keep it a secret for a day, let alone throughout my career. Should I keep it a secret or would it be better to be upfront about it from the start? If I was upfront it would certainly explain all the gaps on my CV.

The job I really wanted was a sleep-in warden at a brand new homeless complex. It housed 40 homeless people and was a place of rehabilitation. They had to pay rent of £3 a week, and for that, got free medical attention, and alcoholic and drug advice. They had to be in the hostel at a certain time or they would be locked out. The hostel was quite lenient and officers would try to find the clients – who signed in and out of the building – permanent accommodation. I stayed over one night for a trial and impressed one of the staff so much that she said she was going to recommend me for the job. A great strain had been lifted from my mind as I had at last discovered what I wanted to do for my working life, and I was one of the fortunate ones. I was going to enjoy my profession and could offer people some comfort. A lot of the homeless are mentally ill so I would be able to identify with them. I would, of course, be careful to keep any rapport I struck up with clients purely professional.

Bipolar, Recovery and NLP

Chapter 10 – Kicked in the head

On 17 March, 2000, I got pissed with Mark and was assaulted by Doorman 419 outside Clapham Grand night club. This really shook me up. I called the police and told them: "I've got manic depression and my head's fucked," but they still took ages to turn up. I felt I had a right to say this as it was true. That bouncer could have fucking killed me. As I was walking off, he did a 360 degree karate kick right into my throat. I was shaken up. He was on the third step when I was on the street. He laughed after he'd done it, saying "Yes." It was a Bruce Lee-style kick and the best I'd ever seen. The police refused to let me and Mark make a statement – we were too drunk, I suppose – and I ended up spending the night round Mark's. He wanted to do the bouncers over with a baseball bat but I wasn't like that anymore.

I told him I wanted the wanker brought to justice. I discovered I wouldn't get much money if it went through court – it would be a head fuck anyway – so instead I went through CICA (Criminal Injuries Compensation Authority) with the help of victim support. This would take a long time but I was prepared to wait. The problem was that the police caught me pissing in the street when they drove up. They seemed to think that we were so pissed we asked for it. I had to prove that this was not the case.

The whole incident was unjust. You can't go round bullying people like that. Doormen are meant to have good communication skills, but the two we came across that night had no communication skills whatsoever. They were just thugs.

It's clear in my mind that this incident triggered a manic episode that proved to be the worst yet. Without the incident, I could have spotted it sooner and taken some pills, avoided hospitalisation and that dreaded suicidal feeling.

The following week my brother came down and he said that I was behaving oddly. For him to say that meant I must have been really fucked. I remember playing squash with him on four different courts for three hours and I wasn't even tired. When I served I would hit the back wall first and I enjoyed humiliating my brother as it was the first time that he had ever played. When we got back to the flat I fried and ate 24 eggs – the amount only someone like Mr. Strong would eat – and washed my hair with a

Bipolar, Recovery and NLP

cold can of Heinz tomato soup. My brother said: *"You've just poured a cold can of soup over your head. Do you realise this? Do you behave like this when Felix is around? My response was: "Me and Felix are good mates." Before I knew it, my brother had gone to see Dom in Clapham and I was rearranging Felix's flat...*

To this day, I'm amazed that my brother never thought of phoning a doctor or even calling my mum or dad and telling them what was happening. Didn't he realise that I was getting ill? Why was his answer to this question to say that he thought I was like that all the time and that Felix just put up with it? I think he was so upset that he didn't know what to do.

Anyway, back at the ranch. In a confused paradise, I basically rearranged all of Felix's books, while putting anything that was black in the bath and throwing anything that was white down the stairs; among other things, I also fixed the cat a fried breakfast and threw all my CDs around the flat (because I thought they were flying saucers that acted as boomerangs). I was also becoming more and more confused as my thoughts became racier. I thought the flat was turning into Noah's ark and I was Noah so I set about my business ... I left the bath water running, made a bridge down the stairs, throwing everything I could find down it, completely trashed my room and started painting Felix's carpet blue. Dom phoned at about seven and said I really did have "serious psychological problems" if I couldn't find him and Harv in the pub.

So, I left my ark and ventured into another world. It was absolutely terrifying, like being spiked with one billion black microdots at the same time. I was so fucking high it felt like acid was crystallising in my blood and I was overdosing a million times. It took me two hours to walk what would normally have taken me less than ten minutes. I kept stopping everywhere thinking that everything was significant. Problem was, I had no fucking idea in what way the things were significant or why they were. That's what freaked me out so much.

I got to Stockwell tube and knew I would be making a crucial mistake on behalf of mankind if I didn't drink three cans of Sprite at the crossroads. I spoke to this Jamaican guy for an hour. He was displaying posters on the floor. He was quite friendly but didn't want any of my Sprites. The only part of the conversation that I

Bipolar, Recovery and NLP

remember is that he said he rode a bike in Jamaica for 12 years. I said that he must have been exhausted. How did he do that without having a break? No wonder black men were such good athletes and nearly always won the 100 metres in the Olympics. We parted on good terms and it took me another two hours to get to a pub in Clapham Common. Thing is, I was in the wrong pub. So I ordered two pints of San Miguel, one for me and one for Sonia who was not even there – although she was looking for me at the time. She was worried that she couldn't get in touch with me as when she had rung Felix he had told her that I had totally messed up his flat.

The San Miguel was really strong. It felt as if I was drinking 200 bottles of Jack Daniels. Apparently, people were trying to get me thrown out of the bar because I kept on going up to everyone and talking gibberish. A sympathetic barwoman saved my bacon. I told her I was really scared, more evidence that you can be conscious that mania is a bad experience even when you are manic (*so all you doctors out there, try and pay more fucking attention to manic depressives who say they feel funny – you never know, you might save them a year's misery and even stop them committing suicide*). She called me a cab but the Ethiopian cab driver hadn't heard of the bar where my brother and Dom were waiting. Anyway, by now it would have been closed so I got him to drop me off at the only place I could get in, and the only place that I could feel safe. This was Rileys' American Pool and Snooker Club on the Wandsworth Road. I was a member there and although I was running out of cash in my wallet, had my visa card.

Once inside, I chose the pro's table and started inventing new games. I thought I was at the Crucible Theatre in Sheffield and that I was the best player in the world. *I placed 10 chairs on top of each other, played with a bare chest because I thought I was in the Brunel Rooms in Swindon ... played on both tables ... and then on the floor ...* I hadn't eaten all day so went out to order the food. I walked out bare-chested and it must have been obvious that I wasn't well ... The French barman walked into the room and asked me what was going on. I said that I was "playing snooker". I said it was OK as "I've got money." He told me quite forcefully to leave and I did so as at the very back of my mind I felt humiliated. I also felt very weak and scared of everything – myself, my thoughts and any form of social contact. Scared of everything that you could possibly imagine. I thought I'd walk back and see Felix. He'd make me feel better. I could trust him maybe ... After all, I'd tidied his flat for him ...

It took a long time to get back to Stockwell tube and I bought my first packet of fags for four years. I chose Embassy No 1 because Adam Rimmer used to smoke them. He had telepathic powers so I thought I'd tune into him and see how he was getting on ... I stopped at Stockwell tube and chose to hang out with the beggars instead of going back to the public school world of Felix. They welcomed me, giving me swigs of their Tenants, Special Brew and Skol Super Strength. I told them of Crucial Brew in Manchester. It was 10%. We talked in great length about blagging, crime, and the strengths and quantities of the cider they would consume. They shared their spliffs with me – the first I'd had in years – and even their fag butts. They were nice people, a little bit scary, a little bit mad, but genuine. I told them about manic depression and they joked about it. This was what I wanted at the time because I was unable to confront my problem. I was too scared, too weak and incapable of doing so. The mania was controlling my mind too much for me to do anything about it. Dionysus was in my head for as long as he wanted to punish me, and any attempt to stop him would be futile.

The police called me over and told me that there had been calls from "members of the public who had been worried about me". In hindsight, I think this was bullshit. They were just trying to stop me hanging around the station, or with the "wrong crowd". I told one of them that I wanted to be a police officer but I couldn't as I had manic depression. A police officer that gave a shit would have got me medical attention, but not these wankers. They just pressurised me into going home.

I asked them for a lift and told them I was scared. One of them just put his hand on my shoulder and told me to go away. Now that was bad policing and this is a clear example of an incident where the Metropolitan Police did not meet up to its responsibility. I realised I had no key to get in at home and when I knocked at the door Felix wouldn't come down. He told me from the kitchen window on the first floor that he would not let me in as I'd ruined his flat. I begged him to let me in as I was scared, and he refused. When I asked him what I was supposed to do he said that it wasn't his problem. Fucking hell, that was one of the worst moments of my life.

I spent hours wandering round Battersea trying to get to Sonia's. I gave someone a fiver so they could get me a taxi and they just fucked off with it. That was all the money that I had on me. I was too ill to think about going to a cashpoint. I tried about 100 times to ring my mum through the operator, but the number didn't work – it wasn't registered. I got one of the numbers the wrong way round and it never occurred to me to mention my stepdad's surname when ringing the operator, as I was too distraught. I waited at Battersea station for ages but there were no trains. I just sat on the platform crying, freezing and wearing a cap that I had found on the track. I don't know what would have happened if a train had come. Don't think I'd have jumped in front of it. Probably would have thought about jumping over it ... or got on it and got even more lost. I constantly thought about Sonia. She cared and she could help. I didn't want to burden her with my mental illness but I had no other option. I phoned her and she was crying, saying that she had met Dom and my brother and had been trying to find me all night but just didn't know where I was. This really touched me – somebody, at last, loved me in a different way. She was true to me and at that moment I became joined to her, gave her my soul. I cried like a baby. I told her I'd get a taxi to her house. I'd been there before a few times but had forgotten where it was. I didn't know where anything was at the time ... *That can be the scariest thing about being manic. It's like being the only member of a universe. Fucking shits you up, man.* She just said to remember High Street Kensington tube and Flat 2 F. She would come out and pay as I had no money. It took me an hour to find a taxi, and I arrived at her house at three in the morning. When I arrived, I told the taxi driver I had no money and he looked well up for a fight. He was a massive black geezer. I told him my girlfriend was paying and when she did I felt relieved but was still fucking scared. Scared that she would leave me, that I wasn't well, and most of all, terrified of the mania that had taken over my psyche. Fuck, I wouldn't commit hubris again. Now I knew my station. I was mortal ... then immortal ... then mortal ... then immortal ... Mania was swinging my balls round again and would continue to do so until the depression finally took over about 10 weeks later.

Bipolar, Recovery and NLP

Someone cared who was not one of my family or one of my friends. Someone new.

When I arrived at Sonia's I was filthy. I was wearing white jeans that were covered in mud. She immediately threw them away, undressed me and ran me a bath. She washed me from head to toe. I was as timid as I was when my key worker had washed me for the first time in Coney Hill. I was incapable of doing it myself. Sonia arranged for us to sleep in the lounge as she still shared a room with three other girls. I thought the four of them were witches who practised necromancy and fronted this by living as dominatrices. Sonia was the head dominatrix and I was blessed to be in the company of such a goddess ... Let alone having her take such good care of me ... I hadn't slept for two days and looked weak and thin. I tried to relax but would do handstands in the sheets and invent new sexual positions. I went to the bathroom and performed the ultimate sacrifice that I knew my goddess would be pleased with. I had a shower and washed my hair and body with dozens of different types of shampoos. With this action, I was cleansing the world of pollution, infidelity and everything else that a politician might have used to gain votes.

I threw Sonia's black leather shoe out of the window, which acted as a metaphorical tightening of a leash around my neck. Now she owned me and I would never be able to escape. That was fine by me because I never wanted to. It was what I had dreamed of all my life. This was belonging to an individual, at last ... but it was scary ... We would be together forever ... and that was great ... but was I doing the right thing ...? I had to complete the ceremony by having a feast. I went into the kitchen and felt extremely naughty looking through all these mistresses' food while they were asleep. I felt as if they were controlling my actions just as Dionysus controlled Pentheus. I was being lured into a world that no other man would have the privilege to see. Dionysus had persuaded Pentheus to dress up as a transvestite to witness Bacchanal Chanting first hand. I, however, was more privileged. I was an abject slave to a mistress. What could be better than that? It was better than scoring a hat trick in a 3-2 win for Manchester United against Liverpool in the FA Cup final.

When I got into Sonia's flat I felt as if I had just escaped from hell. Thing is, I was still in hell when I arrived and would be for several months afterwards. The next morning she took me to my GP who couldn't pinpoint the problem. We waited on two separate occasions for several hours at St. Thomas' Hospital and spoke to a duty psychologist. They couldn't decipher the problem, crack the code. I was too good an actor. I could convince them that I was sane and would start being manic again as soon as we parted company. I was scared of losing my high, scared of being controlled by people who would never know exactly what I was going through. They could never empathise. They just wanted to stick me in a cage, man. Destroy my life again.

All this had taken its toll on Sonia, especially as she had never experienced this kind of thing before. The only way I could become an inpatient was by setting off the fire alarm in the hospital, screaming, shouting and crying that my head was completely fucked. There were no beds in St. Thomas' so they sent me with Sonia and a nurse to Chelsea Charter Clinic in a taxi. This was on the first of April and it wasn't any April fool joke, man.

Sonia soon left as she needed some sleep. She had sacrificed a lot over the previous few days, including missing her second day at a new job because she was looking after me. She told her new boss about the problem straight away, which made it easier for her in the long-term. She needed to rest and at least now had some peace of mind as I was in the right place. They could give me the right drugs and make me better. Sonia had proven that she cared enough to fight and bring our relationship closer together. And this fact became something that meant more and more to me as time went on.

On arriving in Chelsea, I was interviewed by a female doctor. *I thought I was on something like Record Breakers and that Roy Castle was interviewing the man who had changed the world for the better...I was pleased to be interviewed and answered each question politely, coherently, intelligently and in detail. I was proud of my achievement ... Soon I would be awarded for my life struggle, which had cured the world of its imperfection. I looked forward to spending the rest of my life in ecstasy with Sonia. It was nice to be immortal and even nicer to make other people immortal ... It felt great being a saint and that night I had a proper sleep,*

Bipolar, Recovery and NLP

*with the Droperidol that they had given me, for the time since I
was assaulted only two weeks before. I dreamt of my kingdom and
my forthcoming accolades ... the speeches I would make ... and
how I would be modest about the everlasting fame that was due ...
Happy that I had found the partner that would share the special
honours with me ... And we both deserved it because of the old
adage: "What goes around, comes around."* We deserved it
because of all the suffering we'd endured.

My first consultation in the clinic was with my head of security
(in reality, another patient). Paul, from Brixton, told me what it
was like in the ward, what the discipline was like, what the food
was like, when we had to go to sleep, etc. He laughed at my
directness and charisma and I knew he would be good at his job.
He had a fourth dan in karate and wasn't scared of anyone.

I walked into the hospital lounge where somebody was sat
watching TV. (Shaking of hands.)

"All right, mate", I said.

"All right", said Paul.

"What you watching on TV?"

"The news."

"I'll be on there soon when I stop the nuclear war that's
coming."

"I think I'll join ya."

"What's it like round here?"

"It's all right. The grub's good. They let you have a smoke.
You know what I mean? Gotta leave here at 12 though which is
shit. You got a telly in your room?"

"No."

"You wanna ask them. They'll get you one. Then you can see
yourself on the telly. Saving the world wasn't it?"

"That's right. Where are you from?"

"Brixton."

"You can look after yourself then?" I asked. Paul nodded his
head, smiling. I offered him a cigarette.

"Cheers mate."

"I'm Jase. What's your name?"

"Paul."

"What are the staff like?"

"All right, apart from the wanker that's on tonight."

187

Bipolar, Recovery and NLP

"That big bloke in the corridor?"

"Yeah. I'd like to give him some of my knuckles."

"With fists the size of yours I reckon he'd be in trouble." Paul laughs.

"You're all right you are. Funny. I like that."

"How did you get that bruise?" I pointed at the blood on Paul's knuckles.

"Training."

"Training in what?"

Paul stretches and yawns. "I'm going to sleep. You all right?"

"Yes, thanks."

"See you tomorrow. Try and get some sleep you nutter."

"Would do but I gotta stop the war. Night."

Paul leaves the room laughing.

I still had my own room, and although I was still manic I didn't feel as confident in my new surroundings as I did when I painted my landlord's carpet blue.

I had several visitors in hospital. Sonia came almost every day. My brother's friend Shaun, Dom, Mark, and his friend Carolyn who also had manic depression *(there are other victims that live outside hospital walls, you know)*, and mum and dad. Brad phoned (we eventually became close again, as we had been so many years before) and Felix came which was very forgiving of him. Ed from college came as well. He was now working as a news journalist. He was also an inspiring writer and lent me his brother's laptop so that I could enter the BBC talent Sitcom competition 2000. This meant a great deal to me. Ed had been through a torrid time. His brother had killed himself the previous year during a severe bout of schizophrenia. He had also had to deal with the death of his mother from cancer in 1999.

Ed had been through so much shit that I felt a close affinity with him. He was also the first bisexual friend that I had and, as my friendship with him developed, I empathised more and more in my life and writing with gay issues and minority groups. This fed my appetite for sociological studies. He became a very good friend, and the first writer I had met who I could talk to about the art of writing without wanting to slit their throat. He was also extremely intelligent and it was refreshing to have intellectual and artistic conversations with somebody who was never pretentious.

Bipolar, Recovery and NLP

Anyway. My friends put up with me talking a load of gibberish while I was manic. They said that I wouldn't let them speak and that I had grandiose thoughts. I told my brother that I was going to play rugby for England so he bought me a rugby ball, and I rang up Wasps rugby club for a trial. They didn't reply. I even left a message for Gloucester Rugby club telling them who they should pick for their next team. It was a combination of all the best players that I had played with. Half of them didn't even play rugby anymore.

I wasn't very popular on the ward. My mania, intellectualising and vanity were too much for people to handle. I was smoking 40 Embassy tabs a day and the only time people were nice to me was when they were blagging one. Fucking using bastards. I would bore people by telling them I would be a famous writer. I would handle my illness and everyone else's by writing about the experiences we'd all had.

My arrogance even surpassed Tim's, and he was the most popular person on the ward. Tim was 31, wealthy, trendy, an artist and a manic-depressive on ECT. Our personalities clashed when we were in the group, but when we were alone we got on really well. Sometimes, I would go into his room and check out his CD collection. We would listen to Moby and various dance tunes. I would try and bring him out of his depression but he usually preferred not to talk about it. He told me that the consultant I was under, Dr.Tannock, had been his consultant for five years and was the best doctor he had ever had. Tim had been court-marshalled in the army when he was 26, for beating up his sergeant. His paintings were brilliant and he had sold some for a few thousand pounds each. At first glance, they looked beautiful but the closer you looked, the eerier they became. What brought us together was our medication. He was changing from seven years of Sodium Valporate to Lithium and I was changing from seven years of Lithium on to Sodium Valporate. With this in mind, we gave each other advice on how to cope with the medication. It was as if we were swapping lives. Sometimes, he would get anxious and need solitude. That was OK with me. I respected his privacy and was glad that I wasn't on ECT for two reasons. Firstly, it made me feel better because it hadn't been suggested for me, and secondly, I was terrified at the thought of it. I imagined it as an electrical rewiring of the brain. This felt unnatural even though it was popular with consultants.

When I'm manic I can come across as being insensitive. This isn't intentional, though, it's really a subconscious cry for help. A rare time I was shown kindness in hospital was when several patients were watching the film *American Pie* on video in the sitting room. I was bawling my eyes out saying that the film was cruel as it took the mickey out of people. It reminded me of the girls in junior school calling me moonie addict and the boys parading around chanting that they hated Manchester United. I had forgotten until then how much those two childhood experiences had affected my fears in adulthood. Katie, who was on the ward to cure her heroine addiction, hugged me for most of the film in an attempt to stop me crying. She kept saying that it was OK. "Don't cry, because we care about you. We're all together here. We've got to help each other." I kept saying that the world was a nasty place and that "it's not fair that people hurt each other. It's not fair."

One bloke, Trevor, a mercenary after being in the army, was telling me that "everyone cared about me" and they didn't want me to suffer. They wanted me to get better just like I wanted them to get better. He'd spent eight years in prison for doing an armed robbery on Natwest Bank. He kept his mouth shut, though, and got £20,000 when he got out. What the fuck did he know? His head was mashed. He tried to overdose on pills twice a week and kept having to go to A&E to have his stomach pumped. All he needed was a bird to love him. Every time he saw Sonia he would kiss her twice on the cheek as if he were Spanish. This was the closest to having a bird he ever got when I knew him. Mind you, I only knew him when we were in hospital together. I tried not to be the jealous type as my mum always told me that a girl would wind me up if she knew that I got jealous. There was one time, though, when I had to put my foot down and show that Sonia was my bird and nobody else's. This happened on the arrival of a new neighbour.

Sonia and I were sat together one night on the patio, which consisted of a dozen chairs and was surrounded by an enclosed fence so nobody could escape or jump off and kill themselves. Quite a handsome young man dressed in baggy clothes came outside and asked if he could sit next to us. A nurse followed him but sat by the entrance of the patio and lit a cigarette. Sonia and I

Bipolar, Recovery and NLP

were holding hands and kissing each other. He asked me who I was. I was still manic so I told him I was Snoop Doggy Dogg.

He asked Sonia if he could kiss her. She said he could kiss her on the cheek as a friend. That's how the Spanish kiss so I didn't mind. He kissed her on the cheek and then went to kiss her on the mouth saying that she was his girlfriend. I stood up and shouted "Come on then, motherfucker, you're dead." Several hospital staff came out from nowhere, grabbed hold of him and dragged him away just as I was about to kick fuck out of him. I never saw him again. He must have been transferred to the secure unit in Brixton. That's a bad place, full of convicted Rastas. I unwittingly sent Paul there. One afternoon, he was teaching me some karate and when I punched him my knuckles were bleeding. When a member of staff asked me why I was bleeding I told them, and he was transferred a couple of hours later. You normally got a few days' notice, but not Paul. The staff didn't want that kind of stuff going on. I didn't mind it though – it made the stay more bearable.

In the canteen, I would eat on my own as nobody wanted to sit next to me. They all wanted to sit by Tim. The food was better than in any other loony bin as it was a private hospital, but the environment was just the same. Staff bossed everyone around and didn't really give a shit. Then there was the monotony of chain smoking, cups of tea, medication time, watching television, people screaming and people crying. I felt more like a name and number than a human being. Mum and dad would come up together and that really helped. Sonia would leave me alone to be with them. One day, I upset my mum by saying that I wanted to see dad alone. It was the best day I had ever spent with him. We walked round Chelsea and along the Embankment, talked about how I was going to try and conquer my illness, and sport and life in general. It brought my dad and me closer together. If only it had happened years before, then perhaps the gulf between us and our suffering would have been a lot less. Still, I didn't regret anything. It was a special day.

Sonia and I would take walks around Battersea Park at weekends and cuddle, kiss and flirt beneath the trees. We got closer and closer as the weeks went by. She was starting to mean the world to me. Whatever I was doing, whether eating or brushing my teeth, I would be dreaming about her all the time. She was

Bipolar, Recovery and NLP

becoming more important to my existence than even myself. This was comforting and, in the psychological model of transactional analysis, I was the child and she was the adult. I was unable to cope with my own problems so she coped with them for me. I was very confused at times: seeing her as a mother figure, as a goddess, as an angel as well as a girlfriend. I looked up to her and couldn't believe how strong she was: rushing to see me everyday after work, not having eaten and still with a smile on her face. She never got angry and never got flustered, always 100% what any man could wish of his girlfriend. Then one day I really fucked up.

Now, it wasn't really my fault as I was still manic and wasn't sure what I was doing. Even so, it was one of the biggest regrets of my life, and I wish I could turn the clock back and eradicate it from our past. There was a black girl in hospital suffering from anorexia. Her name was Patricia and she was 17. She knocked on my door one evening, crying, saying that a patient had stopped her getting out of her room and had tried to rape her. She didn't want to tell the staff as she was too scared. I was going to tell the staff when she said that the man hadn't molested her but just physically stopped her leaving the room for a few seconds. I made her promise to tell her dad everything that had happened. She said she didn't know how to so I said I'd write her a poem explaining how to tell him. She asked to have a bath in my room. I said it was OK as I felt responsible for her welfare. She had nobody to help her: her dad was a reggae DJ. *I had an understanding with him (even though we'd never met) just as I had with MC Buzbee. By tuning into each other telepathically we could make the world a better place ... After all, I was God ... and I was wearing the black and gold signet ring of Jesus ... He lived further down the ward ...*

He was a man with manic depression who worshipped me ... He knew that I was special the first moment he laid eyes on me ... I would tell him what to do for the rest of his life. I would tell him how he would serve God. After Patricia had had a bath and dressed herself in private, I read her the poem. She took it and sat down on my bed. I was nervous. I was responsible for her safety, her guardian angel. It was my duty as the white God to look after her while the black God, her father, was away ... She also needed initiating as a healer. Once I showed her how to heal she could heal others. She kissed me on the lips and our mouths were closed for a single moment when the night staff stormed into the room.

Patrick, who was a big black geezer and intimidated every patient in there, said: "He had his dick out." I was fucking angry. A female Irish nurse, who was Patrick's superior, accompanied him. I told her that what he said was bullshit and she must have known it was as she entered the room the same time as him. How could I have got my dick back in, in two seconds? I wasn't even thinking of having sex ... I was God. I didn't need to have sex ... I had a girlfriend ... Patricia left straight away and I told them that I would be making a written complaint. I made the complaint but there was no reply by the director, which there should have been by law.

I told Sonia what happened straight away and she was extremely hurt. What must she have thought? *"How could he be like that when I've taken such good care of him? What a bastard. I love him and he treats me like that. Who the fuck does he think he is? Does he really love me or is he just using me for sex? How ill is he? Did he know what he was doing or not? I don't understand what's going on and I don't want to see him tomorrow. I want to see my friends instead. He's upset me too much. He's broken my heart."*

I don't know why I did what I did. I know that I was very confused and manic and was having grandiose thoughts. I knew I wasn't well and wasn't in a normal state of mind when it happened. Nevertheless, afterwards I felt guilty. How could I keep going in and out of mania like that? It was a really weird sensation. Thing is, with mania, it stays with you like an electric shock. One minute you've got it and the next it paralyses you. You might not be conscious of it but you have it. To quantify my state of mind at the time would require complex psychological analysis, and it may never be solved. It was obvious I was unwell and I will always regret what happened. I just hoped that Sonia could forgive my mania and me. Exactly what made me do it I still don't fucking know. It wasn't me. It was something fucking with my head. Dionysus or someone, but I could never see them.

The next day was the first time I hadn't seen Sonia since I'd been in hospital. I spent the day crying and telling all the patients what had happened. They knew I wasn't well and knew that I loved her and said that our relationship would be OK. They said that she loved me and would forgive me, as it wasn't the way that I would behave if I was well, especially as we looked like we were so close. One of them, Pete, a Millwall fan who was caught with 36 E's after falling off his motorbike, said that he would talk to her for me. He spoke to Sonia in detail saying that she was the only thing I ever talked about. Their chat seemed to stitch things up a bit and a few days later Sean very kindly invited Sonia and I out for an American meal. Sonia hardly said a word and would only eat salad. I realised how much I had upset her and I felt like the devil. It broke both of our hearts and I yearned for them to heal and beat as one again.

With some women, the "treat 'em mean and keep 'em keen" approach works. But with Sonia this wasn't the case. We had a genuine goal and tried hard to make things work. Still, if you're nice to a partner, and let them, they can take you for granted, however much they love you. Likewise, if you sometimes wait until you show your affection they can melt in your hands. Good thing with us was that we melted in each other's hands when we saw each other, as we were in love. We worked hard to overcome problems that got in our way. We could discuss problems without shouting and tried hard to be as rational as possible and make up when the other was sulking or angry. Add that to love at first sight and that's true love.

On 15 May, I was transferred to St. Thomas' hospital, and my high mood mutated into depression. The depression was aggravated by one incident. Tim had hanged himself in his room the previous week. The night he killed himself I'd been playing CDs with him in his room, trying to cheer us both up. At about 11.30pm, I had knocked at his door.

"Hope you don't mind me coming, I felt like listening to some music."

Tim was holding his forehead and looking worried.

"No, it's all right, come in."

"How's about some Fat Boy Slim?"

"All right ... Not too loud, though."

"How you feeling?"

"Fucking shit."

"Like me. ECT treatment going all right?"

"Don't wanna talk about it."

Bipolar, Recovery and NLP

"Sorry."

"It's all right." (Lying down on the side of the bed with his eyes closed.)

"Good tune this. (Sitting back in the chair and crossing my legs.)

"Yeah." (Both sitting, eyes closed, listening to *Talking About My Baby* by Fat Boy Slim. I put it on repeat and we sat there motionless listening to the song twice.)

"I'd better go now. Cheers Tim." (Nods his head, scratches his forehead sharply, looking distressed and shuts the door.)

Fuck, I must have been the last person to see him alive. I kept going over that thought in my mind. Tim was dead. Poor Tim. Could I have done anything that would have prevented his suicide? Was it my fault in anyway for not preventing it? As tragic as it was, I knew it was not much to do with me. He had done what he had to do on his own accord. I had to look after myself man, especially after this. That was it for Tim. His life was over, finished; it had ended just like that. Those fucking bastards didn't look out for him. They could have saved him if they cared, but they didn't.

Tim had had seven of his eight ECT treatments. Maybe they had caused his suicide. They sure as hell didn't fucking prevent it. I mean, the treatment hadn't worked in time. The whole ward was crying and the management brought in extra staff. Now the staff cared but it was too fucking late. Tim was dead. The most popular guy on the ward had done himself in.

I blamed Patrick for intimidating everyone in there. This disciplinarian was a bully and epitomised everything that Tim despised in the army. His attempt to exert control over everyone may well have sent Tim over the edge. Although I was very upset by what happened, I couldn't believe the way that everyone was acting. All the patients were wallowing in self-pity. They were feeling sorry for themselves rather than for Tim. What about his family? How would they have reacted? Wouldn't they have been more affected? Of course they fucking would. I didn't show a lot of emotion. I was asking questions, and had to be told to stop talking as I was upsetting everyone. I wanted to work out why this happened. This wasn't one of those fake suicide attempts after which I had seen so many bandages and bruises. Tim really meant it and did it. Fair play to him – he had got out of the stinking shit hole and would live forever. If he wasn't alive in the afterlife then at least he would live in the memories of all the patients and staff in the hospital, especially with his dramatic exit.

I wondered if I would be next. He was the only person who I had met, that I knew, who had taken Sodium Valporate and Lithium, like me. Was I going to kill myself next? It was about this time that my depression was starting to sink in. Could I be as brave as Tim? Was my predicament anything like his at all? Or was his far more serious? Did he have any option? What made him give up? What was the final straw? All these questions plagued my mind in a room with half a dozen patients crying.

I remember the way I found out. His parents were informed first, and everyone was summoned to the lounge. I knew something was wrong and the first thing I said was: "Where's Tim?" The female patients burst out crying and a male patient, Chris, who had also been in the army, said "We don't know yet, Jay." He held my hand. Katie was talking out loud: "Why don't they fucking tell us? I know he's dead. I know it. He was fine before. He was on one-on-one. They were checking him every 15 minutes. Then they took him off it. And he's killed himself. Fucking bastards, it's their fault. They fucking killed him." I sat down on the side of the chair and said "shit", as the tears rolled from my eyes. It was the staff's duty to inform the parents first, but people knew as they wouldn't let anyone near Tim's room. Tim's death seemed to bring out all the suffering we felt and reminded me of the one million suicides that take place in the world each year.

The director announced, in a sincere fashion, what everyone feared. This was the same man who hadn't responded to my complaint about Patrick. That seemed so trivial now. But was it? I know Tim hated him as well. He was the one who should have been keeping an eye on him. The staff offered extra support. Thing is, most of them weren't trained for it. How could the patients have faith in the staff when most of them felt they were treated like naughty children rather than adults with mental health problems?

The only ones who had shown any compassion before had been an Australian nurse called Greg, who had spent 17 years as an engineer, and a Scottish nurse called Pamela. The rest of them

Bipolar, Recovery and NLP

weren't very nice at all – more concerned about puffing cigarettes and reading the newspaper than healing the mind of a loony. I had a chat with my doctor the same day. She was from South Africa and had compassion. She cared about the people she saw and believed she could help them psychologically as well as medically. Her approach was the complete opposite of Dr. Tannock's, who was 100% rational.

On the morning of Tim's death some of the patients stayed in their rooms and lounge and mourned while others went to art group to write poems in his memory. These would be presented to his parents as a tribute at some later date. Tim's drawings and paintings were on display. One of them was a picture of birds flying over a beautiful sea and blue sky. They looked so free. I looked at the date and saw that it had been drawn only two days before. I remember having to tell a depressed, but quite sophisticated, middle-aged woman called Jean, who was very close to Tim, what had happened. She was devastated and was escorted to her room by a member of staff. The art group was the only creative activity in the hospital apart from a few groups such as "Managing your illness", "Understanding your illness" and "Relaxation". *I'd been painting an ashtray in the colours of the Spanish flag for Sonia for a few weeks. It had "Sonia Te Quiero" written on the one side and "Jason Te Quiero" on the other. It looked cool and I was delighted to discover that Jason and Sonia were practically anagrams. The "I" and "J" can look extremely similar, especially in art. That made my sentiments and gift even more romantic.*

I felt morally obliged not to kill myself as it would be too selfish. I loved Sonia and my family too much and could never hurt them like that. The day was for Tim and I wrote a poem from my heart saying the positive things about meeting him. A dozen of us took it in turns to read our poems, and the therapist wrote a new poem with one line from each on the blackboard. He was a kind man, a Buddhist who believed his work was important to those he was helping, and it was clear that he enjoyed what he was doing. He had excellent people management skills and was very patient with me when I was manic. I was flattered, once, when he said that I was "really quite amazing".

Later in the morning there was a discussion group on how

Bipolar, Recovery and NLP

patients were going to deal with Tim's death. I didn't go because I'd overheard that some people would not welcome me. They didn't want a classicist philosophising about his own anthropological theories in an attempt to make the world a better place. They just wanted to feel their own pity and pull themselves together. Some of them may have wanted a bit more – to find out the root of the problem or blame others – but none of them really had the intelligence to achieve this. They needed someone with a bit of balls. That's why Tim and I didn't get on in a group. He knew that I was the only other person there who had balls. When we were alone, though, we got on great.

Sad thing was I felt closer to him than anyone else in there. I used to wink at him when everyone was at lunch kissing his arse. He used to smile back. The last thing he ever said to me was random: "Do you like Kajagoogoo?" I said "Yeah, they're all right", and he smiled. I didn't like them but I knew that was the answer he was looking for. There was an affinity between the two of us and, for me, that was the saddest thing about him going. I still grieve for his family and resent the hospital, as I see it, for being unable to prevent, and even contributing to, his death.

The memories of Tim surfaced for two reasons. I was worried that I would end up the same, and the woman I had told of his death was transferred to St. Thomas' and insisted on talking about it with me. I was so depressed about everything that talking about his death felt absurd rather than comforting or upsetting. I was becoming devoid of any feeling apart from being low. The resources at St. Thomas' and the staff were worse than at Chelsea. I spoke to Brad on the phone a few times and Al Greenwood, my 60 year-old friend from Wales. I would sit and smoke, staring at Big Ben. I had a great view from my bedroom window although I never appreciated it while I was there. I just thought of Parliament and the Government and how fucked up the treatment of the mentally ill was.

Big Ben certainly reminds me of one event during my stay at St. Thomas'. Right near the beginning when Sonia took me to hospital to get me help, we had sat in the cafe at night looking at the clock and I had imagined myself as the first headline on the BBC's Nine O'Clock news for being responsible for curing manic depression. It was "all in the mind", as George Harrison said in the

Bipolar, Recovery and NLP

Yellow Submarine.

During my time at the hospital, I would often set out on day trips. Sometimes, I would wander around the Millennium Eye among all the tourists although I'd feel more depressed and paranoid as time went by, and return to the ward. There were a couple of excursions I forced myself to go on. A member of staff took two of us to the Tate Modern. The other patient was an annoying Australian woman who'd gone manic and spent all her money shopping in Milan. She would even talk about how great it was to be manic ...Well, I didn't agree with that. Didn't this woman get depressed or anything? I couldn't believe that she treated the illness as if it was some kind of joke.

Two staff escorted several of us to the Aquarium. I wanted to see the Dali and Picasso out of my love for Sonia. People went to the Aquarium as it was better than being alone on the uncarpeted ward. Sonia still visited and we had some nice cuddles on my bed. In Chelsea, we had been caught about to make love by the staff so were more careful in St. Thomas', especially as I was sharing a room. The patient I shared the room with was called Patrick. He was an Irish alcoholic. Fortunately he was never there. Then he ran away. He didn't return so Sonia and I at least had some privacy.

I stayed at Sonia's flat for a weekend, and went to Gloucester to stay with my dad. He was very supportive and the bond between us was strengthening. He knew I was in a terrible state and listened to me when I told him that the depression would get worse. They were reluctant to put me on antidepressants as they could make me high if I wasn't low enough.

...

I will never forgive the hospital for the way they discharged me on 12 June, 2000. A hospital nurse basically discharged me without anywhere to live. Fucking bitch, I wished somebody could put her in my situation. I'd have loved to see her crack up like I did. Who the fuck did she think she was? Margaret Thatcher or something? I'd been evicted from Felix's and had spent a week down the Homeless Person's unit in Brixton. I lived with Sonia for a bit but she was sharing a room with three other girls in a hostel. At the weekend, we had to stay in a hotel at £80 a night because her flatmates didn't want me there. They felt uncomfortable with us smooching around and sleeping together.

After begging and crying for a week, I was offered accommodation in Streatham. I was too ashamed to see my family and, if I did, I might not have the strength to return to London, and Sonia and I might split up. She meant everything to me. If I hadn't been so persistent I would have been out on the streets. The people at the Homeless Persons Unit were wankers. They didn't give me any choice where I lived, kept postponing when I would move, wouldn't answer my questions and generally treated me like a piece of dog shit that they were scraping off a brand new pair of shoes. They were African, didn't speak proper English, seemed far less educated than me and determined what happened with my life!

My Case Officer phoned up Felix and tried to get him to let me move back in with him. This was the most humiliating experience of my life. I was crying on the other end of a bullet- and soundproof screen. This screen, as I understood it, was placed to stop assaults on the staff but symbolised how detached they were from their client's problems. It's one thing being impartial, but if they really don't give a fuck how can they do an effective job? They never believed anything I said, kept losing paperwork and were suspicious and rude despite me being as polite, calm and positive as possible.

When I got to the hostel in Streatham I was relieved to discover that I had my own room. People at the Homeless Person's Unit had told me fuck-all and, as far as I knew, I might have been sharing a room with a dozen crack and smack addicts. The room was small and basic and the area was a dump but at least I didn't have to embarrass myself further by taking refuge with either of my parents and their partners or Sonia and her flatmates. I would rush to see Sonia every afternoon and wait for her in Bayswater.

My mum got me a mobile so she could monitor my mood and so that I could keep in touch with Sonia and my friends. It turned out to be really useful and would help Sonia locate me. I became more and more depressed and would only be happy in Sonia's company. I lived to see her and she must have presumed that I was better than I actually was. I stayed off the alcohol and sank into depression. I saw the tramps outside the hostel drinking cider and wasting their lives away. Everyday I would see the Irish man I had shared a room with in St. Thomas' begging for spare change and drinking the same 8.4% brands of cider that I used to drink in Manchester. Once I spoke to him and he didn't even recognise me. I wasn't going to end up like that. I had some dignity left.

At the time, I begged my psychiatrist to put me on some antidepressants. She would make fleeting remarks when I would say that I felt like jumping in front of a tube or out of a high rise building. I could see that she was trying to snap me out of it but I still think it was unprofessional. She was oriental and I couldn't tell if she was smiling at my predicament or if that was her natural manner.

I remember two occasions when my dad got angry with me. In the garden I told him that I was terrified of losing Sonia as the whole episode may prove to be too much for her to handle. He snapped and said: "For God's sake, she's only a girl." I said that I loved her and he said to pull myself together. The other time was when he gave me a lift to meet my brother and his new girlfriend, Angela, in Gloucester. It was the first time I'd met her. I was talking about how I needed to go on antidepressants but the doctor didn't want to risk it as I could go high. I continued talking about my depression. My dad shouted: "Bloody hell, can't you just snap out of it." I started to cry and said how I felt: I was too weak, I didn't know how much longer I was going to be around ... I just wanted to kill myself ... I was a burden to everyone I knew. I couldn't take it anymore. I didn't care if I was dead or not.

My dad put his arm round my shoulders and patted me on the back. He looked horrified and said: "Jay, I'm there for you anytime day or night, OK?" I could stay with him when I wanted to and for as long as I wanted. He told me that things would be fine, that we could fight through things together. He said that if I didn't get put on antidepressants the next time I saw the psychiatrist then he would phone her and get things sorted.

I often wondered what Sonia would think of my brother and vice versa. It was a pleasure and a relief to discover that they both liked each other. My brother had spent the previous three years setting up his own business. As he became more enlightened, he became more ambitious. He set up a company that sold oil paintings and antiques. His ideas were innovative and he worked day and night to kick start his "empire", as he saw it, but he had a bad credit rating and always had problems getting a loan to fund the business. Therefore, it was always stopping and starting. He did not receive the enthusiasm that he craved for about his business from the family, except from me. I've also given him some valuable contacts along the way. Only time will tell if Dr. Crichton can one day pull it off. If he does not he can see enough beauty in the world to have a happy existence.

Trying to fund his business expenses and his other outgoings, however, he'd constantly badger mum, dad, me, Nan and grandma to lend him money for two reasons. Firstly, he thought he deserved it because of the way they treated him in the past. Secondly, he believed that lending money was the kind of thing that families should do for each other. I tried to stay out of that. I would never take sides when it came to the family. I just told my brother not to ask me again and to spend his money more carefully instead of buying things that he didn't need, all the time. I told him to get his priorities right.

The whole thing stressed me out too much. If I thought about my family too much I would become anxious. When I got anxious, my blood pressure increased. If my blood pressure increased for too long I would start going high. It was clear from the therapy I had gone through that I could cope with just about everything from everyday life except for my family. The memories of them, meeting them and seeing them in the places I used to be so often. I couldn't bear being forced to listen to their criticisms of, or worries about, one another. I wanted good news or no news. I wasn't strong enough to weave all the different strands and threads together.

My brother has such a deep love and compassion for art and beauty that it's sometimes hard to believe. He loves listening to Beethoven, looking at art and reading philosophy. He is remarkably well read and extremely romantic as a lover. He is always there to talk to if I need his help. He doesn't mind if I ring him in the early hours of the morning when I am upset or a bit high. Often, there even seems like there is a metaphysical connection between us because when I ring him up we are thinking of the same thing.

However, he is so interested in objects, the world, and the universe that he tends to speak an awful lot. Therefore, it can be very difficult to get a word in when you are in his company. He has a brilliant mind. Sometimes you just feel like writing down the things he says because they seem to have so much meaning and relevance to your life and the lives of others. He understands how the universe works and why people operate in the way that they do.

But he always goes from one extreme to the other. He can go from being the perfect gentleman to standing at a bar with no money in his pocket. One minute he can be at the proms in a tuxedo waving the Union Jack and behaving as an aristocrat, the next he can be walking round with a scruffy top, a pair of trousers with stains on them and holes in his socks.

Anyway, Angela was a 25 year-old, slim, Glaswegian sculptress whose mother looked after homeless people. When she met Harvey he was 29, and wearing a monk's outfit in the garden. Angela and her mother had come round to try and get my grandmother to take on a reformed prisoner as a lodger. Angela, Harvey and me went out a few times and I was over the moon to see my brother so happy. I wished it could stay like that for him forever. Whatever the outcome, I was grateful to her because she has helped my brother love again. Going out with her had got rid of his misogyny and enabled him to be a romantic again. That meant my brother had got over his previous bad relationships and would find it easier to get another girlfriend in the future if he needed to. Then he wouldn't have to be alone in his old age like my grandma.

Harvey is one poor rich man and heartbroken true love. When I got ill it hit him hard. Funny thing is if we hadn't been through so much we wouldn't be as determined to succeed now. I am at ease with my family now and Harvey will be too, in time. Therefore my mum can stop thinking that "everything is her fault". Please mum, never even think of taking an overdose again because my brother and I are proud of who we are. You can enjoy life. So can dad. You deserve to. Take it from me.

Blood is thicker than water and I love all of my family. You can't choose your family, you just have to put up with them, and as friends come and go families usually stick around. They love you for what you are – not what you can give them or do with them. That's the ideal anyway and it's true most of the time with mine,

Bipolar, Recovery and NLP

thank God.

Anyway, the next time I saw my consultant after meeting my brother's girlfriend she put me on Efexor. This time I was sexually functional and it started working within a few weeks. I had clung on long enough to avoid ending up like Tim. There were times when I thought I was going to crack but the will to live beat the will to die. I told Sonia once that I would have killed myself had it not been for her. It was the most upset I had ever seen her. She said that it was not fair to put that kind of pressure on her. It was as if I was blackmailing her to stay with me. If she left I would kill myself and she would be to blame for my suicide. I was so depressed at the time that I thought what I was saying was true. Humans have a lot of resolve, though. Look how Robert De Niro gets the gooks in the Russian roulette scene in *Deer Hunter*. He's pushed to the limit and comes through it. I wouldn't know if I would have survived without Sonia. Glad I never had to find out. Glad she never had to find out, either.

After four months on the antidepressants my life was bearable again. Sonia and I had our ups and downs but maintained a strong relationship. She went on holiday with her friends to Biarritz and I survived without her. That would have been unthinkable a few months before. My mood improved enough for the two of us to go to Corfu. We hired a car and I enjoyed driving around the snake-like winding roads. I harassed the council, my GP, consultant and psychologist to get me my own flat in Vauxhall. They eventually agreed and by 15 October, 2000 I had my own flat. There was nothing in it but I got a grant for £1,000 from the Social Fund to do the place up. That really helped and I owed a lot to one of the housing officers at the hostel. It was an Asian woman who worked in the office who told me that I could apply for a grant. Without her I wouldn't have known about it, and she was very kind and helped me fill out the form in detail. I saw her several months later and thanked her again. She said that she was glad to see me back on my feet again and pleased that I was "one of their success stories". And there weren't many success stories that came out of that hostel.

Bipolar, Recovery and NLP

Chapter 11 – Dealing with it

So in October 2001, for the first time in my life, I had my own flat and my own space. I took pride in turning an empty house with no carpet or furniture into somewhere that actually expressed my identity. It also helps that it's only a 15 minute walk to the hospital, and on the first floor, meaning it's warm and less likely to be burgled.

Mum and dad came up to help me move in, and dad even helped me paint the lounge magnolia – he knows how good it is to feel secure and comfortable in the area that you live in, as much as I do. It was a new beginning and things were looking up. One thing is for sure, though, I don't think I'd be half as comfortable as I am at present without the time, effort and love that dad showed me when we were doing it up – Christ, I've even taken to DIY.

All in all, my life was getting better. For added peace of mind, the authorities reassured me that I couldn't get evicted from this flat, even if I went out of my mind. I went to my psychologist every two weeks and, after I had come to terms with the stigma attached to going to see a shrink, we undertook an intensive relapse prevention programme. Carol Busch, the aforementioned, is a middle-aged, erudite and extremely intelligent individual who helped me put my life and experiences into perspective. Importantly, we concentrated on identifying the early warning signs that I am going high, that I'm heading for another episode. We covered and examined nine signs in all:

The first sign is *energy*: more energy than normal is a potential danger, as is doing too many things at once and being disorganised, so be aware. The second sign of an impending episode is *sleep*: going to bed one to three hours later than usual, taking longer to get to sleep and sleeping less (five to six hours). Third comes *alcohol*: half a pint of lager makes me feel light-headed and confused and my heart rate increases. My mood changes and I can become depressed, quieter, more irritable, self-confident and grandiose. The fourth sign is *caffeine*: drinking even small amounts of coffee, tea or Coca-Cola make me feel anxious, and my heart rate increases. Five, *diet*: I eat less well with fewer home cooked meals and more fast foods – especially burgers. Sixth sign: *headaches* and *migraines* are more frequent. Seven is

Bipolar, Recovery and NLP

social contact: I become more talkative with friends and strangers, yet more intolerant and critical of others. I make more complaints about poor service. If I feel uncomfortable in social situations, I seek out reassurance by sharing my "crazy" thoughts with others. I worry more about what others think of me. Eight, *loneliness*: I feel increasingly lonely, and increase my contact with old friends and family; I try to make new friends. The final category, *sex*: I become more perverted, submissive and lose touch with reality, fixating myself with mistresses in my imagination.

The work I've done with my psychologist is long-term, and a good place to turn to if things ever became unmanageable. Combined with closely observing my medication levels it plays a key role in avoiding serious episodes and ending up "back in the bin". I will never know how bad my illness is compared to that of others but I'm not prepared to find out. I'm determined to do something about it. The boxer that had been hit so hard that he couldn't get back up has found new strength within himself and through the help of someone else:

Still seein' Sonia
bein' honest with ya
hope we can be together
forever and forever
your love is true to me
as mine will always be
so sorry to hurt you
what was I supposed to do?
hope we can get through it
I was evil when we met
for that I'll always regret
we're so close now
that I've taken this vow
always to be faithful
rather than be so hateful
you've been so loyal
removed my hate with toil
I was scared of life
been through so much strife
now I'm so much stronger
just hang on a little longer

Bipolar, Recovery and NLP

I love you more than anything
our happiness is the key thing
thanks for your help and aid
for that you didn't get paid
I'll never forget your tender love
my wonderful magical dove ...

Through a wonderful woman from a different culture than his own this man has found a kind of humanity that is more sacred than he has ever experienced before. Meeting her and having her stick by him has made him face up to all the pain of his past, and for the first time he can be himself. He has discovered his own identity without the bullshit, and without all the pretentiousness, and whatever the outcome he will always be grateful to her for that. Sonia Fernandez Bascones has helped strengthen the resolve of Jason Pegler.

Pride, determination, frustration, anger and a desire to prevent the majority from bullying others will always give him extra resolve and he will fight on as long as he can. Although an outsider, he still believes he can be victorious in a fight with limitless rounds. Someone has to get knocked out unless both come to their senses and stop fighting.

He is fighting for mental health, fighting for those poor mad bastards who wander around the hospital wards wanting to kill themselves. He is fighting for those people who are immediately prejudiced against because of the colour of their skin. He is fighting for the memory of those Jews that were massacred in the Holocaust. He will relive all the pain from his past over and over again to try and help a fellow sufferer. Maybe he could even help a 17 year-old with manic depression accept their illness long before he had, and then they wouldn't have to go through as much pain as he went through. That, indeed, is his goal, just to help one poor bugger, face up to their serious mental illness and enable them to get on with their life. Then, and only then, will all that reflecting and self-analysis be worthwhile.

Bipolar, Recovery and NLP

Chapter 12 – Jaw trouble

By November 2000 things were looking up. I was getting settled in my flat and, as the days passed, I came to terms with my illness. Some days, of course, were harder than others. After all, I'd been depressed and still had to be careful and conscientious when taking my pills, and be able to identify any change in mood. For example, if I cut the dosage of my antidepressants too soon I'd be too depressed, but if I stayed on them for too long I could go high and relapse. And like any episode, it could prove to be too much, and the last one. Game over – you're history.

I had a supply of Valium to relax me when I was feeling stressed out. I knew I was far more vulnerable than people who didn't have bipolar effective disorder and I knew I would have to live my life in a way that would suit my condition. However, I also knew, importantly, that part of my illness was psychological so I could still live a decent life by refusing to give in. The ball, to a certain extent at least, was in my court. I didn't want to be so much of a hypochondriac that I couldn't fulfil my goals, ambitions and dreams. Each time I got knocked down I would get up again because I was a survivor.

The positive philosophy that I had made for myself was severely tested when I had another episode, or a serious blip as my psychiatrist called it, in December 2000. A noticeable difference this time was that I managed to avoid hospitalisation somehow. I had spotted it sooner than before and, thus, decreased the time of my hellish experience. I was hit just as hard but my relapse prevention work had strengthened my ribs. I tried to be like the great Mohammed Ali when Joe Frazier hit him during their amazing fights. Ali said that Frazier would hit so hard that he couldn't feel anything. His body was totally numb.

The most disturbing fact, in my eyes, was that I'd finished the first draft of my memoir on 30 November, 2000 and suffered a relapse the following week. I had achieved my greatest ambition at that point in my life, yet relapsed almost immediately afterwards. Had writing so much about madness made me mad again? Well, it certainly hadn't helped, had it? I had put myself under a lot of pressure by writing 50,000 words in eight weeks. Considering the

Bipolar, Recovery and NLP

subject matter and my condition I had put myself under a great deal of strain. My mother had warned me but I had been fighting too hard. I'd been fighting too hard to catch up with my millionaire-aiming business friends, Mark, Sean, Felix and my brother. I'd been fighting too hard to catch up with my journalist buddy, Dominic, and ended up falling on my arse. My high level of expectation had been my downfall. I was my own worst enemy, putting myself under stress when it wasn't worth the risk.

The whole experience of writing the memoir had been a roller coaster ride that was different to anything I had previously experienced. I had started writing it in July 1998, the day after I left Barclays Bank where I worked as a Sales and Service Advisor. I'd been working full-time for nine months – six of them with Barclays – and the idea of the memoir came to fruition during that period. As my health improved I wanted to write more and more. I wrote 15,000 words in two weeks and was so upset, drained and enlightened by the end result that I couldn't add to it for two years. By the time I'd returned to it and finished the first draft, though, I'd let sleeping dogs lie. I'd found out more about myself and learned to face up to the bad things that had happened in the past. My anger, frustration, hang-ups, and bitterness had come out of the closet, and the ghosts from Green Lane, the rest of Gloucester, Manchester, and even some of those in London, had flown away. All in all, it had been a cathartic experience.

I saw my psychologist on the same morning and she congratulated me for finishing. I even managed to have a meeting with a junior consultant who educated me about the chemical aspects of the medication I was taking. Unfortunately, though, I would soon end up like Hamlet – taken over by my own antic disposition. Concentrating on the theme of madness had to some extent made me mad again. Mad as a hatter, in fact.

Why else had it happened? Wasn't it simple? My medication wasn't right and needed to be adjusted; it would take time and years of practice to be able to distinguish between feeling happy, or content, and actually going high. I knew I was going to have further relapses and I knew that it would be a long time before I would be able to see it all coming. The fact that, on this occasion, I had managed to spot myself going high and had got help straight away saved me months of hell – and possibly even my life. It saved me from topping myself like the popular Tim from Chelsea Charter Clinic. It saved me from becoming too introverted and giving up. It saved me from being chemically depressed to such an extent that I was a lamb to the slaughter. I'd been saved, but the feeling was just the same, the punch was just as hard and the impact was just the same. I was pitiful, weak and a blubbering wreck. I was like a smack head suffering from withdrawal symptoms and in desperate need of a fix.

Other stressors contributed to me going high again, the most noticeable of which was a massive argument I had with Sonia. We were very close by December 2000 and hardly argued. Sonia prefers to keep things to herself and I was always conscious of discussing things rationally rather than shouting, screaming and hurling abuse as my parents had done. Sonia and Anna (her best friend in London, 20 years-old, from Naples and in the first year of a marketing degree) were desperate to leave the hostel that they had lived in since April 2000. In fact, they had moved in on the same week that I had moved into hospital. I said they could leave the hostel and stay with me for a while until they found a shared house with some other people. I would look after Anna's belongings while she went back to Italy for three weeks. This would save her three weeks rent, and I could also save Sonia a couple of weeks rent as she was going back to Spain to see her family for Christmas. I really wanted to help them out, but as soon as I suggested it I started to get stressed out. I panicked. It may affect my benefit. Wouldn't the flat be too crowded? The flat would be a mess, and I knew that would stress me out just like when I used to clear up the mess of my friends in my room, all those years back when I was on acid.

I spoke to my psychologist who advised me to retract my offer, but I still wanted to help them out. They had been good to me and I wanted to repay their kindness.

On 1 December, 2000, a Friday night, Sonia and I went to a classical concert, Handel's *Messiah*, at a church in Sloane Square. Sonia won tickets through the Metro newspaper. During the interval, I bought Sonia a glass of wine and, while I sipped my orange juice, I asked her and Anna for £20 a week keep while they were staying in the flat with me. I knew I was over-vigilant with money and thought that the payment would compensate for the adjustment that I was making and make them concentrate more on finding a flat.

Sonia went ballistic and we left the church without seeing the rest of the concert. It was particularly upsetting as it had been a romantic evening up until that point. I realised that I had really hurt her pride, and became so frustrated when she wouldn't accept my apology that I shouted at her to fuck off. It was dark, and about ten seconds later I started looking for her but she was nowhere to be seen. I looked for her everywhere, shouting her name in desperation.

I eventually caught up with her back at the hostel in Bayswater at about 11.30pm. I told Anna what had happened and knew that I had upset her as well. I'd hurt her pride and I had done something selfish. Sonia didn't want to speak to me. We eventually went for a walk and she was so disillusioned with our relationship that night that she was considering finishing it. We both cried in the street knowing that things weren't as they should be between us, so I agreed to give her some space.

She agreed to let me stay with her that night and I left early in the morning as I wasn't going to beg her to stay with me like I had begged Meredith. I had my pride too, I thought. I also expected her to come to Dominic's sister's thirthieth birthday party later that evening. It would be nice to see Tara as I hadn't seen her for ages, and it would be a special social occasion where I would be able to introduce Sonia as my girlfriend. Sonia eventually did come and we made up.

Over the next couple of days, I spoke to my mum and dad and told them what had happened and they told me that I was in the wrong. Their judgement was enough for me to admit it.

After I'd finished writing my memoir my mood had become quite elevated as it was such an intense experience. The row with Sonia had increased my anxiety and I had been extremely lively at Tara's party. I'd drunk four bottles of Stella, which had been my limit for two years, but because of the strong medication I was on I was very drunk. I was drunk enough to really show off when dancing. I was dancing to some hip-hop, most notably House of Pain's "Jump Around", and the whole dance floor, around 20 people, were watching and applauding me for about two minutes. James Brown would have been proud of me. I don't think that I

Bipolar, Recovery and NLP

was manic then but this instance illustrates that a manic-depressive has to be very aware when they feel happy – there's a fine line between happiness and the very early stages of mania. I'd managed to keep my alcohol limit to no more than two pints in a day since the night I got kicked by the doorman on 17 March, 2000.

On 4 December I met a guy from New York on Oxford Street. He was working on behalf of Centrepoint for homeless people. He taught film studies at some film school in Bristol and gave me an address where I could have my first screenplay "A Can of Madness" critically reviewed. This eventually cost me £15 but proved to be worthwhile. On Wednesday 6 December, five days after our falling out, I invited Sonia out for a surprise. I booked top quality seats for a ballet about a mermaid in the West End.

We met at seven and I was crying my eyes out. I'd told Sonia that I couldn't go to the ballet with her because I was manic. I was afraid and would be unable to concentrate. I was ill. Fucking hell. Not again. When would this fucking nightmare end? I didn't have the strength. I couldn't go through it again. I was too weak. Why me? Why the fuck did it have to be me? Why the fuck couldn't it be someone else for a change? It wasn't fair. I was so glad that she was there. I don't know what I would have done without her. Without her love I was even more vulnerable. I would be even more useless. A lamb to the slaughter; "Meat is Murder" as Morrissey and the Smiths so aptly put it.

I'd seen my consultant earlier that morning and he had recognised that I was high and gave me some new pills: Diazepam, which is more commonly known as Valium, Risperidone, Zimovane, Droperidol and Procycladine. We'd arranged to meet again on Monday 11 December to see how much the new medicines were bringing me down. From then on Sonia was careful to note when I should take which medication and how much I should take.

I can clearly remember being high. My appointment with Dr. Richard Haslam was at 1pm on Wednesday 6 December, 2001, and I had gone to play squash with Mark in the morning. He lived in a posh flat in Clapham Common and was one of my best mates in London. I told him that I felt high and was worried I was going mad. I broke down in tears and told him that I was losing my mind again. Mark's response was to give me a caring pat on the back and ask me if I wanted a copy of the latest U2 album. The song, "A Beautiful Day", was playing in the background.

Instead of going to play squash straight away Mark set about cooking a superb fried breakfast. He put on MTV, made me a filter coffee and told me to relax. Mark was an excellent cook. He would often mix his coffee with brandy, and take breaks having a few drags on a Marlborough Light. He would therapeutically tidy his flat while cooking. He was 29, nearly four years older than me, and was from a wealthy background. He'd spent most of his life working in marketing and was partial to the odd drink or 10. He liked his pills and was into charlie when he felt like it. At the time he worked for an IT dot com that was really pissing him off because of its lack of ingenuity. By mid 2001 he ran an expanding software company that had been set up by his dad. It was a high pressure job where he was in charge of alot of people. He would often fly to Boston for business meetings but was there for me when I had problems. He moved in with an Irish journalist called Maria. She was good for him. They moved into a flat in Tower Bridge and then to Clapham Junction.

When I was watching MTV at Mark's flat in Clapham Common I practised the diaphragmatic breathing that my psychologist, Carol Busch, had taught me to try and relieve the stress that I felt. It was too late. I was as weak and as fragile as a little baby being raped by a paedophile. I sat down absorbed in the television and watched the most remarkable pop video I had ever seen. It was "Coffee and TV" by Blur and it made me cry and feel the most scared I had ever felt. The video shows a little caricatured carton of milk walking around a dangerous route. He catches sight of a pink female carton of milk and is clearly in love but she is run over by a car as they cross the road to meet each other. A tear of milk drops down his eye when he sees his love flattened and, at the end of the video, he is thrown in the bin by one of the band and is flown up to heaven with the help of an angel. I felt so upset when I saw her run over, and I actually thought that I was the carton of milk that was thrown in the bin. I wasn't happy; I was utterly miserable.

Mark arrived back with the greatest breakfast I had ever seen. It was fit for a king. Sausages, bacon, black pudding, mushrooms, grilled tomatoes, eggs, beans, fried bread, filter coffee and orange juice. I ate it like a tramp at Christmas who had realised they had been invited in for their last warm meal for a long time. I knew that this was a special occasion, and I was aware I would experience months of pain and suffering just as I had during my previous episodes.

Soon afterwards we walked to the squash courts and had a few games. Mark won four games to nil, although I scored about six points a game which wasn't too bad as Mark was pretty good. In fact, he'd captained his university at it.

I couldn't believe what happened next. I discovered I was sat next to Geoffrey from the old TV programme "Rainbow" on the train from Clapham Junction to Waterloo. He looked as pale and ill as I did. I remembered seeing him on an advertisement at about four in the morning a few weeks previously. The advertisement mocked him for not having saved a pension. Maybe Geoffrey was mentally ill as well. That was such a pity. Zippy, George and Bungle hadn't been real people and all that time Geoffrey hadn't known. No wonder he was so depressed now that he had found out.

I managed to get to the hospital in time to see Dr. Haslam. I ran all the way from Waterloo station to St.Thomas'. Dr. Haslam said he could tell I was high before I told him. Well, thank fuck for that. This was the first time ever that a medical professional had spotted that I was high relatively early. He should have been given a medal or something. I cursed the GP I had seen a few weeks before. My usual GP, Dr. Law, had not been there so I saw an Indian doctor. When I told him that I had been feeling high and that I had wanted to reduce my antidepressants, during an emergency-only Saturday morning appointment two weeks before, he told me to go home, chill out and drink some peppermint or camomile tea. Fucking bastard. That was another occasion when the system had let me down. Doctors just didn't listen to me. In hindsight, though, I thought of many reasons why: they didn't have enough time, there were too many patients, they had too much paperwork and they couldn't spend enough time one-on-one with a patient. Instead, they just rushed people through the surgeries. I felt like a clone going through the escalators on the underground at rush hour. The thing is, when some shit happens to you like that, you feel let down. You feel like they don't give a shit about you because you are mentally ill. You feel like you deserve to be ill because you're inferior to others. You don't feel human. You feel like a vagrant; like a useless motherfucker. Like a loser in every possible way.

This was the first time that I had been ill since I had known Dr. Haslam, with whom I had struck up a good rapport. We had had some fascinating scientific, psychological and philosophical discussions. It was the best relationship I had had with a highly qualified medic since Kath Porceddu in Manchester some years earlier. I was in his care and he set about planning his course of action to make me better.

First he put me on Zimovane which was a sleeping tablet. Sleeping is often the first thing to go when you go manic and it's vitally important to get back to a proper sleeping pattern as soon as possible. Then he decided to put me on Rispiridone. This was a typical anti-psychotic that also had mild antidepressant properties. I was to take 7.5mg of Zimovane every night. The Risperidone would start at 1mg twice a day for three days in the morning and the evening. After that it would increase to 2mg twice a day. He set up another back-up in case I still felt high. If I felt high at any time I was to take 5mg of Droperidol and wait half an hour; if I still felt high I could take 5mg of Diazepam, wait and revert back to the Droperidol. Each time I was to take one of these drugs, I had to take 5mg of Procycladine to counter any side effects.

When Sonia took care of me that night I found it difficult to go to sleep. In the morning I still felt high. Sonia took the next two days off work to be with me and escorted me to the hospital. Before we went we decided to go for a fried breakfast. Within five minutes of finishing it I was screaming in pain. My jaw was winding. It was a side effect of the Droperidol. The pain was just as excruciating as when my jaw had winded up in Coney Hill eight years before. I cried now just as I did before.

We rang the hospital and a consultant told me to take Procycladine tablets every five or ten minutes until the pain went away. I took three Procycladine tablets in ten minutes and on the way to Scutari Mental Health Clinic at St. Thomas' hospital the pain finally went away. I could see my jaw unwinding itself rapidly. The Procycladine had had an immediate affect.

215

Bipolar, Recovery and NLP

We were advised to go to A&E and see the Duty Psychiatrist, but we weren't going to do that again. We'd spent two days there, nine months before, and still hadn't got anywhere. We demanded to be seen by someone at Scutari even though we didn't have an appointment. Eventually, we saw a psychiatric nurse called Jo Bowd. She told me I could take one more Proclycladine and to take up to four straight away if I felt any pain in my jaw again. She gave me some more medication, and Sonia and I went back to my flat. Sonia was so strong. I was dumbstruck that she was still with me when I was going to go through all this shit again. A lot of women would have got off the roller coaster rather than psyche themselves up for another ride. I saw another consultant on the next day, 8 December, while Sonia spent a few hours in bed with terrible stomach cramp. She wasn't as invincible as I thought she was – she was human as well and needed to be looked after once in a while just like anyone else.

Over the following week I settled down a bit but was still manic. This was the only time that I had been manic leaving me with no confidence whatsoever. It was turning out to be a completely different – but always harrowing – experience every time. I saw Doctor Haslam on Monday 11 and Wednesday 13 and saw my psychologist, Carol, on the Thursday. We all hoped that through my relapse prevention work I had prevented a serious episode occurring. We hoped that with the drug package Dr. Haslam had put together I could avoid going into hospital. Only time would tell. I was as emotionally weak as an eggshell that had been trampled on by somebody wearing steel-capped Dr. Martens, and Sonia stayed with me every night until I went to Gloucester on 21 December.

Despite my fragile condition I managed to attend a meeting with Victim Support on 12 December at Ladbroke Grove. One volunteer, Caroline, was very sympathetic and helped me fill out my appeal for the incident with the doorman that had taken nine months previously. I was convinced that the incident triggered all the horror that followed in the months afterwards. It was the same as not knowing whether my dad's treatment of my mum or my mum leaving home when I was 14 had affected my life and subsequently triggered off my illness. I don't blame either of them. Parents are only human and they make mistakes too. The most

Bipolar, Recovery and NLP

important thing is that I have. and will continue to have, their support in the future because they love me and I love and respect them.

I can say what I like about my dad's behaviour towards my mum when I was little, but he never left me, he always stuck by me and there was always a room for me there, even if it did turn out to be the little bedroom. There was also always a room at my mum's. I used to stay there a lot when I was at university and I knew I could stay there again despite what my stepdad, Michael, had said when he was pissed up that night. Thing is, I didn't want to stay at either of their homes anymore. I wanted them to come and see me live my new life in London. I was making my own life in London. I had made a decision to stay in London after I had fallen ill the last time, and I had my own flat now.

As the depression took over I became more and more introverted and less and less active. My mood seemed to have slumped to an all time low, and my thought processes became lazy and monosyllabic. I was becoming terribly lonely whenever Sonia wasn't around. Thing is, I would still be terribly unhappy when she was with me, no matter what she said. Sonia had to go to work and I would meet her at the tube station every evening. We put the sofa bed up in the lounge and lay there watching TV all night. We would cuddle each other, praying that the pills would do their job. The moments when I felt the best were when Sonia hugged me as I cried my eyes out and reassured me that I would be OK and that we would be OK. She had to keep on reassuring me that I was not a burden to her and that I would get better one day. I had got better before, and I had been worse before for longer periods and battled through it.

I lost count of the number of times that Sonia echoed these remarks but they never seem to register when you've slumped into depression. You become oblivious to everything. You just want the pain to stop. You want to distract yourself but you can't because depression is like a python grabbing hold of you when you're asleep. It grabs hold of you and it takes a long time and a lot of assistance to get it off without cracking your windpipe.

On 16 December, 2000 it was our anniversary. So much had happened in the 12 months since we had met each other. Sonia had got more than she bargained for, but our love was still strong and she was still fighting for me. Someday, maybe, I want to return her loyalty and love and fight for her, and us if need be, in an equally powerful manner. We went for a Chinese meal in Clapham and, although I was very nervous about going out, we had a beautiful, romantic evening. We both loved the duck and pancakes with Hoi Sin sauce, and we both loved each other.

As I boarded the train at Paddington to Gloucester on 21 December I felt uneasy as I knew I would not see Sonia for over a week. She was going to spend Christmas with her family in Spain. This was the first time we would spend so long apart since we had started going out and, although I would desperately miss her, it was a good test of seeing how much we would miss one another. Sonia flew to Madrid the following day and met up with her family in Burgos. I spent a few days with my dad and saw my Nan, grandmother and brother before going to stay with my mum on Christmas Eve. I was getting worse. I spent most of Christmas Day reading Nietzsche's *Ecce Homo* which describes how he went mad, and read from start to finish a book by John Gray called *Men are from Mars, women are from Venus*. I thought it would help Sonia and me in our relationship. I felt that we were strong, but we had been through so much that I felt it was advisable to look at ways of avoiding any unnecessary problems that may have arisen. I needed to keep her. She was a gem.

My jaw ached on a few occasions and I took the Procycladine accordingly. I always made sure that I carried my drugs on me in case I needed them. It was nice to see my mum and dad but I was so weak and confused that the only spark I had was when I phoned Sonia and said "*Hola, esta Sonia por favor, soy Jason*" or when she called me from a phone box. Then my face as well as my heart would light up. I was happy that she was with her family and tried to keep myself together when speaking to her as I wanted her to enjoy her time.

I desperately wanted to meet her family some day, but this was not the time. Sonia had only told them a couple of months before that she had a boyfriend. They were Catholic so they needed time to get used to the idea. I liked the fact that we were from different backgrounds. It made life more interesting. However, sometimes I felt left out. I feared that they wouldn't accept me when I met them. Sonia had been accepted by all of my family. They all thought that she was great, but what would her family think of me? I mean, I was hardly the model boyfriend. I didn't have a job. I wore baggy trousers and had a mental illness. I couldn't even speak their language and I still picked my blackheads. I was from a different religion. I was a Christian. Even worse, I was a Christian who was probably an atheist when he thought about it. How could Sonia explain to her mum that she was in love with someone like that? How could she persuade her mum, dad and two brothers that she wanted to spend the rest of her life with a man who would hardly understand a word they were saying when they met him?

By the time I returned to London on 27 December I was in a really bad way. I spent the night round Mark's, took my sleeping tablets early and saw Dr. Haslam the next morning. He asked me what had happened and told me that my health had deteriorated. He attributed it to the stress of me seeing all the members of my disjointed family in such a short time. Was it my eccentric brother that had driven me further into the abyss? Had his ingenious mind been too powerful for me to absorb this time? Was I a failed hero like Ajax? Had I been embarrassed at not feeling like the most intelligent person in the room and lost my critical faculties even more because of this fierce psychological competition and rivalry that existed between us? Had an unwitting attempt at overhauling his mania backfired and increased mine? It probably had. Dr. Haslam's drug concoction had also not worked as well as we had both hoped. He couldn't explain why, in detail, as he admitted that psychiatry often had to treat people on a trial and error basis. I had to be patient. I had to hang on in there. I had started an episode and it would take time for it to filter out, unless it took me over for good.

I spent the next day cracking up in front of Mark. As we walked across Clapham Common to Battersea on the icy path, a couple saw that I was upset but ignored me and walked pass with their dog. They were probably mental health nurses. Mark had gone on ahead and I broke up crying my eyes out. I told him that I was fucked. I said that I was depressed and I couldn't fucking handle it. He told me not to worry as Sonia would be back soon. I carried on crying out loud. He didn't know what else to say. Who would? I mean there is nothing that you can say to make a

Bipolar, Recovery and NLP

depressed person feel better. That's the problem.

I rang the hospital on my mobile and tried to get in touch with Dr. Haslam. As usual, he wasn't around. It was like the Coyote trying to get hold of RoadRunner. Fucking impossible. The man was never there and it would take him a week to get back to you, and then he would not get the message or would forget. As my credit ran down, 35p a minute on my Orange "pay as you go phone", one of the secretaries managed to get me through to the head of the Mental Health Department at St. Thomas' Hospital, Dr. Davies. I informed him of my discussion with Dr. Haslam that morning and he said they had discussed my case briefly. That gave me some reassurance knowing that there were two consultants who were concerned about my health.

I was told to go to a chemist and double my antidepressant dosage of Venflafaxine, that I had started that same day, from 75mg to 150mg. The chemist spoke to Dr. Davies on the phone and issued me with the drug. I was still terrified as they told me that the drug would not work for about two weeks. Fuck, how could I last that long man? I was fucked. Mark and I went into a bar next door. He drank a few pints while I had a few orange juices. I couldn't touch the booze at all as it would interfere with the medication. I had to be really careful this time and I had to be resilient for Sonia. She had proved her resilience and loyalty for me so I would do the same for her. I would show her some respect and reveal to her that I could be as responsible as she had been when taking care of me.

Sonia came back on 30 December and I met her at the airport. Months later she told me that she couldn't believe how bad I looked. Anna was away in Italy so I spent the night in the room that they shared. We slept and cuddled for 24 hours. We went back to my house for New Year's Eve. We fell asleep about eight in the evening and at 11.57pm woke up to the Queen song "We Are The Champions". As Big Ben chimed we ate grapes and cuddled each other in the Spanish tradition.

The next six weeks were masked with a terrible depression that clouded over me. All the colour went out of my face, my mind weakened and my personality lost all its charisma. I put on weight, slept in late and was terrified of being on my own. I only avoided hospital because Sonia stayed with me every night. Each evening

Bipolar, Recovery and NLP

after she finished work I would be waiting for her, without fail, at the tube station. I would be at Vauxhall most of the time but sometimes I'd meet her at Fulham Broadway. When we met at Fulham we would plan for Sonia to stay there but I would be so upset that we would get a taxi to my place. Each journey cost £10 and that was a noticeable hole in our financial budgets.

It wasn't really fair on Anna. She had moved to a new house with Sonia and wasn't getting to see much of her at all. (We were both pleased for her when she found herself an Italian boyfriend some months later. His name was Enrico and he was a nice bloke.) As the weeks went by I became so desperate for company that I would ring Anna as soon as I had crawled out of bed and spend as much time as possible with her, waiting for Sonia to come back from work. Anna was very understanding and would make me camomile and fruit tea which I brought round for her and Sonia. She proved to be a very good friend and I was lucky that all my mates stayed on the madness bandwagon with me early in 2001. I needed their empathy and I would always remember their friendship and loyalty at such a crucial time in my depression. Loyalty, love and respect from my friends, girlfriend and family provided me with the backbone to survive. Some credit was due to the barbarian instincts within me, although I was in such a state that I never really noticed these instincts surfacing.

I saw my psychologist, Carol Busch, on 8 January and begged for the session to be extended. She just told me to go to Scutari Clinic or A&E. Fucking hell. She talked all that positive, intellectual talk but when it came to the walk got in her car and brum brum brummed off. I was fucked, she knew I was fucked and, when it boiled down to it, I was just another patient. I wasn't her responsibility, I was just becoming an increased burden on her workload. The person who had been directing my life, thoughts, hopes and aspirations for the previous nine months had let me down. If she let me down like that then that meant anyone could. But was she really letting me down? Was this just another, but more poignant reminder, that I had to assume responsibility for my illness? We had set rules together, but as she said some months later: "Only you know how much you can bend them." I knew I could let myself down if I could not get hold of Dr. Haslam. He was the one who had the authority and expertise to change my medication if I got high.

One positive thing about Dr. Haslam was that he was very proactive whenever we met. The guy was fucking intelligent and he really did give a shit. I knew he had a passion for his research and, when I met him on 23 January, 2001, he wrote down a more detailed plan of action than before to show me how he hoped the drugs were going to stabilise my mood. I was on: Rispiridone 1mg twice a day; Venlafaxine 150mg once a day at dinner time; Sodium Valporate 600mg twice a day; Zopiclone 7.5mg a night. Dr. Haslam ran me through them all. Risperidone had some antidepressant effects but was prescribed to stop me going "high". It was a safety net. Venlafaxine was an antidepressant but ran the risk of making me high. Sodium Valporate was the real safety net for mania and depression. I was to continue on the same drugs and the same amount except increase the Sodium Valporate to 800mg twice a day.

The Risperidone had been added after I had relapsed. This, along with the increase in Valporate, meant that I had less chance of a future relapse. The drugs were experimental and their effectiveness was based on a trial and error basis. Combined with my relapse prevention techniques and finding the right drug combination I could minimalise or even prevent future relapses. I had done well to catch this episode early and extremely well to avoid going into hospital. It was tough but I just had to dig in deep and battle on until the episode had worn itself out.

According to figures published by Mind in July 2001, 40% of people who take antidepressant tablets experience sexual problems. The same is true with other drugs. I had become impotent and, by the end of January 2001, had terrible difficulty obtaining an erection. By February 2001 it was upsetting me so much and contributing to my depression that I told Dr. Haslam. He understood that my sexual dysfunction was affecting my moods, and we agreed to risk taking me off the Risperidone and switched me to two 100mg Quetiapine tablets a day. I was to take one in the morning and one in the afternoon. I could have gone high in the interim but fortunately didn't.

Within two weeks I was able to make love to Sonia again. This helped my mood and gave me some peace of mind. Sonia was incredible. I couldn't believe that she was still with me after she

Bipolar, Recovery and NLP

had experienced so much shit. We went to a couple of Manic Depression Fellowship meetings, and it helped the pair of us talk about the illness with other sufferers and carers. It made us feel that we were not alone. And we weren't alone. Scientists believe that between 1% and 3% of people suffer from it. Bare in mind that 13 million people in the UK are taking anti depressants (Samaritans 2004) and over 1 million people commit suicide every year (World Health Organisation 2002) and you begin to realise the scope of the problem. To some degree we all have mental health issues so why not be open about it and help each other.

Today's patients aren't like those poor sufferers who were thrown in the same prison cells as murderers as Foucault describes in *Madness and Civilisation*. We weren't alone but seeing the group was a sad experience in itself. The literature it collected on manic depression was really out of date. They didn't even have the right phone number or form to become a member. The leader of the MDF group, moreover, was hardly a role model as she admitted having great difficulties with coping with the illness from day to day and had some very peculiar ways of trying to cope with it. She regarded being high as being something special and couldn't accept the horrific side to it. The group itself was, on the whole, very timid and lacked inspiration, direction and positivism. They were scared to open up and when they did they were usually talking about how crap their life had been. They were wallowing in self-pity like I had done over the last seven years.

The strongest character there was an elderly woman of about 65 who had cared for her deceased husband for 30 years. I admired her grit and determination, and Sonia told me that the woman gave her a much needed insight into caring and provided her with even more resolve than she already possessed. Thing is, the old lady always stressed how much of a burden it was to look after her ingenious husband who had a professorship in medical science. That made me fear even more that the drug concoction I'd agreed to take with Dr. Haslam would have to work sooner rather than later or Sonia might fuck off and do one. I didn't want that, but I didn't want Sonia to see me as a burden as this old lady had seen her husband. That's one reason why we didn't go back. However, I was also getting better, and the shock of going there and seeing that life does go on after episodes made me accept it and kick start

Bipolar, Recovery and NLP

my life for the umpteenth time.

Although I was bitterly depressed and very fragile, my doctors, family, friends and Sonia encouraged me to escape from the prison that my home had turned into. Instead of hiding under the sheets in the bedroom then hiding on the sofa bed watching TV, sleeping all afternoon, watching my plants die and overeating, which included three giant Kit Kats a day, I actually went out. I met Dom a few times in Canary Wharf for lunch. He'd been living in Clapham Junction and Clapham South with his girlfriend Tiggy. She was a good influence on him and I was pleased to see him happier than when he was in Stockwell. I went to the cinema in the afternoons. I rescued my plants from certain death, put them closer to the window and they began to grow again.

Sometimes, I'd meet Mark for lunch in Clapham Junction. I also went swimming a few times with him or sometimes on my own. I met Felix for lunch and we became good friends again. Time had healed the wound. He had forgiven me for trashing his flat and I had forgiven him for evicting me. I mean, he had no option really. If my flat had been trashed like that I would have done the same thing. I wouldn't want a manic on the loose in my flat. Would you? When I was meeting Sonia I would get to Vauxhall tube station early and have a coffee. I started reading again. I started doing the Daily Star sports crossword, reading the tabloids, even the Evening Standard, and finally some simple novels.

The episode was fading away and although I had more scars I was used to having scars. I'd been in a lot of fights in my life and was a tough cookie, mentally as well as physically. One of the scariest statistics that I knew about manic depression was that between 13% and 16% of sufferers kill themselves, at sometime in their life, during an episode. Well, it hadn't been my time this time. I really got hold of my relapse prevention, sought to educate myself about the drugs I was taking and to maintain the good rapport that I had built up with my head consultant and psychologist.

Having a strong network of professional support is vital if you want to avoid hospitalisation. Nurses, doctors, whoever's path you cross, it's vital to get the most you can out of the system. Some of them are brilliant people and if you find a good one it's vital to

Bipolar, Recovery and NLP

stick with them if possible. They can help facilitate your struggle with mental illness and make the condition a lot more bearable. You can talk about when you think you are going high and plan with them when to alter your medication. Fine-tuning is essential when dealing with this sort of condition. GPs have to see far too many patients, but the Labour Government is actively recruiting more of them all over the country, during the first 10 years of the millennium. There is far too much bureaucracy in hospitals. Staff are forced to waste endless hours filling out forms and carrying out mundane procedures when they could spend that time giving quality care.

So much needs to be done. Governments need to do more. Mental Health awareness groups like Mind and the Manic Depression Fellowship need to be more proactive. More grants need to be available for people with mental health problems. Society needs to be educated to accept sufferers. The media has a responsibility to behave in a responsible, sensitive and impartial manner when dealing with the mentally ill. If they don't then they must be warned and punished. I am all for a democratic society and freedom of expression, but give people an inch and they'll take a yard. A free press is a great idea in theory but, if it persecutes innocent people, it must be held to account.

So the episode that had started in the middle of December 2000 had ended by the end of February 2001. Phew! Now that was the shortest episode that I'd ever had. I'd spotted one when I'd been with Gina but I'm not really sure whether that was an episode or not as I'd spotted it so soon. That time round, I'd found it hard to return to being a normal human being again, but this time it was much easier. I had my own flat so I knew I wasn't going to get thrown out of anywhere. I wasn't being pressured into anything by anybody as I had my own space. I had the security of being a council tenant, had good friends in London, my family to talk to and a girlfriend that I adored. I was proud of how I had come through another episode and as long as I could avoid getting ill my life was bearable.

Hell, even if I got ill every now and then, I would still have somewhere to live even if I trashed the place. Maybe even one day I could buy the flat? I would always be terrified of losing it but I had accepted what my illness would have in-store for me in the

Bipolar, Recovery and NLP

future and I wasn't bitter about it. I was alive and had two arms and legs. I could see, feel, touch, hear, smell and wasn't in a wheelchair. I wasn't one of those guys in the hundred metres in the Paralympics. I admired those guys, their determination and courage. I wouldn't cringe when I saw them on television as I would have before I was diagnosed with manic depression. I would even go so far to challenge people who took the mickey out of them, which I may not have done if I hadn't been diagnosed. It wasn't my job to protect them, they could do that themselves. I wouldn't feel sorry for them. They didn't want pity, they just wanted to be accepted like everyone else.

Everyone has a dilemma when they see a blind person about to cross a road. Should they offer to help him or her? Surely they look like they need help? I'm happy to help somebody like that but I'd wait until they ask for help. That's not me being selfish. That's me allowing somebody to have their own identity. That's all I want for mentally ill people and other minority groups – to be able to live as themselves in a multiracial and multicultural world.

The clouds eventually cleared, the sky had turned blue and I felt as free as the birds looked in Tim's picture in the art room in Chelsea Charter Clinic. I was still with Sonia. I regained my confidence and managed to interact with people again. I was given an opportunity. The man who believed in me proved to be a great councillor, anthropologist, philosopher and friend. Eventually we went down the gym together. He gave me lots of advice and was a pretty mean boxer. At last I had found someone to fight with who wasn't scared of me. We went boxing and I got fitter as time went by. I guess that the moment I we met signified the end of the latest relapse and a new period of sanity. Even though I finally realised that I went in and out of my mind everyday I'd learnt to live with my illness. I wouldn't know how long my good health would last but each minute would be a precious one and I would try not to take any of them for granted.

My dad helped me improve my flat and set up a great office environment to work in. He really came up trumps. The BBC liked it so much that they made part of a documentary called *Smallpox* in it. I'd sent my first draft to several publishers and one of them wanted to publish it. I had to increase it from 66,000 to 100,000 words and knew that I would when the time was right. I saved up

Bipolar, Recovery and NLP

for a computer and buying it and improving my office area inspired me to continue with my memoir again. I got on the internet, discovered another world, took an extensive computer course to increase my IT skills and plugged my memoir to people who crossed my path (this was from August 2001 until spring 2002, but only when my health permitted it). My life was worth living again and I realised that in one way I was lucky. I had the opportunity to help people who were disadvantaged, especially those who had manic depression. If I could communicate myself to them then maybe they would feel better about themselves. My intention for writing the book would often reverberate in my mind: "Even if I could only help a 17 year-old with manic depression then that would make reliving it time and time again all worthwhile."

I now coped with stressors in an effective manner. My brother came to stay and we both managed to stay calm enough to have a great time together.

Tom also came to stay for a week. He had survived a suicide attempt some months earlier, and I was glad that I had spent some time and even more glad to see that he was back on his feet. He'd split up with Perry, which was a shock to me, and was now a free man, as he put it. His presence made me pause for a moment and think whether Sonia and I were with each other for the right reasons. Were we really doing the right thing? Did we really hope to spend the rest of our lives together? Was it worth working everything out and adapting to accommodate each other's needs? Could she forgive me for what I'd put her through? I knew I needed to give her time, space, love and understanding whenever it was necessary. I would have to listen more and be more considerate. I had to be open to criticism. Although our relationship was up and down and I sometimes felt like a yo-yo I always wanted to fight for her. I never wanted to let her go and, to my delight, she felt the same. We could be rational and sit down and talk about things when other couples couldn't. I was very patient in the months that followed, even listening to her doubts over the relationship.

Then one day in June of 2001, as if by magic, I had a shift in attitudes, although fluctuating in and out of madness was to remain a daily occurrence. I stopped asking questions about my past and just accepted it. I'd realised that I'd come of age and that I wanted to enjoy the present and look forward to the future rather than dwell on the past. I'd finally grown up. I also matured in my attitude to Sonia. I knew she loved me and she knew that I loved her. She knew that I would do whatever was in my power to accommodate her wishes and keep us together. I admitted to myself that what would be would be. If we split up then there were plenty more fish in the sea, but I knew that I had a special catch and felt that I always wanted to keep hold of this one.

Sonia and I saved up and went for a holiday to Barbados in July. It was beautiful. The people were so friendly. I took Sonia jet-skiing and she clung onto my waist saying that I was great as we bumped up and down on the waves. We went on a safari tour and learnt about the whole history of the island. We went out on a catamaran and went swimming with the turtles. We even went snorkelling together and saw the tropical fish in the sea. It was so romantic. The place was so beautiful. The plants and wildlife were more beautiful and wild than anything I had ever seen before. We saw steal-drum bands playing, spent time with the locals and drank coconut milk from coconuts that we had got down from the trees ourselves. It was a much-deserved break for us both and we planned many more together in the future.

Bipolar, Recovery and NLP

Conclusion – Looking forward

It's February 2002 and I haven't exceeded two pints of lager (or the equivalent thereof) in one day for 23 months, but I am still aware of my life struggle with alcoholism:

I have no shame for having a chemical imbalance in the brain
And as I sit and write I don't know how or when I'll go mad again
It could be now, it could be then, if or how it's made worse by society.
Despite the pain and hurt I'll succeed and maintain my sobriety

With my psychologist, Carol Busch, I've also set up my first Action Plan For Life helping me cope with, and respond to, the very early stages of going high. The plan is as follows:

Changes in medication: Stop Venlafaxine, increase Quetiapine, add Diazepam, continue with Sodium Valporate, take, or stop taking, sleeping tablets as appropriate.

Follow sleep rules to improve sleep pattern (go to bed before 1am and get eight hours' sleep).

Reduce stress: use relaxation techniques daily, stop multi-tasking, build quiet periods into each day for chilling out, avoid too much social activity – reduce, or cancel, social engagements if necessary.

Reduce or stop work if necessary. Focus more, when at work, on the job in hand rather than interacting with colleagues.

Use up excess physical or psychological energy by doing some physical exercise, again, when appropriate.

Stop intake of alcohol and caffeine.

Contact GP, psychiatrist and/or psychologist.

Contact close friends and/or family for additional support if needed.

On 3 October 2001 Sonia and I left London and flew off to Bilbao. From there we took the coach to Burgos where I was to meet her family for the first time. They were everything I hoped they would be, and more. They welcomed me with open arms and I felt comfortable and relaxed in their home. Sonia's mum and dad didn't speak English but her brothers could hold a conversation. Although I'd started two Spanish courses in September 2001, and I was keen to experiment with the language, Sonia had to do a lot of translating. We had a brilliant time having tapas; visiting the cathedral, local monastery, shops and cinema; walking along the river and around the historical city. Sonia's mum and sister-in-law were also great cooks which was a bonus.

All the anxiety we had as a couple about whether or not I would be accepted was blown away. They could see that I made Sonia happy. Staying with them also filled a void in my relationship with Sonia. I had a much greater insight into her past and could therefore assess her expectations for the future. The whole experience drew us closer together.

We looked through hundreds of photos together of her brother's wedding, when she was in America, her friends and members of the family. I was touched to see so many people love Sonia like I do. I saw the books that she had read, the things that she had kept in her room, her collection of Walt Disney cartoons and her brilliant drawings, which I knew nothing about before. I saw what she was like before she met me and that made me love her even more. I appreciated again how beautiful she really was.

In the hallway there was a huge picture of her when she was eight years old. To my delight and relief she looked as beautiful then as she does now. We only stayed for three nights but went back for nine days at Christmas. My Spanish is improving, and we get closer as the weeks fly by. We are as close as ever and are true soul mates. Like every couple we have our ups and downs and we don't know what the future holds for us. All we know is that we love each other and that we want to be together.

   ...

On 20 October 2001 my best friend from Manchester, Tom Robertson, was forced to end his life. He was suffering from depression and his pain was too much to bear. This was, and always will be, one of the saddest memories of my life. I wished I could have helped him more but I couldn't reach out far enough. Tom, the guy who had been so strong in helping me and others, did not have enough strength left for himself. I didn't find out until the day of his funeral that he had a mental illness. That meant that all those times he said that he understood how I felt were not just words of comfort but were actually true.

Bipolar, Recovery and NLP

When I write now, sometimes I feel like I am writing for Tom. Through what has happened to Tom I've strengthened my resolve and am more committed than ever to helping people with mental health problems and others that are prejudiced against it. As long as I am able I will never give in. If Tom taught me one thing then that is to never give up what you believe in. We often used to talk about the memoir I was writing and its positive implications on the people I wanted to read it. I remember when he read the first draft. When I asked him what he thought he said with a smile "it's deep". One thing is for certain, whatever happens after its release, whether it's a flop or a best seller, I'll never lose track of why I wrote what I wrote. I wrote it to help people relieve themselves from suffering.

Being a manic-depressive has meant that I've grown up quicker than I wanted to, but I'm glad I lead my life the way I do. I intend to reduce the risk of any serious relapses in the future as much as is humanly possibly and let others read my heart instead of just pouring it out for my own comfort onto a keyboard and computer screen. I practise other mediums: novels, poems, comedy scripts, screenplays, raps, short stories and children's stories. It depends what mood I'm in. I empathise with people who suffer more than the average person does. Whether they're homeless, have Down Syndrome, are starving in Africa or Afghanistan, have been tortured or persecuted because of their beliefs I want to help. The only thing that had any significance in my life apart from Sonia, my family and friends the last time that I was suicidal in hospital was when I was reading Nelson Mandela's *Walk to Freedom*. It put my life in perspective. This hero had gone through more hardship than I had and he had overcome it. Therefore, when the cloud lifted, I could do the same.

Hell, health permitting I could conquer the world ... make it a better place ... be a successful person .... win the Booker Prize ... become an MP ... a member of the cabinet ... Prime Minister ... like Winston Churchill, the manic-depressive like me. A manic-depressive ... I've got more talent ... as I'm God ... better be the pope as well ... to help these mortals attain peace ... set up Chipmunkapublishing ... The Mental Health Publisher... Reduce Stigma and discrimination on mental health... stop the 1 million suicides that are committed every year... Create the world's first mental health brand. Oh, and be an astronaut ... and learn to fly ...

Better stop there for that's a manic mind after all. Wouldn't want to have another episode, now would I? ... And none of you want one ... that includes everyone, believe me.

Curing Madness

By Jason Pegler

The Selected Works of a former manic depressive

"To cure a mental illness is always possible. If you always believe so it will happen. This is how I transformed myself. You too can do the same if you decide to do so". Jason Pegler

Bipolar, Recovery and NLP

Published by
Chipmunkapublishing
PO Box 6872
Brentwood
Essex CM13 1ZT
United Kingdom

First published 2006

A record of this book is in the British Library.

http://www.chipmunkapublishing.com

Bipolar, Recovery and NLP

CONTENTS

"To cure a mental illness is always possible. If you always believe so it will happen. This is how I transformed myself. You too can do the same if you decide to do so".

Jason Pegler 2006

Bipolar, Recovery and NLP

Bipolar, Recovery and NLP

DEDICATION

I want to dedicate this book to Alistair Priestly who I went to school with who so sadly took his own life recently, his family and his friends. I would also like to dedicate this book to my girlfriend, my friends and family who have stuck by me through thick and thin. You have helped provide me with the strength to lead a life in which I am fortunate to be able to focus on my goals to help empower people who have suffered from mental health issues.

I would not feel that this book had any real accuracy or value though, unless I thank one man in particular. That man is a man who I have shaken hands with twice just before walking on fire: the American life coach, Anthony Robbins. From the year 2000 I started reading Anthony Robbins' books and found his work inspiring. By studying his material and applying it to my own life I managed to gain more and more internal strength and my inner voice grew. In September 2004 I finally met him at one of his Power Seminars and it was during these days that I finally decided to come off the psychiatric medication. By the end of 2004 I managed to come off whilst liaising with my psychiatrist and to my delight I have never looked back. My life has improved dramatically since this time and I know I will never be back on this medication or in a mental hospital again, unless I am visiting with the intention of meeting patients and improving the way the services are run.

Ever since this moment I felt motivated to carry on with Curing Madness and as I come to realise the end of this project my cure is complete. This release of positive chi now gives me new found strength to continue dedicating my life, and the life of others, through my work with Chipmunkapublishing the Chipmunka Group and related companies, to harness the largest civil rights movement of all time. Giving a voice to those with "mental health issues", so we can prevent the suffering, humiliation, injustice and abuse that these people and their friends and families face.

Bipolar, Recovery and NLP

Bipolar, Recovery and NLP

INTRODUCTION

I am now completely free from the psychiatric drugs that poisoned my mind, body and soul from the ages of 17 and 29. I was fortunate that I had the willpower not to commit suicide whilst being on them and again fortunate to rebuild my life so I could come off them and never look back. I am not advocating that if you are on medication that you should stop immediately. Read this book first and then re-evaluate your life, find out what your values are and work out your diet, physical exercise and emotional intelligence. Take appropriate advice and then there is no reason why you can't get off them and lead a fantastic life using the pain you once had to help other people in the world.

This book has some real challenges ahead. If I slip into utopian mode please bear with me, such is the nature of a former manic depressive. The mission of this book is to focus on saving the world from itself, most notably to stop the humiliation and stigma of the "mentally ill" and to expose the drug industry and psychiatry for what it really is and provide hope for the future of what it will be replaced by.

Curing madness is the follow up to my autobiography on living with manic depression, A Can of Madness. A Can of Madness is a rollercoaster ride about coming to terms with living with manic depression and making a 90% recovery. It has helped thousands of people realise that they are not the only person in the world, that they go through such amazing highs and lows and enables loved ones to finally see and understand what their partners, friends and family are going through. However, this is still not enough.

Everyday more and more people are being falsely diagnosed with mental illness and being over medicated at the hands of the drug companies. There needs to be a global shift in communication in the "mental health world" as

Bipolar, Recovery and NLP

Martin Luther King did for black rights and Bob Geldof did for Africa.

By writing Curing Madness I am making my personal testimony as a social entrepreneur, rap artist, consultant, publisher, speaker, Chief Executive and Chairman to prove that I was able to cure myself by taking consistent positives steps, and taking massive action. By believing I could get better I actually did. It is my view that anyone who has ever been diagnosed with a mental illness can do the same thing and my duty as a human being to create a system and work with other like minded people who share this vision and are capable of doing something about it.

For me writing Curing Madness is the next step. It is a quantum leap from my previous book. A Can of Madness was said to make Prozac Nation look like a walk in the park. I hope from the deepest part of my soul that Curing Madness will demonstrate that anything in life is possible no matter what your previous psychiatric or social history.

There are two hurdles to overcome. Firstly, pill popping is now so prevalent in our culture that it is already an epidemic. This action must be replaced by looking for alternative therapies; most notably people must be given the best tools such as practising NLP, hypnosis and being encouraged to raise their self esteem and expectations of their own lives. The great work of practitioners like Anthony Robbins and Paul McKenna must be brought inside systems such as schools and the NHS. We must go a stage further than Robbins and McKenna and make these services free across society so that these systems are intertwined into our culture. I believe passionately that the work that I am doing is central in achieving this purpose. History will tell us the answer.

Secondly, there has been thousands of years of psychological and now psychiatric oppression in most places on the planet and people who are different or have mental health issues have never had a voice. By using my own personal testimony I make myself an example of how the world is changing in this regard and how people have moved from their own disempowered self to thinking and empowering others.

My mission is a utopian one and can best be understood by studying the diagram below.

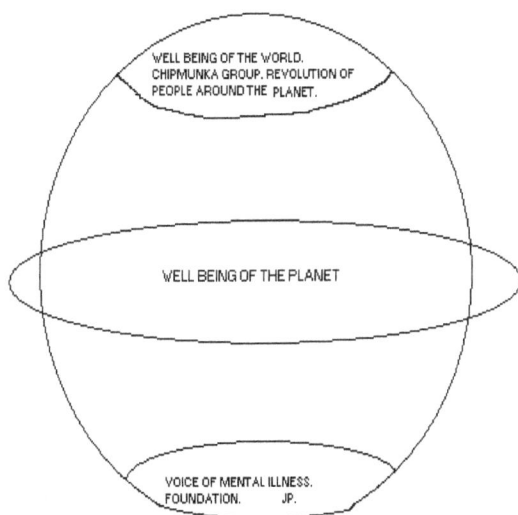

WELL BEING OF THE WORLD. CHIPMUNKA GROUP. REVOLUTION OF PEOPLE AROUND THE PLANET.

WELL BEING OF THE PLANET

VOICE OF MENTAL ILLNESS. FOUNDATION. JP.

Figure 1.1

The diagram above illustrates how I can achieve my utopian goal. My main work goal in life is to reduce the humiliation of people with mental illness. I visualize this goal working so I can place it in the well being section in the diagram above.

241

Bipolar, Recovery and NLP

To achieve my goal I use a variety of steps. At the bottom of the diagram I put in the small steps. For example, in this section I would include the Chipmunka Foundation (see www.chipmunkafoundation.org: Registered charity number 1109537). The fact we help people with mental illness and the fact that I as an individual have had manic depression gives me credibility in this area.

In my view the steps at the bottom of figure 1.1 are necessary steps towards the utopian goal. The big steps would be the Chipmunka Group, including Chipmunkapublishing. The fact that I set up Chipmunkapublishing as the Mental Health Publisher enabled me to set up the Chipmunka Foundation. Even if the Chipmunka Foundation achieves its mission and becomes the most effective and significant mental health charity in the world it will not become a bigger influence than Chipmunkapublishing or the Chipmunka Group as they were the catalyst for it.

Bipolar, Recovery and NLP

The Chipmunka Group is a social entrepreneurship and philanthropic model that enables the Foundation to grow organically. Resources from the Group "The World's first Mental Health brand" are pumped into the Foundation. The Chipmunka Group generates its own revenue.....and actively supports the Foundation. It also gives opportunities to people with mental health issues to become self-employed, social entrepreneurs and show that people with mental health issues can achieve anything that they believe is possible therefore creating the world's first mental health celebrities.

The charity in itself, although it can transcend economies in a humanitarian context does not in an economic, political or socioeconomic sense.

The Chipmunka Group itself has the same mission as the Foundation but uses economic forces to take a bigger step. Therefore, all parts of the

Bipolar, Recovery and NLP

Chipmunka Group would go above the goal cylinder because of their economic potential.

The fact that my life's mission is to help people with mental illness is also in my eyes a small step. By October 2005 Chipmunkapublishing alone receives more web traffic than any other mental health organization in UK with over 15,000 visitors every week. This is because we are giving people a voice, an opportunity to have their voices heard in a world where they are discriminated against.

The reason why I have put helping people with mental illness as a small step is simple. I deliberately used the wrong language. There is no such thing as mental illness really[1]. It is a manufactured term set up as a form of social control as governments do not generally want people to think for themselves. I believe that they also want people to fit the selfish motives of

---

[1] For further reading read "The Necessity of Madness by John Breeding published by Chipmunkapublishing.

psychiatry and drug companies to condemn and make money out of people taking medication that they profit from.

The big step here is to improve the well being of people on the planet. The real voice here is changing the term mental illness and turning it into well being. If people see the issue as well being there will be no taboo. They will realize that mental illness affects everyone. Then they will be more inclined to talk about mental health and then more likely to help a homeless person when they see one and not just give them a handout that will more than likely be spent on drugs, but talk to them or give them an opportunity to get employed and manage their own life or money or offer them appropriate support[2].

The other advantage of using well being is also the mindset of the person with the "mental health

---

[2] The Big Issue set up in 1991 to empower homeless people has pioneered this social phenomenon.

issue." They will see their state as something that can be felt by more people or even anyone.

Then they can see a way out, change their mindset and cure themselves. With this paradigm shift[3] the drug companies and psychiatrists influence on the world will lessen, their grips will loosen and new well being ......will be developed creating a healthier happier world.

The final small step I would like to discuss is the fact that I as a former manic depressive have credibility in the area of "reducing the humiliation of people with mental illness."

By the time I'd set up Chipmunkapublishing in April 2002 and launched my autobiography on living with manic depression "A Can of Madness". I knew that my story was an example of someone who was prepared to face up to what being

---

[3] 'paradigm shift' a term used by Stephen R Covey author of The 7 habits of Highly Effective People.

diagnosed with a mental illness meant in the eyes of society. In fact what motivated me to write it was to stop the humiliation and suffering of another 17 year old with manic depression.

This is because I went through it first when I was 17 and it is only natural to want to stop someone else going through the same point that you went through. This is a natural human instinct. I am no different than any other human being. This is precisely why my own experience is a small step in the universe. My experience planted the seeds for Chipmunkapublishing, the Chipmunka Group and the Foundation and is my driving force for realising my goal to eliminate global humiliation. It is my passion that makes me get up buzzing every day and commit more and shapes my belief systems and well being. I am only one person.

The goal I have is to stop the humiliation of anyone who has been told they have a mental illness because this is an ideal. It is something that in my eyes should not occur in the 21st Century or should have ever occurred in history. This is a utopian goal but one that I believe is possible. The big step here would be a crowd of people stepping out as I have done and using mental health as a positive thus creating a paradigm shift. This would require millions of people stepping up around the world and saying why the humiliation of mental illness is wrong. This like anything only receives real credibility and revolutionary status if it is led and controlled by the "sufferers" themselves, by the people who went through it. The goal is beyond my own ego, it's beyond the Chipmunka Group. It's about millions of people all around the world being brave enough to stand up for what they believe as human beings and having the mental strength to give back and take on the responsibility of giving others an opportunity to empower themselves for the well being of the world and the planet. This is for all of our sakes; for the future well being of everyone on the planet; for our children and our children's children, for people in the 3rd world, so we live on a humanitarian world. So we can live in a world of peace and a world without global warming.

Let's go into more detail about the Brand. A brand is needed to bring all this to the public domain. When I set up Chipmunkapublishing it was a great idea but just the first thing that happened. Let me explain by talking about my own experiences. When I was 17 I had been in a mental hospital for six weeks[4], thinking that I was god and that my life was football manager the computer game. Typical of feeling high you may say. From the age of 17 when I came down from mania I had an epiphany. The moment I became aware I was living in a mental hospital I had a shocking feeling of humiliation and guilt in my heart, body and soul. Humiliation that all those realisations I had were not true in the "real world" and guilt that I couldn't have cared less about people who were in 'mental institutions' until I was actually in one myself. Immediately I had a life long mission. The first was to make a Hollywood blockbuster movie about my own life to explain the previously unimaginable humiliation that I felt, because this was the only way that I would ever psychoanalyse myself and heal 100%. Secondly, I now had a new insight into the pain, humiliation and suffering of others and I wanted to stop another 17 year old from going through the same pain and indeed anyone else that I could possibly help.

So, writing and Publishing were the first things that happened in the public domain. Now there are so many things going on that I am actually creating the world's first mental health brand. When you think of Computer Software you think of Microsoft, when you think of Music you think of Sony, when you think of mental health and want you to think

---

[4] This was the first of 5 psychiatric admissions between 1993 and 2000.

of well being instead and then think of Chipmunka. You can use NLP techniques, honesty, marketing; it doesn't matter as long as your intentions are true to yourself and you feel comfortable with it. Being diagnosed with manic depression made me more sensitive as a human being and gave me the opportunity to make a choice, and I chose to help other people. It's a natural response and is, I believe, an example of the humanitarian nature in all of us.

So with the economic and humanitarian models working in tandem the charity and social corporate models have the opportunity to squeeze together and create this utopia. This is the mission. Let's see what's been happening over the last few years and draw some inspiration first before we get to the nuts and bolts later on.

Well, since 1969 there has been a campaign led by the Citizens Campaign for Human Rights to kill psychiatry. A noble aim, supported by 9 and a half million scientologists worldwide, including Tom Cruise and John Travolta. I have a lot of sympathy with their view as they report the truth but they fail to provide the ultimate alternative that will replace psychiatry when they aim to dethrone it by 2010. They attack psychiatrists head on as they have blood on their hands, because the drugs companies that so cleverly force the world to take drugs for their own gain are too hard to dismantle without taking away their foundation i.e. the drug pushers and sellers. The psychiatrists. This is brave beyond belief, and necessary, but Mr Hubbard missed one thing. An organisation cannot change the world, nor can an individual. It is the people within it that shape what happens in the world. So the rise of the madman is inevitable and my mission in life is to facilitate this process in the most forceful way that I can. Then more lives can be saved and we will all accept openly that we are all a little big crazy.

I am convinced that the rise of the mental health sufferer is the biggest civil rights movement of all time. This could also be described as a social evolution. The social evolution that is taking place I believe is more important than mass world communication, terrorism and third world debt together. The fact that it actually connects all of these grave problems together will become apparent by the end of this book. More and more people are becoming aware of this. By 2050 the humiliation that mental illness brings will have disappeared. Then the one million people who commit suicide every year will be understood. The humiliation that those diagnosed with a mental illness feel will have disappeared, as the world is finally honest enough to admit that we are all equally vulnerable and it is for the benefit of the human race to always be open about our mental health and emotional problems. Madness will have been cured. The term mental illness will be redundant and Hubbard's and my mission will be complete.

A logical first step is to look at Hollywood liberalism itself. Let us analyse this in a simple form so that we all understand it. Think of the film As Good As it Gets starring Jack Nicholson. This is a film about a writer with Obsessive Compulsive Disorder but is never presented in this fashion in the public domain. It is advertised as being about a Reclusive writer. The Obsessive Compulsive Disorder is the comic element. If the film were called "The Man with Obsessive Compulsive Disorder" instead, then would empathy for this condition in society be raised to a higher level? Would this lead to a greater increase in empathy of the real suffering of people, who endure this kind of condition in the public's consciousness? If so then why not promote As Good As It Gets as a film about Obsessive Compulsive Disorder?

1) Because it would not be appealing to the eye and it wouldn't sell? Possibly. People go to the cinema to be entertained and to switch off. They want to forget problems and go into a dream like state. Looking at recent films like Fahrenheit 9/11, serious documentary film makers have now proven that

there is room for them to have a voice, and a real impact on the way that the world thinks.

2) Because comedy itself acts on a subliminal level and is often more serious than tragedy? Maybe. Just ask a comedian what drew them to the profession, and analyse the mood swings of any comedian. There is a fine line between comedy and madness and they are often intertwined. A genius like Paul Merton (A comedian from England, for any American friends reading this) has been open about his manic depression since the early 90's. Think how many people he has helped just by announcing that. A lot. Think for a minute… if he starred in his own autobiography on manic depression in a Hollywood blockbuster… What a positive impact on mental health that would have. Also if Paul Merton can achieve this why can't I or you for that matter. Think how many people we could empower with mental health issues then.

3) Another reason why we don't promote As Good As it Gets as a film about "Obsessive Compulsive Disorder" is that there is no objective proof that this condition exists. It is a manufactured term like any other mental illness. The American Professor whose book I have published on behalf of Chipmunkapublishing, John Breeding, is exactly right when he says that "Philosophically madness is a social construct and psychiatry is a form of social control that is unrivalled since the Nazi's genocide of the Jews". Any intelligent Buddhist or spiritual healer should be able to articulate the value to one's health in understanding this line of thought. Although this is not yet a practical solution for us all, as people still find it difficult to create creative flows all of the time. However more and more people around the world understand this line of thought as the social evolution of curing madness takes place. You have begun to understand as you have read this far. If

only the owners of GlaxoSmithKline, Astra Zeneca, Wyeth and Sanofi Synthelabo admitted this. Think how many people we could help.

4) The film As Good As it Gets is also not promoted as a film about OCD (we can now call it this for convenience) because world economics and drug companies are already doing this job for us. I'm not necessarily agreeing with this, just mentioning it as a possibility. The instant response here would be: "drugs help people like that so it is not our problem, and I do not want to be associated with somebody with Obsessive Compulsive Disorder anyway as that would cause stress in my life. Also if I get too close to it and understand it too well I may realise that I have it myself and so do people in my family. Then I will need medication and have to take pills for that on top of my Prozac. That would affect my drinking and nicotine patches".

5) Jack Nicholson is already the greatest madman on earth. How else would he be the most successful Hollywood actor of all time? (If you look at Oscar nominations he is). He is the man from One Flew Over the Cuckoo's Nest. There is no need to redefine him as a madman when the status quo has already been conditioned into unwittingly understanding his public persona. He has been deliberately typecast by the inner circle of Hollywood's major players to enlighten the world about what it is like to suffer from madness as people still identify him with that film.

All five points raise the level of awareness of mental health. Now let's take it a step further. As Good As it Gets is a powerful film that creates empathy for people with mental health problems and reduces stigma and discrimination against the mentally ill in the media and society. It helps to break down the taboo of mental health and stops people who need help being seen as axe wielding maniacs that go round killing others because they forgot to take their medication.

A Beautiful Mind has arguably done much the same thing. It shows so accurately the goings on and sufferings of the mind of a schizophrenic. The realisation when the audience sees that the star is actually mad is one of the most powerful moments in the history of cinema. It is the closest description to my own realisation and reflection of my manic rituals that I have ever seen, or even imagined, on the big screen and it is my goal to change the way Hollywood thinks and depicts the mental health of us all, so that must be a compliment (this drive within me is not to gratify my own ego or even to psychoanalyze myself but a humanitarian sensitivity to want to help other people).

Hollywood is such a powerful medium as it takes royal status in our consumerist culture. Film is such a powerful medium as it is everywhere, in and around us, what people model themselves on, idolise and daydream about being. It is on such a global scale. The moment in a great piece of cinema can live with us forever and change the way we think about something. This can of course be done directly and on a subliminal level. For Russell Crowe (who appeared in A Beautiful Mind) perhaps it was even too much. I wonder was that why he punched that producer? Because he was so emotionally involved with that character that he did not want the words of his character edited. He had become like the *Freddie in The Nightmare On Elm Street* but for a good reason, to help people with mental illness. A Beautiful Mind broke new ground but could have gone even further if it had covered the major character's homosexuality or implied that the medication was part of the problem. Still there is only so much you can do with one movie.

As for the social evolution, visualise what is known by few as The Mental Health Movement i.e. people campaigning for equality for people with mental ill health –

Bipolar, Recovery and NLP

e.g. people with manic depression, schizophrenia, obsessive compulsive disorder, severe personality disorder. Compare the mental health movement to The Gay and Lesbian Movement for a moment.

In 1986 when I was eleven I noticed that Gayn and Lesbian culture was not accepted. By the time I was nineteen in 1994 it was part of the social norm. In fact it was cool to be gay once people realised that HIV wasn't a gay disease. By 2054 it will be cool to have manic depression. Let's hope that by 2104 nobody will have a mental illness. According to the World Health Organisation by 2020 suicide will be the second most common form of death. Figures are on the increase world wide so my predictions for 2104 could well become realised. Makes drug companies money so we're all bound to have something right?

The most natural way to get to this utopia for people who have experienced mental health issues is to fight for their civil liberties (as they have been doing quite noticeably since the 1960s, but not on a scale sufficient enough for the whole world to take any real notice) to be open about their own mental health issues.

As I was diagnosed with manic depression in 1993 I see both everything and nothing as a mental health issue. I have accepted what happened and overcome the humiliation, and as a result managed to cure myself. I realised that there was no mental health issue except the one created by society and my own mind and unconscious fears, insecurities and desires. I spend my life convincing others that everything is a mental health issue so that the taboo of mental health is broken down and that they realise that everything and nothing is a mental health issue at the same time. Once their unconscious fears have left, then the social evolution takes another step forward. That is what I am doing on a subliminal level. At a grassroots level I will always be open about my "condition" and encourage others to come out of the closet and be proud of who and what they are. Leaders are needed throughout the world to stand up and speak out.

Just because someone has manic depression or something similar doesn't mean that they should feel embarrassed. In fact experiencing madness, like any kind of struggle, gives an individual a greater capacity to bounce back and become a stronger person. Overcoming madness in particular gives you the potential power to help other people who go through the same experience. There is no greater feeling in the world than this, except for maybe true love, and having children. Once you help more and more people you begin to realise that you can in fact prevent the pain and suffering of others, you can avoid that negative state and feeling of isolation, humiliation, confusion and nothingness that being labelled and experiencing a mental illness brings.

Let's examine another two case studies/metaphors for the social evolution. Visualise Frank Bruno and Mike Tyson. Both former heavyweight champions of the world and both have been described as mad. Mike Tyson's madness has almost been an endearing part of his character. Mike's madness was part of his persona as the greatest knockout puncher in the most macho sport in the modern world. The madness in him (I remember fondly his cameo performance in the film Black and White where he quotes Nietzsche when giving some advice to his friend), his fighting, his training is part of the Tyson package. This is an example that madness is something that fascinates people, but not something that they want to get too close too. There are many people who admire Tyson and a few who say they would go in a ring with him, but a minute number when it actually boils down to it. Just imagine the fear of the madness when stepping in with Tyson when he was at his best. Like putting a psychiatric patient in a straight jacket, or having a meeting with your psychiatrist in a ward round for those of you who are more informed of the power imbalance in the psychiatric model. No chance and not therapeutic.

Bipolar, Recovery and NLP

Now let's look at Bruno. He's a public hero. Britain's most loved man in many ways. In 2004 Frank Bruno was devastatingly taken into a psychiatric unit near to his home in Essex. The Sun had headlines of "Loony Bruno", as Britain's hero had become one of the institutionalised mentally ill. Marjorie Wallace MBE from SANE the most skilful PR mental health strategist of her generation from a mental health charity in the UK managed to have the tabloid change its headlines before the morning paper. What significance did this day bring. A very sad time for Frank Bruno, his friends and family of course, but this day will be looked back on again as a historic moment in 20 years time and onwards.

The day a public hero fell from grace and became one of the mentally ill. That was one of me, one of who I was. If it could happen to someone as loved as Frank Bruno then the rest of Britain would finally empathise and begin to understand what people with mental health issues go through. It would cease to be a taboo. It would be part of the social norm. Only a matter of time. For people would be forced to realise that their own mental health is perilously close to going over the edge.

Imagine this shift in consciousness doubling in size that day and doubling every subsequent month as the Bruno effect began to influence society. Then, improved communication amongst friends after work about their own mental health. Not embarrassed to talk about this anymore. Frank Bruno went through it; everyone likes Frank so I can talk about it and vice versa. Then this historical shift takes effect. If you believe in it, it will happen. Positive chi spreads.

Within fifty years a generation of people have began talking about their own mental health and it becomes as normal as watching a game of football in your home on SKY five years ago i.e. year after year it becomes more commonplace as people have gone before and it becomes

Bipolar, Recovery and NLP

more acceptable (in the case of mental health) and more affordable in the case of SKY SPORTS. Mental health becomes a commodity, a brand, like Virgin Records was the first and then 250 Virgin Companies followed to form the Virgin Brand. The same will happen with mental health.

My vision is that this will happen in the brand of Chipmunka. Why? Because everyday I take massive action[5] to do this, I am totally committed to it. Before I embark upon my vision further I would like to emphasize that the need to develop it does not come out of gratifying my own ego, fame or fortune but the understanding to follow on a humanitarian and anthropological impulse, an inevitable development in man/woman kind, where life will be a recognised Global Mental Health Brand. My intention is not to repeat any other activities that are going on in the Mental Health Movements throughout the world but to have them plug in to each other so that they can all achieve maximum effect and work together to reduce suffering in the world. There is also nobody doing it the way that Chipmunka does it. We give people a voice as they tell their own story. It is not my role to care for people who have had mental illness. The mental health sector in the UK, and globally, has been doing this for the past 40 years. Its very premise is redundant. Anyone who understands the massive benefits of Neuro Linguistic Programming and newer more advanced techniques will understand that it comes from the individual. It is only the individual that can snap themselves out of a mental ill health mindset.

There is nobody doing it like Chipmunka. We produce products where people tell their own story. They have the voice. They are the leaders of their own destiny. Chipmunka is just the mechanism by which they do it. We are like their football agent. We positively discriminate in their favour.

---

[5] The phrase 'massive action' is used by Anthony Robbins. For an introduction to motivational speaker Anthony Robbins read Unlimited Power, Published by Simon and Schuster 1989.

Bipolar, Recovery and NLP

On closer evidence it becomes apparent that the odds are stacked in Chipmunka's favour. It is impossible to usurp the pioneering body of something. The universe doesn't work like that. This can only be a good thing for society and people in general. With the raising of awareness of such a brand, more people get the help that they need. They do not feel as isolated as they were. They can rejoin society again.

Bipolar, Recovery and NLP

Bipolar, Recovery and NLP

CHAPTER ONE

CANS OF MADNESS

Episode 1: The Play

**"I began writing a play of fiction when I was 19 years old about my first manic episode because I did not have the 'mental strength' to write this drama in the first person due to the humiliation that society made me feel and because of the way I self manifested my mental illness".
The experiences of Will are my own experiences in real life.**

Jason Pegler

Will is a tall, confident, charismatic individual with a rather worn look about him. Smithers is his surname - walking round his apartment with big hand movements.

WILL: It's about time something went right. Could have been a millionaire by now or something, but no - stuck in that rut. Trapped in the world of man, the people aren't so bad; it's the governments, the media and religion that are to blame. The masses are nice enough, just boring, of course annoying, frustrating and aggravating, but so is life. Nothing everlasting except death. Only thing that's worth remembering is madness. A can of madness. It's in a class of its own. [Sets up a beer bong] A glass of its own, a jug, a jar, a crate, an offie, a wholesale, a world... [He necks the beer bong] There isn't any way out, at least there shouldn't be. That's the tragedy.

Flashback to 4 years previous at a rave with some friends; Will is rushing, looks at glen and cookie three times. Camera close up, firstly on Will and secondly on his mates. 30 seconds long accompanied to music.

NEIL: Coming up on those pills man. Absolutely off it. Me and Cookie are going to chill out "you'll be all right"- Yeh it's sorted here.
The club is hard-core like a cavern. A triangular dance floor with a balcony upstairs - everybody's fucked. Local DJs at the front are kicking it.

WILL'S HEAD: The music's getting louder. Will's coming up. Off it all right! He's the craziest fucker in there all right. He's so fucked he stomps all the way up the stairs round the whole fucking club.

WILL: all right mate

WILL'S HEAD: He shakes some fuckers hand whose been imitating him all night.
WILL: He's banging downstairs again. Can't even see. Will walks forward stomping from the back left to the middle right of the club. "Where's the MC?" [Louder] "Where's the MC?" [The dodgy looking sounds-man points towards the left. Will walks diagonally left and finds the MC].

WILL: [To some big fuck by the decks]. Say to Lomas that Johnny from 109 says hi.

BIG FUCK: What?

WILL: Say to Lomas that Johnny from 109 says hi.

BIG FUCK: Alright mate. [Hands Will a nice pill].

Will goes to the front of the club and stomps alarmingly robotically for five minutes. The club's night is over but not Will's, he's still fucked. Now this lads been e'd up before right, but he's always been highly charged you see. The Mc's Bacchanal like chant of hardcore becomes absorbed into Wills head.

Bipolar, Recovery and NLP

WILL'S HEAD: Back At Will's mate's house everyone's off it, right. They're all chilled out, but this fuckers stomping 'til ten in the morning, then he's smoking spliff and necking vodka.

WILL'S HEAD: Next night's a Saturday and there's another party. This one's more pretentious, but still just as crazy. Fifteen hundred fuckers poncing about. Will's still stomping his head off, right.

The screen goes blank and a scream is heard. Aaaaaaaaahhhhhgg! The scream symbolises the plight of Will. Four hours later Will is woken up. He's taken into the bathroom by David, undressed and given a bath. Will does not speak he's confused and embarrassed. He is bathed by David, his head soaked with a flannel to clean the bruise. The water drains away and a towel is put round him, afterwards. Now Cookie and Glen are there and they're going with the flow, nothing too noticeable like, just chilling. Now, 20 hours stomping is enough to do anyone's head in, but not Will's. A five minute massage and he does not give a fuck. Only thing is two days later Will aint come down. In fact, two weeks later he's not come down but gone up, gone up so much he's in the bleeding local mental asylum for assaulting his brother. He's not sectioned right, but when the authorities ask him what he wants to do, he says he'll go.

They take him down the hospital for a brain scan and the daft twat thinks he's having his hair cut. He's taken down the cells 'cause they don't know what to do. After head butting the cell door for three hours continuously and left with a lump the size of a tennis ball on his head, they section him and take him down the bin. Yet this fucker, although he's in a straight jacket in the back of a police van, still thinks he's going off to a rave right. What are they gonna do with him? It's dark when he gets there and desolate. Only one night nurse there. Exhausted, Will goes to sleep. He's screaming 'cause his prick hurts. They've given him some drug, see.

NIGHT NURSE: It'll be o.k. Will. [She's holding his hand]. Come on Will, let's go to bed.

She takes him up to some dormitory and undresses him. Will curls up and goes to sleep.

Next morning at 8.00am this alarm sounds and within 30 seconds several Zombies are off to clean their teeth.

DAVID (MORNING NURSE): Nudging Will. Come on Will, wake up...Wake up.

LISA (A NURSE): [Calls to David from the corridor, but not in the room].Is he not coming up then?

DAVID: No. We'll leave him as it's his first day.

LISA: You sure?

DAVID: Yeh, there's no harm in that.

David cleans his teeth.

Four minutes later Will is in the lounge. The lounge is rectangular with seats for twenty people facing a large television. Separated by some bookshelves another half dozen seats are visible for those who want some more privacy. In the kitchen area, at the end of the hall is a table-tennis table. A gap in the wall where the food is dealt out and an old piano gives a physicality and nostalgia to the kitchen.

All is observed by the employees of the institution. They take it in turns to look out through the gap in their wall, one of the nurse's called Marge, is sat watching the TV with the others.

The following characters are shown interacting in the lounge:

A granny named Doris sits nearest the telly. She knits and chain-smokes. Adjacent is Phyllis, an identical old woman who is prone to knitting more and smoking less.

Graham is more of a loner at sixty years old. He's chain-smoking roll ups, has yellow and brown fingers and tends to bite his nails nervously. Graham is miserable, nostalgic and plays the piano. He has the tendency to talk incessantly to himself about old things such as the school he used to go to, the music he's heard and books he's read. When he's nervous he rests his head on his neck and bangs his knees up and down.

Bipolar, Recovery and NLP

Stevie is fat, gay and over friendly; he sulks if nobody notices him. Stevie has a high pitched voice wears a pink cap back to front and wears luminous clothing. He looks more like a cartoon than a real person.

Terry moves a lot, to sit in different seats. Terry usually keeps quiet. He's a big bloke, an ex-skinhead, a tough nut who spends most of his time blagging cigarettes and looking at his knuckles. He gets into gardening eventually.

Lee attempted suicide. A volatile character, one minute he's laughing and the next minute he's devastated.

Nigel, on the same day his wife left him, he lost his job and admitted he was an alcoholic.

Marie is a fifty year old sophisticated lady. She's a part-time writer and is well spoken. Marie seems 'all together' but, is very depressed.

Martha is a 30 year old black chick with glasses. She has contradictory characteristics: pretty, friendly, talkative, nosey, stressed, neurotic and argumentative.

Bipolar, Recovery and NLP

Simon is a university lecturer. He is in some sort of a relationship with Martha. He can be very arrogant and judgmental, but he is also very honest and an interesting personality. Simon wears glasses, is smartly dressed and has messy brown hair and crazy eyes.

Julian can be found with his legs bouncing nervously. He's either shouting 'Man. United' continuously or doesn't say anything for weeks.

Mark is a schizophrenic, he never speaks and is good at chess.

Martha, Simon, Stevie and Nigel all exit. Lee leaves the lounge, but then comes back. Winnie and Scott enter.

Will walks around in front of the television and calls each of them, in turn, a hardcore DJ.

WILL: You're Lomas, you're Carl Cox. Nice to meet you Stu Allen and you must be Top Buzz. I'm the MC, the muther fucking MC. Alrigghtt.

Will walks out of the lounge towards the nurse's room and meets David.

WILL: You're MC Tunes. I'm MC Will.

DAVID: Your mother and brother are here to see you.

WILL: HI MC Lennie! I'm MC Will. Come into the quiet room.

DOMINIC (Will's Brother): What's the quiet room? [Dominic has a broken nose].

WILL: It's just through here. [He signals to ten yards past the nurse's room]. Look at this lot. Isn't it great? Loads of it? Where's the DJ? Where's the DJ?

DAVID: If you make a mess Will, you're going to have to clear it up.

WILL: No, MC Lennie's gonna clear it all up. Ain't ya.

DAVID: [Talking to Dominic] He's pretty bad as you can see, but they all come in like this and they do get better. [Signalling to Will] Your brother's not going to clear it up Will. You'll have to, once you've finished.

WILL`S MUM: Is it drugs?

DAVID: We don't know yet. That's what it seems

to be, but it's more complicated than that, it could be anything. Drugs are almost certainly part of it.

WILL: I'm the DJ, where's the MC? There you are!

DAVID: Stop it, that's enough now Will.

Will has thrown a stereo on the floor. Games, puzzles and all their pieces scatter over the ground.

WILL: You're going to clear it up [motioning to Dominic].

DAVID: No he's not. Why should he? You did it.

WILL: I know you're going to clear it up.

DAVID: Leave him tidying up and we'll have a chat.

WILL: This is the quiet room.

DOMINIC: [Smiling] I know…The quiet room.

The audiences' attention is drawn to shrieking in the background.

BACKGROUND VOICE: Get off o' me. Get off o' me right. You're dirty right. Get off o' me. Free me. Free me. Save me God. Get off o' me. Right, leave me alone. Who do you think you are? Give me a cigarette!

Bipolar, Recovery and NLP

MARGE: What do you say?

WINNIE: Right.

MARGE: What's the magic word Winnie?

WINNIE: Please. [Takes the cigarette] Give me a fucking cigarette.

MARGE: That's not very nice, I gave you a cigarette and you say that. That's disgusting. Give me the cigarette back!

WINNIE: No... Ha, ha, ha. [She pulls a funny face].

MARGE: Did you see what Winnie did David?

DAVID: Yerh, that wasn't very nice, was it Winnie?

Will sits down, near where Graham usually is, and smokes a cigarette whilst hiding his packet.

MARGE: You can have the cigarette Winnie, I don't mind. It's dinner time in a minute anyway. Doris, will you help me serve out today's lunch?

Doris puts her knitting down and advances to the kitchen. Will observes this looking through the bookcase.

Will rushes to the canteen and is at the front of the queue. He is given a huge lunch and eats it all. By the time he reaches the pudding, he just sticks his mouth in it and eats the sponge cake with custard in one mouthful. His mother and brother look on with a look of horror, but are glad that he is, at least, eating.

At nine o'clock in the evening all Will's visitors have to leave. Thirty seconds of music here… Scene moves into the kitchen area.

DAVID: Would you like a game of table tennis then Will?

WILL: Give us a bat then.

DAVID: [There is dark lighting] When you beat me you can leave here.

Will gasps. He has now realised that he is living in a mental asylum. David wins quite easily, playing intelligently, cleverly and defensively. Will's not very co-ordinated at the moment.

It is now a few weeks later, Cookie is sat next to a cationic Will. There is quite surreal lighting. Will suddenly tries to speak but there is a pang in his jaw. He's crying from the pain. It is the worst moment of Cookie's life; his mate has turned into a cabbage, a fucking vegetable. Cookie's eyes are watering and he breaks down and cries on his way out.

Apart from his family, Cookie and Glen are Will's most frequent visitors. They seem to take it in turns visiting him and they brighten up Will's day. Glen helps a lot because he has just stopped pinging up billy. He knows what it's like being off your twat as he's still off his twat.

GLEN: Sorry I'm a bit late, I went down the gym.

WILL: It's alright

GLEN: I've put on twelve pounds in the last two weeks.

Will raises his eyebrows with sincere acknowledgement.

GLEN: I'm doing one hundred and fifty pounds on the bench press now.

Will raises his eyebrows once more, but this time a little higher.

WILL: How many repetitions?

GLEN: Ten. I'll be squatting eventually.

WILL: Yeah?

GLEN: I was thinking about me and Taylor earlier, on me way up 'ere. Them times in the squat were mad... Mad Will. I was staring out of a window right, and Taylor prodded me saying I'd been staring out that window for four hours. I thought I'd just been glancing at it.

WILL: You're madder than me. [Smiling]

GLEN: Remember that time round your house and your gran turned up. [Laughing] I'll never forget that. Cookie answered the door and ran up the stairs terrified of her 'e was. [Will smoke's a cigarette] We all 'ad them trips and that wiz. You 'ad to get to France the next mornin'.

I'll never forget the time you sparked out Graham Burgess. [Laughing louder] We all went round there on acid. You asked him to come out, so you could have a word with 'im, and decked 'im and started bootin his head in. He knew you woz gonna hit 'im but 'ey still came out.

WILL: Ey put his feet up in my kitchen. I had to hit him.

Bipolar, Recovery and NLP

GLEN: What about that time when you knocked that copper over the 'ed. I couldn't stop laughing when you told us. Only you'd ran back in the van, you loon. Did you knock 'im out?

WILL: I pegged it and looked around thirty seconds later, he was crawling to someone's door to get 'elp. Worst thing was when Cookie threw away the CB I could have flogged that down the car boot sale. Well, at least I never got caught. I'd have ended up in borstal.

GLEN: What about when we did that shit bomb, with Jon's shit in that bag? I'd love to av seen the look on their faces when they saw it all over their patio windows.

You know, Fantasia was the best night of my life. What was it we 'ad? ....Doesn't matter, you know when I was down the squat I had a quarter in one ping. None of them down there 'ad as much as that, not even Johnny.

WILL: You're madder than me.

GLEN: Wanna game of table tennis, nutter?

WILL: Yeah.

Bipolar, Recovery and NLP

They walk through the lounge of zombies into the kitchen area. Will's back is against the zombies and Glen is against the far wall. Will may look rather drug induced but his table tennis has improved whilst being locked in a vacancy. The ball shoots from side to side. Each shot looks a winner, but the other player is able to carry on. Rather like that scene in Terminator two when Arnold Schwarzenegger cripples the other Terminator with a shotgun, but the injured party is miraculously transformed and continues the chase with the utmost ease.

The score is 3-2 to Will and he serves like one of the Wongs in the Wanderers, throwing the ball three feet in the air and cutting it. Here the score appears on the screen to give the audience a sense of participation and continues until the game is finished.

Five all and Glen tries a smash, which lands in the middle of the lounge. Nearly in tears of laughter he retrieves the ball, 5-6 to Will.

Bipolar, Recovery and NLP

Serving like Tommy out of 'Goodfellas' - return like Joe Pesci's death in 'Casino'.5-7. Serve like the policeman spitting on Larry Fishburne's mate in 'King Of New York' – response: he licks it up 5-8. Serve like a baseball swinger in the 'Warriors'. It's out 5-9. Serve like fat fucker loser in 'Full Metal Jacket' and returned like he ends up, a psychopath, 5-10. 11-5 classic Johnny Woo serve with perfect oriental direction. 11-6, Carling getting beaten up in 'Scum'. 12-6 smashed like Begbie in 'Trainspotting', unfortunately. 13-6, spin like agent Kuyon in the 'Usual Suspects'. 13-7, like Spartacus almost gets away with but doesn't quite. 7-14. Escape shot like Robert de Niro in the Russian roulette scene in 'Deer Hunter'. 7-15, as cool as Mr. Blonde in 'Reservoir Dogs'. 8-15, as helpless as John Travolta is when shot in 'Pulp Fiction'. 9-15, as sly as 'Dirty Rotten Scoundrels'. 9-16, as cool as Matt Dillon in the 'Flamingo Kid'. 16-10, missed serve. 16-11, four shots a piece, overpowered defensive shot. 16-12, the longest rally of the game and a fabulous winning smash.

17-12. Spin serve wins point. 17-13. Bad serve. 13-18. Bad serve. 14-18. Serve not returned hits the net. 14-19, fourth shot hits corner. 15-19, serve not returned. 16-19, serve not returned. 20-16. Eleventh shot smash. 20-17, bad serve. 21-17. Third shot of rally is a majestic back spin on the forehand which wins the game.

They both place their bats on the table. Glen sits in the lounge. Will grabs the ping pong balls, walks into the kitchen and puts them in the microwave where they soon explode.

GLEN: What did you do with them?

WILL: Put them in the microwave.

Glen laughs. Will proceeds to smoke a cigarette.

GLEN: I'll have to go in a minute; I've got a date tonight.

Will looks upset.

WILL: It's alright.

GLEN: I'll come tomorrow though, after I've been down the gym, same time. [Will offers Glen a cigarette]. No thanks Will I haven't smoked a cigarette for three and half weeks now... 'The Krays' is on tonight.

WILL: Yeh.

GLEN: Remember when we 'ad them mushrooms round your 'ouse. I couldn't count the money to get in the taxi and I had lunch with your old chap and Catherine. [Mad frown and laugh at the same time]. Them were the days. [Looking at his watch] Better be off then. See ya tomorrow mate.

They shake in mutual agreement of the next meeting. Will sees Glen out.

GLEN: See you tomorrow Will. [Raising his eyebrows]

Will is sitting in the rectangular quiet room. He is vigorously banging his feet up and down and chain smoking whilst listening to hardcore techno. Cookie walks in and acknowledges the frenzied repetitive beat immediately.

COOKIE: Alright Will. There's somebody to see you. [Lydney pops his head round the door]

Bipolar, Recovery and NLP

LYDNEY: Alright Will. [Lydney is dressed like a DJ and behaves accordingly. His persona is flamboyant and jocular].

Will and Lydney join in male bonding, hugging of course, silly.

COOKIE: Oh by the way Will, I've got some stuff for you. Some chocolate and some pop.

WILL: I don't want that crap.

COOKIE: Well if you don't want me to bring anything then I won't.

LYDNEY: So how long you been crazy, Will? Noh, only joking. What you doing in here Will? You've gotta get out of this place. Everybody's crazy in here. This bloke on the way in right, he looked like a ghost. No seriously man, I thought he was a ghost. In fact, I still think he is a ghost.

Lydney still offers Will a cigarette. Will takes one although he has a plentiful supply.

Man you've got your own cigarettes. Still... doesn't matter this once, does it? As long as it's just once. Still at least you're not as bad off as Steve. You're not going to believe what he did Will. Check this out man. This is the funniest thing you're ever going to hear. Man, your not going to believe this. [Cookie laughs]. Poor Steve... He's in his room right. Oh by the way nobody else knows this right. Well nobody's supposed to know. But it's so funny man. It's soooooo funny, I have to tell it. Listen to this right, Will. Steevo is in is room right, you know he can't pull any birds right. Well he's got hold of this battery operated vibrator right, from his sister's room. It was a present from her boyfriend for her birthday. Anyway, he's got hold of this vibrator right and he's fiddling around with it.

He puts some cream on it. The next bit's disgusting man, don't say I didn't warn you. He sticks it up his arse hole and switches it on full speed. Now this cream was the wrong sort of cream, coz he electrocutes himself. Some time later his sister opens his door probably wondering where her toy has gone, as her boyfriend is working late and her brother's lying there unconscious with her precious vibrator up his arse. He had to go to the hospital and stay there overnight for his drunken antics and ribald buffoonery. Now if I go round there, his sister won't speak to 'im. She hasn't spoken to him since, poor cow. Now what do you think of that?

Will seems to have been listening tentatively but is rather sedated and frowns whilst reaching for one of his own cigarettes.

I thought that would 'av cheered you up? It certainly cheered me up.

COOKIE: Anyone else been to see you today Will?

WILL: Yeh, Glen.

LYDNEY: I haven't seen Glen for ages. How is old Glen?

COOKIE: ...He's alright. He's stopped injecting now. He goes down the gym most nights.

LYDNEY: I remember old Glen. Everything that kid did, he always did it to excess. He was dead against drugs for ages, wasn't he? Then he ended up being the one who pinged up. Yep, he's a nutter. He's always been a nutter. Remember when he came round when we had those strawberries? He had a funny look on 'im then, as though he didn't approve or something.

COOKIE: He soon made up for it though didn't he.

LYDNEY: Anyone up for a game of table tennis. I'm gonna whip ya Will.

They proceed into the lounge and Will goes into the kitchen to get a glass of water for Lydney. Cookie has the pop. Cookie and Lydney are playing when Will goes back into the kitchen. He makes a cup of tea with milk in it.

One of Nigel's visitors is just coming out of the kitchen and says hello to Will. Will gives a somewhat muted acknowledgement. Suddenly, Will pours the cup of tea over this middle-aged man's head. The man curses loudly and David rushes in. He looks physically threatening and asks Will to give an explanation for his behaviour.

NIGEL'S VISITOR: It doesn't matter; it wasn't boiling, just warm.

DAVID: But that's not on.

NIGEL'S VISITOR: It doesn't matter, leave it. He's only a young lad for Christ's sake. Look at him.

Bipolar, Recovery and NLP

Cookie and Lydney look on intensely. Cookie puts his hands in front of his eyes in disbelief whilst Lydney shakes his head. That's the last time Lydney's going to visit.

DAVID: Lads I think you'd better go; it's almost nine o'clock anyway.

Lydney and Cookie look at Will. Will stares through them.

LYDNEY: Alright if we go now Will?

COOKIE: I'll come back and see you tomorrow Will.

WILL: [Shakes hands with Cookie]. Yeh, thanks for coming.

The next morning Will is sat down in the lounge smoking a cigarette bored, depressed, lonesome, frustrated, irritated and spaced out. His father walks in.

WILL`S DAD: Hiya, Will.

Will picks up the chair opposite him and runs with it, hurling it through the window.

WILL: Aaaaaahhhhhhhgggghhhh.

Will's Dad goes bright red and begins to cry whilst Will glares at him. Sat in the room between the quiet room and the lounge Will is chatting to an old woman who looks uncannily healthy. It's his grandmother. She hands him two different packets of cigarettes which he grabs eagerly.

WILL: Everyone's doing my head in.

OLD WOMAN: What do you mean 'doing your head in'? Do I do your head in?

WILL: Yeh. You do my head in... Everyone does my head in.

The old woman looks hurt and her lips start to quiver accordingly.

OLD WOMAN: You've never told me that I do your head in. Do I always do your head in?

WILL: Not always. It's this place that does my head in.

OLD WOMAN: I know it does but, I don't do your head in, do I?

WILL: Everybody does my head in. Not just you. My head's done in. Look at it. I'm doing my head in.

OLD WOMAN: I'd better go now.

WILL: O.K. Thanks for the cigarettes.

OLD WOMAN: It's O.K.

The woman leaves rather abruptly and is obviously very upset. Will seems rather annoyed as he did not mean to upset her, but he is glad that he has some more cigarettes to pass away his repression and boredom.

Will is alone in the quiet room dancing his head off to some hardcore- the rave that never was, but should have been. Glen walks in, glad that Will's off his head having a laugh. He mimics a hardcore night of a rush coming on, whilst heading for the tape deck.

GLEN: Wicked tune. Alright Will. Check this tape out you've gotta hear it. It's mental.

WILL: Yeh?

GLEN: Listen to this... Ever dreamt about a nuclear war?

Glen is smiling and nodding his head in little movements. The music starts, it's mad transcendental brain altering techno...Glen gradually turns up the volume and gives quicker and more violent nods of his head. Glen lights a cigarette sits down and starts dancing with it. Will continues being mental.

WILL: Nuff man dead fiddi I know.

GLEN: Come with us and go with the flow.

Glen turns the sound down and Will, still happy but not ecstatic, sits down and takes one of the cigarettes that Glen is offering.

GLEN: What d'ya think then? [Will smiles]. It's my maddest tape at the moment. I play it every night. You can 'av this I've made a copy for ya.

WILL: Thanks Glen.

GLEN: It's alright mate. How are ya then?

WILL: Bored until you cum.

GLEN: You're looking betta… Not so spaced out. Alright if I 'av a glass of water?

WILL: Water?

GLEN: Yeh, I'm thirsty from today's gym session [Stretching]. Pretty knackered actually.

Bipolar, Recovery and NLP

Glen's looking at Will, who gets up and walks through the room of his bin colleagues. He retrieves two plastic beakers, as they are pretty small glasses, and fills them up with water. Will drinks one of them and fills it up again and walks past his fellow bin acquaintances, glancing at them watching the telly intensely.

Terry asks if Will has any cigarettes. Will shakes his head. He's thinking 'my fucking hands are occupied anyway you stupid cunt. How could I even give you a cigarette without spilling the two glasses of water'? Of course, Terry is rather self obsessed and doesn't give a fuck about anyone else. Something that is inevitable when you are crazy, you enter a world of your own and find it more interesting than the world which you have apparently left.

Will gives Glen the glasses of water.

GLEN: Cheers mate, there's two glasses?

WILL: You said you were thirsty.

Will leaves the room and ventures into the bathroom. He marches into each cubicle removing

287

the toilet rolls from the holders and drops them into the toilets. Will then goes to the toilet feeling satisfied that he has completed his mindless daily ritual.

Will leaves the toilet, walks past the room Glen is in and advances towards his bedroom, which is on the ground floor as he has been rather disturbed lately. It is the only bedroom on the ward and kept for the, seemingly, most ill patient so they don't bother themselves or any of the other patients on the ward.

Sick of this military regime, Will has an idea. He goes back into the quiet room and opens the curtains, which lets the sun in. Will places a rucksack on his left shoulder filled with clothes and carries a handful of clothes in the other hand.

GLEN: What are you doing? [Laughing and still recovering from pinging up, Glen watches Will put on several pairs of socks, jeans and jumpers].

WILL: I'm going.

GLEN: [Hysterically] Where you going?

WILL: I don't know, but I'm going somewhere.

Bipolar, Recovery and NLP

Glen erupts with laughter and can't stop. Will has put on all the clothes that he possibly can, puts the rest in the rucksack and walks around the room looking like he's been on steroids for five years.

GLEN: Do you know where you're going yet?

WILL: Out of here. [Will walks out of the quiet room and into the staff room]

I'm getting out of here. [Will walks into the lounge]

I'm getting out of here. [Will walks back into the quiet room]

WILL: I told you I was getting out of here.

Glen explodes with laughter once more and Will sits down.

Will is sat on a bench inside the hospitals grounds. Birds are singing and Will is accompanied by his brother Dominic and the old woman, his grandmother.

OLD WOMAN: Do you want a sandwich?

WILL: I'm sick of it 'ere.

DOMINIC: Would you like a sandwich?

OLD WOMAN: Oh shut up Dominic. Can't you see he's upset? [Dominic raises his eyebrows vehemently]. What's wrong darling?

WILL: I'm just sick of it.

OLD WOMAN: I know it won't be long now. This horrible nightmare's nearly over.

Dominic accordingly relaxes his eyebrows.

WILL: I'm so bored.

OLD WOMAN: Can't you read or something?

WILL: I can't concentrate for more than five minutes.

OLD WOMAN: Isn't there something you can do? Some sort of hobby or exercise to keep you engaged?

WILL: There is circuit training in the mornings but it starts at 8.00am.

OLD WOMAN: It might do you well to get up in the morning.

DOMINIC: Mornings? Yes. There's nothing wrong with getting up early in the mornings, you know you can see the hills, the sky and the postman if you get up early enough.

Bipolar, Recovery and NLP

OLD WOMAN: Yes it might be just the thing you need, to get up early in the morning, get you back into some routine. Take it from me if you've got no routine then you've got nothing to get up for and nothing to do. If there's nothing for you to do then you're, more often than not, going to be bored or depressed.

WILL: Maybe.

OLD WOMAN: It's not a maybe, take it from me. Do what I say Will and believe me, you will feel better. If not, then at least you've given it a try and at least you've tried something different.

DOMINIC: You've put a bit of weight on as well you know bro.

Slapping Will in the chest, his brother smiles and Will's attempt at smiling is also partly successful.

OLD WOMAN: You could cut down on your cigarettes as well you know? But that's for you to decide. There's no hurry. I smoked for over sixty years and I still gave up you know.

Will, we had better get off. Dominic has got to sign on and I've got to get some vegetables from the market. You'll look back on this whole experience one day and realise that it's strengthened you mentally. You will, I promise. Believe me. You wait and see. Goodbye darling, we shall come and see you tomorrow. [She kisses him, Dominic and Will shake hands]. Take it easy. [Smiling, but more as a forced grin]

WILL: *See you later bro.*

DOMINIC: *Later bro.*

Next morning sure enough Will is off to do some exercise. It's about time really; he's been a miserable, lazy and headshot bastard for quite a while now. It's not necessarily his fault, but he's at last bucked up his ideas and decided to do something positive. It doesn't matter how trivial a thing he is doing, but it's important that he's made a decision to do something.

He has a brief conversation with Marge about him being up so early. The simpleton is only trying to do her job but reminds Will how many of the simpleton's ramblings he is forced to deal with everyday.

The song 'Football's coming home' is in the background and commentary is heard with the ensuing game.

Will arrives at the gym first. Soon, a couple of other zombies are queuing up outside the same door, when what looks like two junior school teachers appear. They both, a man and a woman, greet everyone with bland, vagrant and condescending 'hellos'. Will wants to puke. Will was once the school rugby captain of his grammar school and top goal scorer in his previous football career. He is, therefore, dumbfounded at the thought of a ten pounds overweight slob, bouncing a plastic football, believing he can teach Will anything about anything. Even worse for Will, the obese instructor proceeds to introduce himself, but reminds Will that he is a newcomer. He then adds that he hopes Will would choose to continue to go to his fitness classes.

Bipolar, Recovery and NLP

The door is un-padlocked and opened. The zombies start kicking the football around as the two trainers attempt to gather them round in a circle. The effort is successful, but only as successful as it would be for a gym teacher to control a bunch of eleven year olds, with his militaristic tactics and accompanying whistle.

The exercises are for retards. Standing up, with one's feet apart, one bends over and tries to touch the ground keeping one's legs straight and one's fingers stretched. This is repeated three times at the front then back to the starting position; three times in the middle and three times underneath one's thighs. Everybody then proceeds to roll their shoulders vigorously forwards, then a break and the reverse procedure. The next loosener is to roll one's head round and round.

Having missed out other stretches some may deem important, the overweight instructor picks teams. Will, somewhat bewildered, stretches his ankles by rolling them either side and loosens his calves by putting one foot in front of the other and bending the front leg forward. Then intentionally catching the woman instructor's eye he stretches his back by putting his hands behind his back and pushing his hands up.

There are three people on Will's team and four on the other. The woman instructor leaves. She has only come to open the gym and gloat on and be offended by, psychotic penises, which can't even threaten the frigid bitch, as their beholders are mentally deranged for the foreseeable future.

The game starts as most football games start. A simple tap and the receiver tries to run past the opposing team and score on his own. In a fluke, passing one man, the attacker is floored by a good crunching tackle by Will's team mate. He then coolly passes back to the keeper who is rather slow but just manages to get the ball to Will. Will goes past two men and thumps the ball wide. Confronted by Fat-trainer-ma', who thinks he put Will off, Will is told he was unlucky.

WILL`S HEAD: How am I supposed to score with that fucking shite ball anyway? It's fucked. Just like me and this lot, all of them. I might as well kick a boulder of the same size. I got more chance of scoring with that. I could get more power behind it! The other team scores a flukey goal. One of those goals that have a lucky ricochet and the scorer actually thinks he's a good player. Not even for one moment can he admit of his spawn.

Fat-trainer-man gives a smug grin and Will, in his trance like state, feels like a supplicant. Spurred on by going a goal down, Will's team give new meaning to what should be a John Wayne saying: 'Something good usually comes out of something bad'. They equalise immediately with what actually looked like and was, a good team goal. Two passes, a one two and a tackle maniac zombie-man side foots it past the goalkeeper.

At the restart, the opposition start how the rest of football matches start. Two passes and back to the goalkeeper. A feckless kick. Will intercepts, his shot rebounds off the goalie and trainer-man puts the ball into an empty net.

Bipolar, Recovery and NLP

WILL`S HEAD: The goalie had come out, you see, that's the thing when it's rush goalie, you get knackered and get caught if you lose possession.

Fifteen more minutes and Will's team lose 4-3, but with three men that's not bad. The ball's so shite that nobody could score, especially Will. He had plenty of opportunities, but just could not score.

FOOTBALL COMMENTATOR: They've finished for the day and they're sweating like rapists. In fact, they would be rapists if they had the guts and could get away with it. Bet that's what it is to some of the women bin members, that's why they broke down. That's why they broke up. Up or down, does it really matter, there's still no way out.

Next time we see Will, he's in the lounge with two new faces. Lee and Neil are two older friends both none the wiser. They're both able to take a cynical, satirical and constantly hysterical view to Will's clinical insanity.

NEIL: You're not mad. At least you're conscious of what's happening.

Bipolar, Recovery and NLP

LEE: You're crazy. [Laughing] You're crazy and you always have been. Crazy… Fucking Crazy.

Both of them laugh incessantly. Will's happy to see both of them but frowns, speechless with his mouth open.

NEIL: No, seriously you'll be alright. You're no crazier than me nor Lee, you're just the one it happened to, that's all. Don't worry about it.

LEE: Yerh, don't worry about it you cocksucker. I know people who're crazier than you.

NEIL: Yerh, your brother.

LEE: Dominic.

NEIL: Now he's really fucked.

Both continue laughing incessantly, just like a double comedy act. Except, they're not aiming to be funny, they're sad, predictable, selfish psychopaths. Nevertheless, they brighten up Will's day and always have done. There's a real intensity with them, not like with Cookie and Glen. That's more relaxed. Here there's no such thing as respect. The rules are, there ain`t no rules.

Bipolar, Recovery and NLP

Amidst the riotous laughter Will's mother walks in with a muted and concerned smile.

WILL: Hi mum.

NEIL: Don't worry, we're not corrupting him or feeding him any drugs or anything. Not that these people don't seem to think so that is. I guess you've heard that they thought I was giving him drugs? As if. My Dad came up and had a right go at them. Anyway how are you?

WILL'S MUM: Alright thank you Neil. How are you Lee?

LEE: Oh, I'm alright.

WILL'S MUM: Don't worry, I won't tell anyone that you were here. Not anyone in particular.

LEE: [Sarcastically] thank you.

NEIL: Is the person in question Mr. Smithers, by any chance here? Does he still wish to... how can I put it? Want to have a quick word with you Lee?

LEE: I think he wants more than a quick word, more like a brawl or something.

Bipolar, Recovery and NLP

Will's mother nods her head.

NEIL: Well, it's not surprising that after Will sang songs all day about Lee being a drugs dealer, that he wants to give you a jolly good old boot, old boy. What have you got to say to that Will? Eh?

WILL: I was only telling the truth. Anyway I can't really remember it.

Will runs out of cigarettes and looks rather startled as a result.

NEIL: Well, we'd better be off anyway. We're playing tennis this afternoon. Bet I'll win. Still you've got to play against someone, haven't you? Hurry back to normal Will and we'll have a game, you can borrow my racket... See you later and don't worry about it. You're alright, just the same as us really... Goodbye to Will's Mum.

WILL: See ya Neil. See ya Lee.

WILL`S MUM: Shall we get some cigarettes from the shop?

WILLL: Which shop? The shop inside the hospital?

Bipolar, Recovery and NLP

As Neil and Lee exit, Lee distracted by one of the inmates, proceeds to miss the open door and walk into the wall, bashing his head.

LEE: You see what you've done to me Will? I'll be in here next and not just coming to see you.

Lee starts a mad cackle which is rhythmically accompanied by Neil. The two howling wolves leave.

Will's MOTHER: You o.k.?

WILL: Yeh.

MUM: Lee didn't do your head in?

WILL: No.

MUM: Good.

WILL: It was good to see them.

MUM: I`m sure it was.

WILL: You alright?

MUM: Yes dear, why shouldn't I be?

WILL: Just asking.

MUM: Don't be silly

WILL: I`m not. [Smiling]

MUM: They'll keep you in for longer if you're silly.

[Will groans vigorously but quietly]

Bipolar, Recovery and NLP

MUM: Are we going to the shop then? [Grabbing her handbag]

She begins to rise and Will is slow, but uniform, in his effort to stand up. Some pensive music begins as Will is sulking, looking at the floor.

MUM: Coming then? What are we going to get?

They walk outside of the lounge and through the door. There is only a left turning and they walk down a corridor, which has a painting on the right hand side of the wall. The painting on the wallpaper covers the length of the whole corridor. Green trees, birds and blue sky represent an idyllic landscape yet look grossly out of place in such a madhouse. Will walks down the corridor with his palms brushing the painting. His mother looks round and asks:

MUM: What are you doing?

WILL: Painting.

A kind, but forced smile reaches her face as the doors of the corridor confront her. A forceful nudge opens the door, but only just. The next corridor is brighter and seems twice as wide. Yet the corridor's lighting is in the wrong place and it is actually dark. The seeming brightness is only for a nanosecond. The corridor has no windows. Twenty yards on the right hand side is a door but the camera is drawn to somebody who is twenty yards away from the end of the corridor, when Will and his mum walk in. The camera zooms in and concentrates on this overweight bloke in jeans and trainers smoking a cigarette. Then a sound is heard in the background which is the shop door opening.

The shop is three metres wide and three metres long. Will has less than three metres on the shop floor. The cashier in the shop is a sweet looking girl whom Will thinks is beautiful and mistakes for some E headed tart. Will grabs some Lucozade and proceeds to smother it in his left arm. Then he gets a Bounty bar, a Mars bar, two cans of Sprite and four packets of crisps.

WILL`S MUM: How about some cigarettes as well?

Will knows what cigarettes he wants, low tar Silk Cut, but his attention is drawn to the girl behind the counter. He cannot contemplate the room, which reeks of civilisation yet, is in bin surroundings. It was even more alien without the lemon and lime colouring of the rooms. Irritably alien, as Will is constantly reminded of societies conventions. If he would have been left in his own enlightening madness then he would have no worries or misgivings, in fact, he would be deliriously happy. Eventually he speaks.

WILL: Twenty Marlborough Lights.

WILL'S MUM: Make it forty.

Will look's at his mother in sombre thankful tone. The girl reaches over her right hand side for two packs of Marlborough Lights and she puts them on the desk.

WILL: Thanks but make it one pack.

MUM: Good. Are you going to those fitness classes again tomorrow? Do you want to go for a coffee now?

GIRL: That's on the house. Don't tell anyone.

Before hearing the price of the items, a crescendo of mind blowing techno is heard, the producer at Universe. The camera zooms in on Will's right wrist, which is violently shaking. The camera subsequently zooms into his head and then inside of his brain. (Bad Taste style)

Bipolar, Recovery and NLP

Will is having a flashback. Surreal camera work is needed for this scene, therefore, no sense of time. Lydney and Glen are in a room. The curtains are open and flowers are in the background amidst a sloping driveway. The lounge is rectangular. There are two sofa chairs on the left hand side and a settee on the opposite corner. A television forms a right angled triangle. The sun shines through the window.

LYDNEY: Man, nothing happens, we've been conned just face it.

WILL: What time was it?

LYDNEY: We've been waiting for nearly two hours now. It's only supposed to take an hour.

WILL AND LYDNEY: Did you see that?

WILL: What?

LYDNEY: What d`you see man? What d`you see man?

WILL: The wall's breathing.

LYDNEY: Seriously.

WILL: Yerh.

LYDNEY: Noooo way. Nooo way. I saw the same thing, that's amazing really amazing. We've been sat here for two hours and seen nothing. Then suddenly bang. [Lydney gives a mad cackle] Wow they're moving.

Lydney is sat on the left hand side on the floor. Will is sat to his right, behind Lydney. Will motions to respond to Lydney`s remarks but then gulps, refrains from conversation and has suddenly fully realised that he's on his first trip and

Bipolar, Recovery and NLP

it has nowhere nearly ended yet. All the colours in the room have become more colourful since they came up.

LYDNEY: Woooow! The curtains are moving. See those patterns on the curtains. Look!

WILL: Lydney? [somewhat pensively]

LYDNEY: Not now Will, their zigzagging. Oh my god. This is great. Ha, ha, ha, ha. I don't believe it.

In the background a ringing is heard. It's the phone.

LYDNEY: Is that the phone? Nooo, is it? I've got to go and see if that's the phone. Wooohoo. Oh my god, that is the phone. Go on, pick it up. See who it is. Go on.

Will picks up the phone and suddenly looks dumbfounded. Glen is on the other end of the phone.

GLEN: Alright Will? Will rapidly hands the phone over to Lydney.

WILL: Speak to him. I can't speak to him; he'll do my head in.

LYDNEY: No way, you speak to him. I'm not speaking to him. I'm having a great time. I`m not gonna spoil it. I'm going back in the lounge. You can speak to him.

GLEN: Will is anyone there? Will?

WILL: ...Strawberries man

GLEN: Strawberries is that what you said? ....What do you mean strawberries?

WILL: Nothing Glen.

Bipolar, Recovery and NLP

GLEN: You said strawberries.

WILL: No reason, I just said it.

GLEN: Yeh right.

WILL: No seriously. We've just had some Spliff.

GLEN: Yeh? [Interrogatively]

WILL: Yeh, were fucked. Come round if you want.

GLEN: Well, I dunno. I might do. I might see you later I might not.

WILL: Yeh.

GLEN: I might see you later, I might not.

WILL: Yeh.

GLEN: I might see you later then.

WILL: Yeh. Bye.

The conversation ends. By now Will is paranoid as hell. Lydney is not a sympathetic ear. Lydney advances towards Will and stops in front of him.

LYDNEY: I can't believe you told him we were on acid. He doesn't like drugs much, old Glen, does he Will?

WILL: I never told him we were on acid

LYDNEY: He knows though it's obvious.

WILL: Do you think he'll come round?

Bipolar, Recovery and NLP

LYDNEY: Of course he'll come round, he's nosey.

Will is even more distraught and rings up Gavin.

WILL: Gavin. Listen right I`m on acid and it's doing my head in right. I've just spoken to Glen and I've told him we're stoned, but I don't think he's bought it. Come round if you want, but stop him coming round here. Please.

GAVIN: Alright. I'll see what I can do. [Laughing] Who are you there with?

WILL: Don't bring him round Gavin, please.

GAVIN: Alright. [Laughing] I'll see what I can do.

WILL: Are you coming round then?

GAVIN: Yeh, I'll see you in a bit.

WILL: You sure?

GAVIN: Yeh. [Laughing] See ya in a bit.

Lydney shouts from the lounge.

LYDNEY: Come and look at these curtains Will, they got mad patterns on them, look.

Will floats into the lounge almost.

Woow Ha ha ha ha ha ha hab ha. Wonder if I can get traces yet. Do you know what, I reckon I can. [Lydney moves his hands up from the armchair and waves them rapidly] Woow aaaaahhhhh. Wooow haaaaahaahaa. This is unbelievable, unbelievable! Watch it, hi-ya... hi-ya.... hwooah hwoooah. I love acid. I`m gonna take tonnes of it. My mates are all lightweights not to have taken more.

Bipolar, Recovery and NLP

The doorbell rings and Will glides towards the front door opening it. Gavin and Glen are stood there. Gavin gives a cheesy grin whilst Glen looks aggravated.

Then Will is back in the bin, a euphemism for mental asylum of course, having a coffee and do-nought in the canteen. Will feels absurdly normal. He didn't know this place existed. His mother's theme of conversation tries to analyse how happy she is that Will is getting better. Unfortunately for Will, narking inside of his mind is the exact moment when he first entered this room.

WILL`S HEAD: One night in the bin the Krays had just finished and Will was sat with Terry. They all heard a thud, at least I think they all did.

JULIAN: Why don't you go and investigate Will?

Will look's for Terry's approval, who nods his head.

TERRY: Yeh go on Will.

Will walks out into the corridor. The painting can just be seen along the wall. He opens the door and comes to a right hand turning. Five yards on there is a closed green door. Will looks under the door and can see an empty room that looks like a large dentist's surgery. With increased ringing in Will's ears he focuses on the bed in the middle of the room. A metal bed without a blanket, Will can see two metal zigzagged strips hanging from the ceiling, or so it appears anyhow.

Will takes some tapes from out of his pocket and throws them down a metal drain which is right next to him. He breaks them in half. Before doing so he looks under the door imagining somebody bolted to the bed. He goes into a controlled frenzy, pulling his hair he gets up from the floor and heads further down the corridor. At the end of the next corridor on the right hand side is another door. This time it's red. He walks into the same canteen that he's eating his do-nought in. Straight ahead is where you get served. Towards the left are chairs. Will proceeds to piss on the coffee machine. He then picks up a broom and smashes the fuck out of the canteen. He only needs to hit things once, as they either smash to pieces or fall to the ground. Just starting to relax he puts a can in the microwave. By the time it has blown up he is sat on the canteen desk top, smoking a cigarette, completely calm and at peace. Night nurse two enters.

NIGHT NURSE 2: What the bloody hell you doin?

He pushes Will, and then continues to nudge him out of the room. Will concedes and the screen switches back to Will sitting back in the canteen, smoking a cigarette the do-nought and coffee finished. His mother's cup is nearly full. She's just finished a sentence.

WILL'S MUM: Out soon you know?

WILL: What?

WILL'S MUM: They're thinking of letting you out soon, you know? But they don't want you to get ill again, like last time. You're seeing Dr. Bailey again tomorrow.

In the doctor's office, which happens is also the quiet room.

DR.BAILEY: Hello Will. How are you?

WILL: Bored.

DR.BAILEY: I know it must be frustrating for you. How do you feel in yourself?

Bipolar, Recovery and NLP

WILL: Bored, lonely, tired, drugged up, smothered, excited and claustrophobic.

DR.BAILEY: Excited what makes you feel excited?

WILL: The thought of getting out.

DR.BAILEY: And that makes you feel excited, does it?

WILL: Well, nervous actually.

DR.BAILEY: Nervous?

WILL: Yes.

DR.BAILEY: What are you nervous of exactly?

WILL: People laughing at me.

DR.BAILEY: What makes you think people will laugh at you?

WILL: Because, I've been in here.

DR.BAILEY: What if they don't know that you've been in here?

WILL: Then I can still feel them laughing, almost.

DR.BAILEY: Why?

WILL: Because, I know I've been in here

DR.BAILEY: Well that's what I'm here for. To help you come to terms with what has happened to you and to help you, to help yourself to feel better, if I can.

WILL: Feel better?

Bipolar, Recovery and NLP

DR.BAILEY: Well, yes. I'm here to make you feel better and if you want me for anything else than I'll try and help you with that as well. Or if you want me just to talk with you, then I'm here for that as well and only that if you wish.

WILL: I don't mind talking to you.

DR.BAILEY: Well, thank you and why is that, do you think?

WILL: Because, I can say something daft and you laugh.

DR.BAILEY: Well, thank you, I think? I'd like to hope that I only laugh when it's funny, that I get the joke, O.K? Oh by the way, I forgot to say, I have to go a bit earlier today. I'll still have time to speak to Dr. Godray though. Anyway, we still have some time to talk. What would you like to talk about? Is there anything in particular?

WILL: Yes.

DR.BAILEY: And what would that be?

WILL: What do you think? They'll let me go?

DR.BAILEY: You mean let you go back home? Well, that's what I shall speak to Dr. Godray about this afternoon. Hopefully, if you keep progressing and getting better, next time we see each other it will be you coming to see me, not the other way round.

WILL: Would that be next week?

DR.BAILEY: Yes, if that's o.k. with you and it's o.k. with Dr. Godray then that's what we can all work towards very soon.

WILL: Yes.

DR.BAILEY: It's O.K. with you?

Bipolar, Recovery and NLP

WILL: Yerh.

DR.BAILEY: Good then, fingers crossed. Is there anything else that you would like to talk about?

WILL: No.

DR. BAILEY: Well I'm sure you've been through the worst of it now. In fact you seem perfectly fine to me. What has been a bad dream can now be an awakening, if you choose to call it that. If you don't then it's no problem whatsoever. Oh, is that the time already? I'll go and speak to Dr. Godray now then and see what he says. You wait here if you like? That's it, have a cigarette, I shan't be long. If you're not in here when I get back I'm sure I'll find you.

Will lights a cigarette and walks into the staff room with it.

DAVID: You're not allowed in here Will, especially not with a cigarette. Will stays still. But... as you're going soon we'll let you off for a change. Dr. Bailey chatting to Dr. Godray now is he? Shall we have that game of table tennis then?

Will's eyes roll from right to left. They walk into the communal hall and start playing table tennis.

DAVID: Which side do you want Will mate?

Will shakes his head.

DAVID: Alright if I choose then? Will nods in agreement.

They start playing. In the first rally, David hits the ball into the lounge; Will runs into the centre of the room and picks up the ping pong ball. They play whilst Will smokes his cigarette and start scoring when he puts it out. Will wins the game

Bipolar, Recovery and NLP

quite comfortably. With six months practice this is not a great surprise.

DAVID: Looks like you've done it. Advancing towards Will and shaking his hand. Well done mate. Hardcore uproar right?

Will smiles nervously.

DAVID: Let's go in the staff room and have a cup of tea Will.

They walk towards the staff room. Will glances at the telly on the way and looks at the routine way in which everybody is sat glued to it.

TERRY: Have you got a cigarette Will?

Terry takes the cigarette and puts it on his ear. Will stands observing him whilst David goes back into the staff room to make coffee. Terry has tattoos on his fingers and one of an Asp on his arm. He sits down bouncing his legs up and down, then frowns, and holds his unlit cigarette at both ends. He stares at the cigarette turning it round with his left hand, and then puts it back onto his ear. Will then walks off. His back is turned when Terry calls him. Will turns round and Terry says Thanks.
Will now walks into the staff room and sits down. Lisa is in the staff room as well.

LISA: David's just told me that you're going soon Will. What d'you think about that then? Pleased I bet? Fed up of us old fogies in here then?

DAVID: Here's your coffee. I should think you'll be glad to see yourself out of here Will. We're all sick of the sight of you anyway. No... only joking!

WILL: Hardcore uproar.

Bipolar, Recovery and NLP

LISA: What's that mean? Hardcore uproar?

DAVID: It's Will's invention, it just took him a while to wait for it to happen that's all.

LISA: Oh I see now

WILL: Hardcore uproar.

Dr. Godray and Dr. Bailey enter the little room. Dr. Godray is a tall man with a blue suit. He's very sensible looking. Dr. Godray smiles at everyone, nods his head at David and winks at Will.

DR. GODRAY: Bye and see you next week Will...oh, and by the way, that's at my office not yours.

Will gives a tentative sigh of relief.

DAVID: Shall we go into the interview room then Will, for our last chat.

They walk in the small room and sit down.

DAVID: So you're out in a few days?

WILL: Yep.

DAVID: What are you going to do with yourself then, as soon as you get out?

WILL: Go to McDonalds.

DAVID: And have a Big Mac meal?

WILL: Yep, with super size fries.

Bipolar, Recovery and NLP

DAVID: What are you going to do with your life?

WILL: Nothing. Just study.

DAVID: What are you going to do to yourself?

WILL: Nothing. Get drunk

DAVID: You gonna take drugs again?

WILL: Don't know.

DAVID: You going to come back here again?

WILL: No way.

DAVID: Never?

WILL: Not for a long time anyway and then only once.

DAVID: You don't want to be here anyway. You've got your whole life in front of you. Haven't you? You should be out having a laugh, get yourself a girlfriend or something, not stuck up in here.

WILL: You're stuck in here.

DAVID: Yeh, but I go home at night. You don't. So have you thought about what you're going to do in the years to come?

WILL: Yes.

DAVID: Thought so. Copper?

WILL: No.

DAVID: Drug dealer?

WILL: No way.

Bipolar, Recovery and NLP

DAVID: You going to be famous then?

WILL: Yeh.

DAVID: Write a movie or something?

WILL: That's right.

DAVID: Yeh good. That's it then. Get out of here! I never want to see you again unless it's when you're visiting. I'm on holiday as from tonight, you see.

Will gets up opens the door and hears David say his name and then say 'hardcore uproar' once more. Will smiles and carries on walking to see the girl of his dreams in the club of his dreams. Jacques Lacan could not make this scene anymore realistic. The MC is heard chanting "hardcore, you know the score". Will is now dressed up in his rave gear with cool shades on. He walks to where the girl is dancing. With his bare top half he walks next to her on the stage. He is just about to start dancing when she stops and gives him a massage. The melodic piano tune song of bye bye sugar pie is heard and Will is in ecstasy.

The room at the start of the film is shown again. Will is pouring two vodkas with black Russian. He gives one to his wife and says "alright Honey". It is the same girl that gave him the massage in the club.

CHAPTER TWO

MADNESS IN GREEK TRAGEDY

"This dissertation is submitted in accordance with the regulations for the Part II examination in the Honours school of Classical Studies, University of Manchester".

Jason Pegler 1998.

The dissertation I wrote at University although it is on the theme of Madness in Greek Tragedy is another example of how I tried to understand my own insanity by looking at the history of madness and not facing up to my own life.

Jason Pegler December 2005.

Bipolar, Recovery and NLP

Bipolar, Recovery and NLP

1. INTRODUCTION

2. WHAT CONSTITUTES MADNESS IN GREEK TRAGEDY?

3. THE MADNESS OF ORESTES

4. THE MADNESS OF AJAX

5. THE MADNESS OF AGAVE

6. THE MADNESS OF HERAKLES

7. THE THEME OF MADNESS IN TRAGEDY

8. WHAT CONSTITUES MADNESS TODAY?

9. CONCLUSION

Bipolar, Recovery and NLP

Bipolar, Recovery and NLP

INTRODUCTION

Before focusing on madness in Greek Tragedy I shall discuss the phenomenon of the madman in general. If someone is driving down the road and a car pulls out in front of them that person might be inclined to refer to the other person as crazy, or a lunatic, or a madman. This is a matter-of-fact reference to madness. However, problems arise when people say things that they do not mean and when they judge something that they do not understand.

The driver that name calls is guilty of contributing to both of these problems. Firstly, he does not mean that the other driver is clinically insane although he literally says that he is. Secondly, and more importantly, who does he think he is in categorising somebody like that? Of course, he judges in a moment of anger but would not a real madman be upset in the way that he is viewed? Although he should he would probably not, for if he was mad at the time of hearing the remark he would view it differently than a sane man. Still the madman does not deserve derogatory remarks. For being mad is difficult enough as it is. The remark is not directed at the madman but it is an example of society's hostile view towards the insane.

Fortunately, seventeenth century France saw a revolution in society's treatment of the mad[6]. For the first time institutions were built exclusively for the mentally ill. The madman no longer always had to share cells with criminals or suffer humiliation on the streets but joined others in safe houses for the mad.[7]

---

[6] Michael Foucault discusses this in his study of "Madness and Civilisation" (1967).

[7] This interpretation in its generalisation leads Jacques Derrida to the conclusion that Foucault's attempt to identify the history of madness is an impossible task (Derrida and Deconstruction page 202).

Bipolar, Recovery and NLP

Psychiatry set about trying to find a cure for madness, for ancient Greek culture and modern societies generally accepted that there was something wrong with being mad. Madness is an undesirable state to be in, I have been there myself, and I know what it is like[8]. The madman is different from the sane man and whilst attitudes to madness are becoming less prejudiced, the mentally ill are still regarded as an enigma. The natural fear of being mad oneself is the reason for any hostile portrayal by a real person. In Tragedy any hostile portrayal is rectified as it induces pathos. Only in the last fifty years in Britain has attempted suicide not been a criminal offence. The only time mentally ill people seem to be discussed in the news is under extreme circumstances. They may have killed someone with a machete or have been brain damaged by taking the wrong kind of medication. Whilst the reports may point out that the patient was not looked after properly, the horrific events may be misinterpreted and force the viewer to misunderstand the madman. The Media give a chilling representation of the madman and so does Greek Tragedy. Of course, they do not aim to give a sympathetic account of the madman and there is no reason why they should except for a humanitarian one. Madness in the context of Greek Tragedy is fascinating and gives a revealing insight into the history of the insane.

WHAT CONSTITUTES MADNESS IN GREEK TRAGEDY?

The thirty one Greek Tragedies that are extant from the thousand or so that were written are sufficient in quantity for a modern reader to be able to identify and define madness within the genre. Madness in Greek Tragedy is caused by an external force. Specifically a god brings about Madness in one of two ways. The god induces madness always as the punishment of an individual for their own hubris or the hubris of one of their relatives. Herakles is

---

[8] The author suffers from bipolar effective disorder, more commonly known as manic depression.

Bipolar, Recovery and NLP

made mad by Hera, while Ajax is made mad by Athena. Once they are mad both victims lose the ability for rational thought. The madman is deluded and out of control, and does things that he would not normally do.

The madmen and women in Greek Tragedy are not aware of what they are doing but think that they are. When they recover from their frenzied state they regret what they have done. Terrible deeds are done by the madman, deeds that can only be those of someone that is out of their wits.

They cannot be forgiven and cannot forgive themselves for what they have done unwittingly. If they survive, then the experience will haunt them for the rest of their lives. If they do not, then the ordeal was simply too much.

Being mad itself is depicted as evil. Mad behaviour is led by demonic forces whether actions have justification or not. Orestes may kill his mother as a means of revenge. Different levels of madness are represented by playwrights. For example, Aeschylus makes the Furies only 'haunt' Orestes (Cite), whilst Sophocles makes them drive Orestes mad (Cite). Whilst vengeance contributes to Orestes' state in Aeschylus and Ajax's state in the Ajax (Cite), Euripides goes further and makes madness entirely external. Agave has no reason to kill her son; she does so because she is possessed by some Bacchic frenzy.

The madman is perceived as having contracted some kind of terrible disease. This leads to ridicule and humiliation. Teucer and Ajax are characters who experience this. Still there is a positive aspect to the treatment of madness in Greek Tragedy. For example, the reference to the mad, being part of a divine language (Ajax L243f) as they are like a "frenzied god not a man" places the madman on a superhuman level. This simile refers to a state of existence that a normal human being cannot achieve. The presentation of the madman as something out of the ordinary and extraordinary is something which remains consistent throughout Tragedy.

The function of the madman in Tragedy in my view is to extend Aristotle's standard realms of catharsis. Madness is a very powerful concept and Aeschylus, Sophocles and Euripides all benefit from addressing the theme of madness. There is possibly nothing worse that man can experience and therefore madness is the perfect medium for tragedy. When Agave holds her son's head thinking it is the head of a lion the devastation that madness can bring makes the spectator's stomach crawl. She is completely oblivious to what she has done. Only a madman (or madwoman) can do such a thing, the most grotesque and shocking moments of Greek Tragedy take the form of the mad experience.

Despite a wonderment and awe that soon transforms itself into fear, hate and condemnation, there is an attempt to cure these mad folk. Cadmus manages to cure Agave from her madness and his actions are similar to those of modern psychiatric techniques.

Although there is pity for the characters it is often forgotten as the characters assume a different identity when they are mad. Their behaviour is unwitting and the state of frenzy takes away their humanity. An educated reader is able to distinguish between the representation of madness in a realistic and in a bad light. Tragedy consistently presents madness in a realistic light. It explores the vulnerability of those that are mad and those that are affected by it. It evokes the fundamental point that madness is an isolated as well as an altered state of mind. The coming in, and out of it, are separate from the moments of insanity.

There is frequently in Tragedy reference to characters before, during and after their madness. Madness is easier to identify if there is something to compare it to. The normally conscientious and heroic Herakles would of course not kill his children if he were sane. Mad behaviour in Greek Tragedy is so intense that it leaps out from the text. When Ajax mistakenly tortures sheep instead of men anyone in their right mind would realise that he is at that moment a madman.

There is no reason to focus on whether people in Tragedy are rightly or wrongly regarded and treated as mad. For constant moralising detracts from the facts. There is also no need always to try and determine what constitutes madness in Greek Tragedy for madness in a sense defines itself, and it is what it is as the gods demand or enforce it. A mortal cannot escape suffering and a madman is constantly regarded as being in an abominable state. The madman is physically repulsive[9]. He vomits black bile and has overbearing rage in his eyes.

Madness is the consequence of Hubris. This occurs when an individual or member of a character's family is punished by the gods for being too arrogant. Ajax rejects Athena's advice and is therefore made mad for being guilty of hubris. There is no arguing with this, it just happens. Madness is part of fate in Greek Tragedy. The madman has nowhere to run or hide. He cannot recall the frenzied state and when he escapes from it he will not consciously be able to get back to it[10]. Instead he has to cope with the trauma and the consequences of his actions. Some cope better than others. Depending on the situation some characters can recover from it, others are engulfed by it.

An analysis of four characters already mentioned Orestes, Ajax, Agave and Herakles will identify why each

[9] Ruth Padel in her book "In And Out Of Mind" is fascinated by the physical manifestations of the madman in Tragedy.

[10] The reference to a madman wishing to get back to the mad state is interesting for two reasons. Firstly a return to madness makes the madman forget the present. Secondly, in Tragedy madwomen are given godlike powers (Agave and the Maenads). Here lies the positive aspect to madness in Greek tragedy.

becomes mad, what they do exactly, and how they cope with being mad, as well as with what they have done.

Bipolar, Recovery and NLP

THE MADNESS OF ORESTES

Now follows the treatment of Orestes by Aeschylus and Euripides. Firstly, Aeschylus and the Libation Bearers: Electra claims that the recognition scene is madness as it causes so much pain (L211). Madness is always associated with some kind of pain. The traumatic state of Orestes is worsened by the Furies. As he kills his mother the Furies haunt the murderer. They are visible only to Orestes with their "eyes burning, grim brows working over you in the dark - the dark sword of the dead!" (L290). Although they avenge the death of Agamemnon, who is slain by Clytemnestra, their presentation is similar to that of Satan and his devil worshippers[11]. With such powerful enemies Orestes falls into the abyss. The theme of darkness which goes hand in hand with vengeance is part of what might constitute madness but not sufficient to make someone mad on his or her own. For example, the Orestes of Aeschylus is in a sense in the dark as he alone sees the Furies and enacts vengeance by killing Aegisthus but is able to maintain a sane mind.

Mad people are blind to what they do when they are mad. The leader tells Orestes that "The blood's still wet on your hands. It puts a kind of frenzy in you" (1055). Here is proof that the moment he kills his mother he is in a sense mad. This is not clear cut madness as Orestes does not lose consciousness of what he is doing. He does, however, hallucinate as the Furies are present in the text. So this shows that the character has one of the symptoms of madness. What else made him adhere to "this murderous hate, this Fury?" (1075). The house of Atreus is an infectious, disease ridden place. Orestes and his family are all victims of a curse put on them. This curse is contagious and Orestes catches its symptoms. For example, if his

---

[11] Satan is a concept that is developed after the date of the text and is mentioned as an appropriate form of communication between ancient Greek Tragedy and the modern viewer.

Bipolar, Recovery and NLP

mother kills his father then vengeance demands Orestes to commit matricide.

In the Eumenides Orestes is cured. He is protected by Apollo who tells him to kill Clytemnestra (L200). Apollo drives back the Furies with his bow and arrows (175-8). Apollo says that the Furies' "manhunt of Orestes is unjust" (L219). Their pursuit of him multiplies their pains (L224).

It is the shrieking frenzy, the hymn of fury that causes pain to Orestes and the Furies themselves (L330 + L343). This hymn of fury as an external force is something that deities older than the gods cannot escape. Symptoms for the Furies are black froth erupting from their lungs (L180)[12]. There is no indication in Aeschylus where this suffering comes from except that it is fate punishing Orestes' grandfather Atreus (L1066LB). It is part of the curse on the house of Atreus. Still it is ultimately in the control of the new deities. The Gods rid Orestes of his torment as he has suffered enough. Orestes is the figure closest to being a madman that is explicitly treated and cured by the gods (L767Euminides). He is freed from guilt but is most definitely not mad in Aeschylus.

The cure of Orestes lies in the need for the new judicial system to supplant that of the old. His recovery provides the mechanism to impose the Olympian gods ahead of the weary old deities, the furies, and with it come the law makers of torment. The law itself can be described as fate which supplies the origins of any manic or schizophrenic state for any character of Tragedy.

---

[12] Here Padel comments on the physical manifestations of the madman (throughout the text). Her categorising of all madmen having these physical attributes is misleading as Orestes in Aeschylus fits her definition of madness but is not actually mad. Her work exemplifies the danger of giving absolutes in critical theory.

Bipolar, Recovery and NLP

The Orestes of Euripides, however, is mad. He is punished with madness for slaying his mother (L37+400). Electra tells us this madness is "heaven-inflicted" (L844). He is pursued by the Furies, who are physically repulsive "gazing blood, horrid with snakes" (L256). Tyndarus points out that Orestes is "hated by the gods" for killing his mother (L531). He realises that it was "unholy" to slay his mother (L545). There are also suggestions that his madness is infectious when he speaks to Pylades, "take care how thou art partner of my madness" (L790).

The Orestes of Euripides is a character who is in need of more careful attention. His "grievous malady" (L36) causes him to lie at his sister's feet (L87). He is physically exhausted and weak (L228). He cannot control his madness that comes in fits (L227). He was deluded by the gods when slaying Helen (L1589). His eyes roll when he raves with madness (L839). This Orestes is madder than in Aeschylus. His madness is infectious and incurable. He kills Clytemnestra and Helen and is only just prevented from killing Hermione. Apollo's forcing of Orestes to marry Hermione does not cure him from madness for he still suffers (L1681). The god enacts destiny (L1654), and although Orestes has a future there is no indication that he is relieved from his madness.

The chorus want the madness to stop (L332-3) as they want the suffering to stop in the Libation Bearers (1067f). They are unable to do anything about it. Insanity corrupts men as does war and comes from within. Only the gods can enforce it. This makes the suffering of the madman and those observing him more tragic as they are helpless to prevent what is inevitable.

Orestes borders on madness as he is always haunted by the Furies. Their sick and frenzied hounding is sufficient to make any mortal question his or her sanity. Orestes is never in control of his actions. He may have a justified reason for killing his mother but he is ultimately an unwitting contributor to fate. His appearance borders on the schizophrenic[13], with delusions and the witnessing of horrible evil creatures suffocating his existence. In Aeschylus and Euripides his relation to other people in the text is symptomatic of a schizophrenic as only he has delusions.

As Cassandra is the misunderstood prophet, Orestes alone suffers from the wrath of the Furies. He has nowhere to run or hide. Within the conventions of Greek Tragedy his character's suffering produces catharsis and adds to plot detail. In Euripides he can be said to have had a horrific mental breakdown caused by external circumstance. For other characters within the play cannot see the Furies and do not understand what Orestes is going through. His ability to maintain consciousness despite the persistent harping of the Furies reveals him to be a character that is mentally strong and resilient.

However, the damage is already done. Vengeance forces him to kill his mother and he will never recover from this terrible crime. Like Oedipus he commits matricide which is one of the worst crimes imaginable (L886LibationBearers). Apollo possesses him in order to carry out the matricide as he could not do it with a sane mind. His family is not exempt from hubris, however. The House of Atreus is damned by the gods when Thyestes eats his children. They carry out the fate of Orestes.

He is motivated by the external force that he can never control. He discovers that Apollo made him kill his mother only after he has done it. Still, if he had known at the time of the event what he was doing resistance to the will of Apollo would have been equally futile. Of course he has a certain justification for committing matricide so may not have wished to refrain if he had been sane. This identifies a

---

[13] Medical conditions were not recognised in the same way in ancient Greek culture as they are by some today, but the work of Euripides inevitably evokes comparisons with modern illnesses.

problem with discussing insanity which is that it drives one into moral speculation as it is such a powerful subject.

All mortals in Greek Tragedy have to bow to the superior gods. The problem for the Orestes of Euripides is that his submission to the external force allows madness to come to the fore. He is released from his madness. Orestes could have been permanently insane or killed himself. The conventions of Greek Tragedy, uses madness for its own means. It explores the consequences, causes, nature and modes of madness as it sees fit. As regards to the madness of Euripides' Orestes, he withstands it, is given it, is not responsible for it and experiences different types of it. He is a victim of demonic forces that are part of an unjust world. His response to it is a brave one and to be admired.

Euripides continued the treatment of Orestes where Aeschylus left off. Euripides made his Orestes mad and by doing so induced more suffering and pathos in his treatment.

Bipolar, Recovery and NLP

THE MADNESS OF AJAX

The Ajax of Sophocles describes a madman who cannot cope with the consequences of his madness. Ajax is so disturbed at having been mad that he stabs himself to death (L866). He leaves his family and friends behind (L855). Humiliation is the reason for his suicide. He says "look at my shame" (L366) and "I am their laughing stock" (L455). Ajax feels that all of Greece will laugh at him for killing sheep when he meant to kill Agamemnon and his company. This would qualify him as a paranoid schizophrenic today. He suffers from hallucinations and fears the worst possible scenario which is suicide.

In course of the play Ajax loses his heroic code of honour. The tragic hero must "bring back honour for my father". His failure to win Achilles' belt and act of hubris make suicide his only way to "die with honour" (L478). His suicide will show his bravery and restore him to the heroic hall of fame.
Unlike Orestes, Ajax is guilty of hubris. He tells Athena:

I'll do anything you ask - except change my plans for Odysseus.

Athena appears to accept what Ajax says but we already know that she has "warped his sight". She hates him as he "thought himself an equal of the Gods" (L777). As the paranoid schizophrenic when depressed would feel that he is an embarrassment to society because he has manic thoughts and delusions,[14] Ajax must be made to feel the same way for his inflated opinion of himself[15]. He is not a god, only a mortal that is too arrogant for his own good. He has offended those that are superior to him so must be punished in a fitting manner. He is made an example of. "Athena's broken toy" (401) makes a slaughter house full of sheep instead of men (L55). To effect his humiliation Athena turns his brain with wild thoughts of revenge (L51).

As with Agave, Tecmessa gives a fascinating insight on madness. She says of Ajax that he was happier when he was mad (L270). The trauma of coping with the actions of his madness is too much to bear. The moments of madness themselves are enjoyable although they are disfunctional. Ajax is happy as long as he maintains madness. As soon as he comes out of it he is forced to face the real world and deal with the terrible events of his madness. Ajax is not given the opportunity to deal only with returning to reality. With madness regarded as a terrible affliction he will always blame his madness for the predicament that he is in (which is of course true). However, he does not deny it but faces up to it immediately, for Ajax is no coward but is a man of bravery. His tragedy is that through being mad he has lost his honour.

Only madness could have driven him to do such things (L181). Madness even induces fear in one of the most intelligent and caring characters in the whole of Greek Tragedy. Odysseus tells Athena that he will not face the madman (L82).

Poor Ajax is left in limbo. What can he do? He feels that society is against him. He feels that the gods are against him. People do not understand what he has been

---

[14] The author comes to this conclusion based on patients that he has met in various mental institutions.

[15] Simon Bennett "Mind and Madness in Ancient Greece" (p93) refers to divine agencies driving the protagonist mad. This provides the most humane treatment of Madness (of all the texts that I have read on madness in Greek Tragedy)

Bipolar, Recovery and NLP

through. Once one of the noblest of the Greeks, he loses so much dignity that he chooses to end his life. His suicide is presented as brave and tragic. There are no gods on his side. He leaves his wife, son and comrades, whom he loves very much. He refuses to ask for any sympathy. Instead he goes quietly and takes his own life. Brave in life and brave in death (L1337). The one flaw of hubris is sufficient to destroy him and devastate those that are close to him.

The Herakles in Euripides' Herakles manages to live on after realising that he has killed his children. He has divine help, unlike Ajax. The suggestion that there is honour in suicide is extraordinarily advanced in my view[16]: As recently as in the early twentieth century suicide was a criminal offence and frequently viewed as the 'easy way out'. People are as scared of suicide and madness today as they were in Greek tragedy. This is why they condemn it. In Ajax suicide is his decision and is part of his destiny.

Madness instigates his suicide. The madness is external, although he unwittingly contributes to it. His ordeal demonstrates man's powerlessness against fate. This is also true in Oedipus Tyrannus, where patricide and marrying one's mother is inevitable. Ajax's pride makes him succumb to the wrath of Athena. His choice of suicide is a way of the tragedian characterising Ajax as somebody who cannot cope with madness. As victim of overbearing external forces and traumatic circumstances his suicide is realistic.

Others suffer from Ajax's madness. Teucer is ridiculed, spat at, harrassed and threatened for being the "brother of a madman and a traitor" (L720f). The chorus of the followers of Ajax when discovering his death are so upset that they might as well be dead (L900). As Ajax is no longer there to

---

[16] Large sections of modern culture view suicide as a cowardly act. See the final act of the play Hedda Gabler by Henrik Ibsen. Throughout the play the motives for and reaction to suicide are the underlying themes. Hedda shoots herself in the final act like Ajax because she feels trapped. She chooses suicide as her escape.

protect them Tecmessa worries that she and her son will be slaves to Agamemnon (L944).

The situation when Ajax has recovered from his madness is significant as it shows the damage which mad behaviour can cause. It suggests two paradoxes, either that the madman is not alone but feels he is, or that he is alone and does not feel like he is. For example, Ajax kills himself since he feels he is alone, but in fact his family and friends are in a sense with him. They are on his side. If his family is not with him he imagines people to be ridiculing him.

Sophocles has presented madness and its consequences in a realistic manner which is similar to modern psychiatric thought. Ajax unfortunately refuses to treat himself so that he can recover. Odysseus gives back Ajax some dignity by saving his burial rights. Having a proper burial is an essential part of showing respect to those who have died in ancient Greek culture.

Tecmessa's references to Ajax being possessed (L218) and acting like a "frenzied god" are reminiscent of the constant hounding that Orestes had to endure. The chorus do not know whether Ajax is mad again or whether he is horrified at what his madness has done to him (L337). They soon discover it is the latter. The madness of Ajax is more damaging than that of Euripides' Orestes as it leads ultimately to death. Orestes' madness comes in fits and is equally as traumatic, but it is managed. With the actions of madness that Ajax has done his loyalty to the heroic code makes him kill himself. Society would say his fate is tragic. Existentialists could argue that Ajax is lucky to escape a finite existence and obtain the inevitability of death[17].

Whatever interpretation is held regarding the fate of Ajax, he is a tragic hero whose pride is his weakness. This

---

[17] Jean Paul Sartre is, as far as I know, the pioneer of thought expressed in this manner. This view derives from the reading of Speech and Language in Psychoanalysis by Jacques Lacan.

weakness is the reason for his suffering in the play. His madness is the consequence of his act of hubris. Odysseus finds a way to save his reputation but Ajax still remains notoriously mad. Pride is a fault of all men though, and Athena's victim is merely privy to fate which determines the action of the goddess. As if it were a disease, madness engulfs him and he is unable to prevent it from ruining him.

The character of Ajax presents a realistic response to madness. It is so powerful that nobody is able to cope with what it does. There is no necessity to speculate what kind of madness Ajax suffers from as these diagnoses are neither part of Greek Tragedy nor ancient Greek culture. However, he can be described as being on a high one minute and then on a low the next. This pattern of behaviour is similar to that of the manic depressive. Many kinds of mental illness can induce this kind of dysfunctional behaviour. As soon as Ajax is out of his mind he is recognisably mad and when he is in his mind he is sane.[18] Therefore Ajax fails to manage the illness that inflicts him. Sophocles demonstrates the worst possible scenario that madness causes. Madness is so overpowering that it can lead a hero to commit suicide. This is where Sophocles' treatment of madness is unique.

All other madmen in Greek Tragedy survive to mourn the consequences of their mad actions. Bearing this in mind, it becomes frustrating that hundreds of Greek Tragedies are missing. With the plays that have been restored Sophocles and not Euripides deals with the suicide of a madman. The reputation of Euripides as a radical Tragedian therefore is not merely because he chooses the most disastrous consequences of madness.

Sophocles also chooses not to describe Ajax coming out of his madness. This is a significant difference

---

[18] Here the title of Ruth Padel's book "In and Out of Mind" is the most appropriate language for losing and recovering one's sanity.

from Euripides, who analyses the recovery of Herakles and Agave very closely.

Bipolar, Recovery and NLP

THE MADNESS OF AGAVE

There is no doubt that the visual images of the madman (madwoman in this case) in the Bacchae of Euripides are the most disturbing in the whole of Greek tragedy[19]. How is a mother to react when she realises that she has hunted her son and holds his head and not that of a lion? If she loves her son as Agave clearly does she will be devastated (L1279-1288). Killing one's child is at the very least equally disturbing for Agave as the matricide of Orestes. It is possibly more disturbing for Agave as she has no motive for killing her son unlike the vengeful Orestes. The viewer is voyeur of much more graphic detail than the murder itself (in the Bacchae). This naturally adds to the visual effect in the play and induces more pathos.

She cannot remember her actions during the Bacchic frenzy (L1294-5). Madness is a punishment for slandering and ultimately causing the death of Semele, the mother of Dionysus (L1297). Agave and her sisters are made mad as a means of revenge for Dionysus (L26).

Ajax's acceptance of Athena as a deity shows that Sophocles does not go as far as Euripides. Regarding the treatment of madness, Euripides makes the denial of Dionysus the act of hubris. Pentheus had no idea that Dionysus was a god. The fate of Pentheus is grim because he refuses to worship Dionysus (L44). The play shows the prevailing theme that humans are powerless to prevent the punishment that a god enacts.

---

[19] I disagree with Bennett (M&Mp124f), who believes that *Ajax* is the most visual treatment of madness. Ajax is unique in that he kills himself, but there is no imagery as powerful as Agave holding aloft the head of her son or ripping his body apart in the *Ajax*.

Bipolar, Recovery and NLP

The consequences of Agave's madness are that she will be parted from her father (L1363) and forced into exile (1368). So madness is once again responsible for isolating individuals and is portrayed as a contagious disease that nobody in their right mind wants to catch. Pentheus catches the disease and can only then die from it. Agave's response to having killed Pentheus is in my view rather abrupt[20]. The lines after her realisation are sadly missing (L1301f). Still she is clearly in untold grief, mourning, disbelief and horror at what she has done (L1279-88).

Agave is not to blame for her mad actions as she did them unwittingly. She is responsible for offending Dionysus but is human and therefore prone to make mistakes. The mad episode has totally ruined her life. She must seek another identity elsewhere for her act of hubris. Her punishment is too severe as Dionysus agrees (L1347).

However, Zeus is described as ordaining that offending the gods makes the punishment suitable if not desirable (L1348).

As a result of her madness Cadmus and her sisters must be exiled (L1352). Pentheus cannot be given a respectable funeral. Although there is a lacuna after lines 1300, the previous line describes Agave asking whether the body is torn limb from limb or not? The answer is most definitely yes. There is a detailed scene earlier that shows how the body of Pentheus is ripped to pieces. She grabs his left arm, places her foot against his ribs and tears his shoulder out of its socket (1127).

Agave has graver consequences to deal with than the quick stabbing of Orestes or the torturing of sheep of Ajax. She has to deal with the fact that she kills her son, tortures him, holds his head apart from its body and rips his

---

[20] What she does to Pentheus is so tragic that the subject could cover an entire play.

whole body to shreds. This is a disgusting thought, nauseous to anyone in their right mind, and can only be performed by someone who is out of their mind. However, each madman has their own problems to face; Orestes has the Furies haunting him, whilst Ajax has his heroic honour amongst other things to consider.

All Agave's suffering derives from offending Dionysus and the gods. For denying that Dionysus is a god (L45) he makes the women involved mad by joining in Bacchanal worship (L32). This frenzy singles out Agave amongst the women who refuse to worship and pour libations to the god. When Dionysus says that he will reveal himself as a god (L47) this is an indication that hell will break loose.

The prologue makes it quite clear that Dionysus' principal victim is Pentheus (L47). Throughout the text there are warnings that you must "honour the gods" (L1010) otherwise you will be "stung by madness by Dionysus" (L118). The play explores Pentheus changing from a sane character to a character who is mad. Dionysus invades his personality making him see the god turn into a bull as he tries to lock him up. The Bacchae is unique in tragedy as the treatment of Pentheus and Dionysus provides the only extensive interaction between the agency and the victim of madness[21]. This interaction shows that Dionysus is an embodiment of the unconscious impulses and fears of Pentheus[22]. For example, the dress making scene describes the god encouraging the manly Pentheus to dress up as a woman so that he can view the worship of the Maenads (L810f). The man who could not put on female garb (L836) has his mind altered by the god and becomes fascinated by how he looks when he is dressed as a woman. He wonders whether he looks like his mother (L924) and notices if a curl is out of place (L930). Pentheus is clearly mad at this point as he

---

[21] See Simon Bennett, Mind & Madness, pages 115-116.
[22] See Simon Bennett, Mind & Madness, pages 113-122.

sees "two suns and a double Thebes" (L918) and Dionysus as a bull (L920). The presentation of Pentheus emphasizes that in madness delusion is accompanied by a blurring of the self and the other, a confusion of personal identity.

Teiresias says that a man is a bad citizen if he lacks sanity (L271). This comment suggests that madness is an undesirable state abhorred by those in their right mind. The mad Bacchanals are a terrifying bunch with their cries of ecstasy (L149 + L156). Pentheus is terrified at the thought of being caught by them. However, more significantly, Teiresias notices that "that which is manic possesses great mantic powers". This introduces a positive element of madness within the play. The messenger's speech describes the quiet of the Bacchic women and their peaceful occupations (L677-774). The madness of Agave is consistent in the psychological order in which the madness of Pentheus is described and has a different emphasis. She too is driven mad by Dionysus but by absorption into the Maenads as opposed to personal interaction with the god. The Maenads are able to express their femininity by worshipping Dionysus when they nurse young animals. They are more powerful than armed men with their thyrsoi but as the thiasos revolves around a male leader they lack penis power and the prerogatives of men[23]. Pentheus breaks down because he is unable to accept a feminine side of himself that lacks power (L310); the women are dependant upon a male no matter how effeminate he may be. Therefore group ecstasy becomes madness because the Bacchic ecstasy does not resolve underlying conflict. The theme of group madness is exclusive to the Bacchae.

The Maenads are presented as perfectly peaceful and in harmony with nature until they are interfered with. Dionysus gives the Bacchanals great strength. How else can they pull a huge tree out of the ground? (L1110). These women drink honey and milk, wear fawnskins, hissing

---

[23] See Simon Bennett, Mind & Madness page 119.

snakes and hold clubs. They attack everything they see when they are in a state of frenzy. Their behaviour is due to their denial of Dionysus and therefore because of their hubris. They are the tools of his vengeance.

The good sense of Teiresias is shown when he refuses the demands of Pentheus and the chorus to go against the god:

For you are most grievously mad - beyond the cure of drugs, and yet your sickness must be due to them (L326-7)

Teiresias knows that you should not "raise arms against a god" (L789). He realises that the gods are better than mortals and he will never be guilty of hubris. His behaviour demonstrates that madness is a grim state that nobody wishes to experience. He would be of the opinion that once Pentheus is mad he is doomed (L44). Dionysus is the instigator (L305) and is directly responsible for the suffering of the mad Pentheus and Agave. Dionysus claims that he follows the law of his father Zeus who has to carry out fate as it is set out before him (L1348). This shows Dionysus on the defensive as he shifts responsibility onto Zeus in order to rid himself of guilt. This behaviour exemplifies the presentation of Dionysus as an imperfect god in the play. It also reveals that Euripides is more critical of the gods in their enforcement of madness than Sophocles.

Agave suffers from various types of madness, although Greek Tragedy does not distinguish between them. Her mood is high when she joins in the festivities of the Bacchanals only for her mood to be lowered when she comes out of the manic state[24]. The events of the Bacchae show that tragic events are problems that mortals have to deal with. The play criticises the god's handling of madness as a punishment implying that it is too severe. It incorporates

---

[24] The use of modern terminology of high and low mood is expanded here from the discussion on Ajax on p17.

positive and negative aspects of madness in a realistic manner.

Bipolar, Recovery and NLP

THE MADNESS OF HERAKLES

There is no explicit reference that madness will invade Herakles until Iris speaks (L823). Herakles is not mad until the second half of the play. Madness is so powerful that time is of little significance in inducing pathos upon the plight of a madman. Sophocles makes Ajax dead half way through the play whilst Euripides makes Agave mad throughout the Bacchae. Each play has its own style in presenting madness. However, the mad appearance of Herakles is the central theme of the play.

No other mad tragic figure except Herakles kills his wife and offspring. Is there anything more precious to a man than the well being of his wife and children? Will his removal of them all show his world falling apart? Will he end up like Ajax? Yes, yes and no respectively. He suffers great torment for what he has done but lives to tell the tale.

Facing up to the murder of his wife and three children are the immediate consequences of the madness of Herakles. These catastrophes are presented in a way worse than that which Orestes and Ajax have to endure, and are on a par with the devastated Agave, for Herakles kills more than one person that he loves. He feels responsible for murdering four of the closest people to him. Before the murders sympathy is increased for Herakles when he mentions that everyone adores children (L638). The misery that his madness induces also satisfies the wrath of Hera (L830) and resolves her vengeance.

The main problem for Herakles is trying to cope with what he has done. His father has to point out the terrible deeds, as the murderer has no idea what he has done when he first comes out of the frenzied state. The response of Herakles is one of total anguish (L1132). He asks whether he was possessed or if it was his own doing (L1142). Either way his first thought when he realises the effect of what he has done, is to kill himself (L1147). Like Ajax he contemplates suicide and hides himself in shame at the

Bipolar, Recovery and NLP

terrible atrocities that his madness has done (L1159). It is mostly the remarkable loyalty of Theseus but also that of his father which makes Herakles choose to live (L1219 + 1399). Ajax has the support of the chorus and his family but is unable to step out from his responsibilities under the heroic code.

Thanks to the loyalty of his friend, Herakles is able to stand although his limbs have seized up (L1396). This pathetic moment reveals a realistic cure to someone who is mad. In effect, good friends can help you conquer the terrible affliction. This emphasis is specifically Euripidean. Amphtryion helps Herakles as Cadmus helps Agave come to terms with the consequences of her madness. Sophocles does not attempt to bring Ajax out of madness directly but instead makes Tecmessa describe his recovery (L306f). Euripides' treatment of Herakles choosing to live on avoiding suicide is a fundamental concept of psychotherapy[25]. However, in Greek Tragedy madness has already left Herakles enabling him to recover.

Herakles is not responsible for the murders as they stem from the madness that is inflicted upon him (L1187). He knows himself that he is hated by Hera (L1264). His denial of what Zeus is, is the reason for carrying out labours and rebuttal of him as his father shows that the man whom Amphitryon hails as being as capable of saving his family as his godly father is guilty of hubris.

He has the curse of the Furies (L1077) like Orestes. He celebrates his madness in a similar way to Agave in the Bacchae. He rejoices in Bacchic ritual dancing to the mad frenzy of the pipe (L878). The Bacchic madness is so strong

---

[25] Shirley Barlow presents this phenomenon in her introduction on Herakles 1996. Its relevance here is not to challenge that the madness of Herakles is enacted as is always the case in tragedy by *hubris* but to make the modern psychiatric point that chemical conditions and psychological states are both equally significant causes of mental illness.

Bipolar, Recovery and NLP

(L898) that he is only freed from it by being physically knocked out by Athena (L1005). The chorus tell us that the madness is fated (L1024) and Iris reveals that Hera is responsible. The law of gods makes certain that Hera's anger will be felt by Herakles. Only by this treatment can gods show that they are superior to mortals (L840). Fate comes before Hera's decision for vengeance. Nobody is responsible. The spectator knows that madness occurs from within Tragedy.

Fate dominates the cause and nature of madness. Madness is a form of punishment. Madmen have no control whether they are mad or not. Herakles is punished but his character is strong enough to survive it. He passes the test that a god lays out in front of him where Ajax fails. The first episode of Herakles coincides with the murders whilst his emphatic recovery is the end of his madness.

His mad episode is an unwitting one. Lyssa points out that he will not realise that he has killed his children until her madness leaves him (L863). The nature of his madness is so upsetting that she remarks how she is against it (L858). This sympathy from a god is exclusive to the Herakles. Apollo in the Orestes shows a little sympathy for mankind in preventing Orestes from committing another murder but this is ultimately so he can be worshipped. Herakles is privy to the actions of Lyssa, she must follow the law set by Hera who enacts fate for Zeus. Herakles suffers in similar ways to Orestes, Ajax and Agave. His eyes are poisoned (L866) and froth falls out of his mouth (L934). He hallucinates believing that his children are those of Eurystheus (L969).

He is not in his right mind. He has had a history of mental anguish, for he has not only had to endure the ten labours which would drive any sane man wild but also when he was only a baby Hera sent frightening serpents to kill him (L1266). His madness is so intense that on his return from it he is not sure who is his father nor is he familiar with anything at all (L1106). It pollutes him and those around him

346

Bipolar, Recovery and NLP

(L1398). The fact that madness can make a man who has been to Hades and killed the dreaded Cerberus (L609) wish to turn himself into stone (L1395) shows how vulnerable mortals are.

The essence of Tragedy makes it inevitable that it is a nightmarish event which constitutes his madness. Herakles becomes deranged as soon as the gods enforce it. He has no awareness or control over what his madness does. He shows every aspect of the deranged mental asylum archetype. He is off his head, loony and a nutter. He enjoys the experience giving a maniacal laugh (L935). This shows a solitary positive aspect to his madness. His state of delusion at this moment in the text is enjoyable; however, it does not compensate for the ensuing horrific consequences of the experience. He wrestles with people that are not there (L959). His madness is so intense that it takes a violent strike by Athena with a stone to rid him of it.

His return from madness guides him through what has happened to him and makes him face up to it. It is realistic and is a pioneer for modern Clinical Psychology. The questions Herakles raises about what constitutes his madness are answered and put into context by Amphitryion. In this way he is guided back into accepting what he has done to his family. All the madmen and women in Tragedy are released from madness once their punishment is complete. The characters of Euripides cope with the aftermath of madness better than the characters of anyone else. It is not my prerogative to discuss whether characters of Euripides reach higher levels of madness or are the most resourceful in tragedy but Agave and Herakles are certainly thicker skinned than Ajax.

Bipolar, Recovery and NLP

THE THEME OF MADNESS IN TRAGEDY

Always as a form of punishment madness is immediately recognised as something that is bad for you. It is therefore an undesirable state. Just as a Christian fears Hell the characters of Tragedy are terrified of what madness induces individuals to do (L261Ajax). Madmen are not blamed for what they have done. For example the chorus in Ajax mourn the suicide of Ajax and claim that they might as well die with him (L900). Also in the Bacchae, Agave tears Pentheus to pieces but she is not blamed by her father for killing his grandson. Cadmus feels deep grief for his daughter (L1217) and assists her to come out of her madness (L1277). Madness is such a powerful medium in Tragedy that it tears people apart and brings people together in mourning.

The Tragedians utilise madness as a powerful theme to induce empathy for their characters and the society that they write about as a whole. Characters are sometimes more tragic if they appear to be mad. Therefore Tragedy is frequently more powerful if it explores madness. What can be more tragic for the spectator than seeing the actor's world destroyed by the actor? The answer is nothing as the involvement of the spectator does not go any further than empathy for the actor. The question also elucidates the all - important Aristotelian distinction between the spectator and actor - we see someone else seeing himself destroying his own world. The actor is not in control of his actions and neither is the character especially when he is mad.

The madman feels guilt as he feels responsible for his actions. However his mad actions stem from hubris which is part of fate. The gods punish the relations of an individual if they do not wish merely to condemn the guilty party. For example Herakles is wounded by the gods as a child and he is not made mad because of hubris. The vengeance of Hera is the reason for his psychotic frenzy which is part of his destiny. Even the goddess herself serves Zeus. Zeus may have ordained that mortals are to be punished if they have unsettled the gods but he can only postpone fate not change it.

Characters that commit acts such as hubris do so because they make mistakes. As they are mortal they will keep on making mistakes. The characters' behaviour, identity, beliefs and actions are only consistent in their inconsistency. The only thing consistent about the madman in Tragedy is that he suffers tremendous pain. The inevitability of grief and death in Tragedy evokes what is an almost existentialist ideology. As the Greeks did not believe in the after-life in the fifth century BC this is a remarkably advanced perception within Tragedy. The existentialist comparison is more suitable to Tragedy than elsewhere in Greek literature. There is no time for the hero dying the heroic death as Hector does in the Iliad and for him to perform heroic tasks within Tragedy as it explores the characters' identities and sufferings in such a profound manner. The serious nature of Tragedy urges the spectator to think and reflect on telling circumstances.

What better way is there to show characters suffering than through madness? There is no better way as madness is unique in presenting characters that suffer. It makes them do things that the sane person would not even dream of doing and also makes them deal with the consequences of their actions.

Modern metaphors of madness such as Hell and the abyss add to the curiosity of what it is like to be mad. An analysis of the happy delusions of Ajax torturing Agamemnon's men and Agave's celebrations at slaughtering Pentheus show that the moments of madness themselves are not undesirable. When a character returns from the abyss they can not believe what they have done and have no way of changing it. By causing such regret in the character the author is able to manipulate the emotions of the spectator.

There are notable distinctions between Greek Tragedians. Sophocles omits Ajax coming out of madness and makes Athena describe it instead (L306). This shows the horror that madness can cause both the character and the spectator. Euripides deals with it directly in detail slowly bringing Herakles back into the real world via dialogue (L1106f) and Agave likewise (L1277). Sophocles' treatment lacks the psychological advances of the later fifth century BC. Although it was produced earlier than Aeschylus' Oresteia (458BC) the Ajax (mid440sBC) comes before the teaching of rhetoric of Gorgias (427BC). As one of the pioneers of Sophistry Gorgias sought expediency of action and denied the absolute moral actions of the earlier part of the fifth century[26]. Euripides benefits from the likes of Gorgias as Herakles (430-420BC) and the Bacchae (406BC) were produced during the first generations of Sophistic thought. As the seminal figure of epistemology Gorgias' thoughts are evoked in Euripides' text. How do Agave and Herakles know that they are mad? They have to be told in stages by Cadmus and Amphitryion. The moment when they realise that they are or have been mad they recover from their madness. For this reason Euripides' treatment of madness is the most sophisticated of the Greek Tragedians.

There are parameters to madness in Greek Tragedy. Fate carries out what happens and madness fits within this context. The madness of characters in Tragedy is presented with empathy and pathos and each individual is cured. Herakles avoids permanently remaining mad which is a bloody pollution (L1398) and when cured goes into exile. This evokes the humiliating fate for distinguished people in Ancient Greece as does the exile of Agave. For characters

---

[26] See Greece and Rome *The Birth of Western Civilization* page 83.

of such noble background as Agave and Herakles exile is a tragic outcome.

Only several of the thirty-one remaining plays use the theme of madness in depth. There are other plays that come close to inducing madness on their characters. The experiences of Deianera in Sophocles' Women of Trachis and Electra in Electra are both so distressing that they border on madness but they do not fit the criteria for madness as they are not guilty of hubris which means that they are not made mad as a punishment by a god. Their characters therefore lack the intensity which madness gives to a character such as Agave.

Madness is always presented as a form of divine influence that creates violence. As violence is a fundamental part of madness and its effects the tragedian is able to use it to impose a greater dramatic effect on the spectator.

Madmen are cured and helped when they return from their madness throughout Greek Tragedy. Orestes is pardoned (In Aeschylus) and has Menelaus for company (Euripides). Agave can go into exile with her sisters. Herakles is looked after by Theseus. Even Ajax comes out of his madness and is helped by Tecmessa and the chorus. Although he dies he receives a proper burial which salvages his reputation within the context of an ancient Greek culture. The brain of the mad character is permanently altered but this is what constitutes the best Tragedy.

Madness is presented as part of fate for individuals who have gone against the rites of a god. The behaviour of the mad character is inevitable and it is unfitting to draw their actions into moral speculation. For the mad character does things as he does them not because he should do them. It is also inevitable that the madman cannot be presented and received in a completely objective fashion. This draws critics into speculation, such as whether it is right that Orestes should be deprived of his humanity in Euripides' play. [27]

All the characters of Tragedy carry some of the same symptoms. Delusions, manic states, racy thoughts, depression, violent outbursts and paranoia.[28] They all contemplate suicide although Ajax is the only one that goes ahead with it. He suffers in a specific way as does each character of the same attire. Madness occurs due to reasons outside of the individual's control. Only in the aftermath does the actor deal with it as the spectator tries to digest the text.

---

[27] This is an assertion openly made by T.A. Buckley in his introduction to the translation of Euripides in 1887 and exemplifies the arid moral speculation of critics prior to modern deconstructive theory.

[28] These symptoms are identical to those experienced by sufferers of Bipolar effective disorder today emphasizing that the presentation of madness in Tragedy is realistic.

Bipolar, Recovery and NLP

WHAT CONSTITUES MADNESS TODAY?

As the presentation of madness in Greek Tragedy is realistic what constitutes madness today is essentially the same as what it constitutes in Greek Tragedy. The difference lies in that madness in Greek Tragedy is governed by a law. In tragedy madness has a starting point and finishing point that is determined by a god. Madness today is identified as deriving from a combination of a chemical or psychological origin and we can only speculate on the nature of madness. For example bipolar effective disorder is believed to occur due to a lack of salt in the blood. When Lithium is taken as requested to counter-act the salt deficiency the individual concerned may still suffer from manic episodes. Therefore Psychotherapy searches for any destructive part of the individual's past that might be deemed as a contributor to their madness so that they can change the behaviour of the individual in a positive manner in order to remain sane.

Madness today is also categorised into different types of madness. There is no schizophrenic, manic depressive or psychotic in tragedy. Psychological advances in the last two and a half thousand years provide new interpretations on the texts (Herakles and the Bacchae) where Herakles and Agave are talked out of their madness by Amphitryion and Cadmus. Although there are different presentations of madness in Tragedy the dramatists do not distinguish between different types.[29] Herakles is recognisably mad as a

---

[29] There is no attempt to assimilate modern types of madness to characters in Greek Tragedy here as it is not entirely appropriate modern types of madness are not within the text.

character whether one describes him as a madman or a particular kind of madman. For madness, is as easily identified today, as it is in Tragedy.

The madman is defined by stereotypes. When Jack Nicholson walks into the dormitory near the end of "One Flew Over the Cuckoos Nest" having been lobotomised with his mouth wide open, eyes contorted, arms aloft and shaking his head from side to side, he has the same symptoms as a madman in Tragedy. Today, as it is in Tragedy, anything that is undesirable and not the doing of a sane man is the action of a madman.

The madman today may become the chronic patient of a mental asylum. There is no such safe house for the madman of Tragedy and no such place in Ancient Greek culture.[30] There is therefore a greater recognition today that the madman needs help. However, characters like Cadmus and Amphitryion in Tragedy are clearly sympathetic and assist those who are mad.

As the madman's mind leaves him he is excluded from the society which he is part of. Throughout history the madman has been abandoned. Ships from England would take mad people in boats to Australia in exile of them. The criminal was abandoned and left on his own for months as a punishment to see if solitude would drive him mad. The madman's identity remains a taboo subject, or cause for ridicule. This kind of hostility towards the madman stems from the fear of being mad oneself.

A madman stands out from the convention of society whilst he is mad as this is the very essence of madness. He

---

[30] If any critical text would mention the existence of mental asylums in ancient Greece it would be The Greeks and the Irrational and it does not. This book is the main influence on modern discussions of madness in Greek Tragedy. In my view its style lacks the critical accuracy of modern literary thought.

is out of his wits and unable to communicate with others in a world of his own. Tragedy explores madness in the same way and also identifies the parameters in which the madman will behave. It explains that madness is the dark side of man's mortality and the role of madness has not changed today.

Bipolar, Recovery and NLP

CONCLUSION

It is a basic premise of Tragedy and ancient Greek culture in general that no-one can handle the experience of madness. It is also a prime function of Tragedy to enable at least an approximation to emotive identification with people of different experience. This function as regards the experience of madness is best carried out by Euripides. Aeschylus does not actually misunderstand[31] and Sophocles understands exactly what madness makes a character do but neither can provide an effective positive aspect to it. It is only Herakles and Agave that are nurtured out of their madness. These pathetic moments represent the basis of modern treatments of Psychotherapy and confirm Euripides as the superior poet on the theme of madness in Greek Tragedy.

Those who are mad in Tragedy are possessed by an undesirable state. Characters kill themselves, their wives, mothers and children because of madness. The presentation of such terrible events invites the spectator to interpret that the madman needs to be sympathised with if not cared for. Their physical disabilities of sight, foaming at the mouth and seizures present accurately the horrors of being mad. However, the most painful part of the mad experience is coming out of it. This is precisely what is demonstrated in the Bacchae when Agave is holding the head of her son. The fact that Sophocles does not describe Ajax coming out of madness directly is the most striking difference between him and Euripides.[32]

---

[31] This judgement of Aeschylus is because, as stated earlier, none of his character's not even Orestes are mad.

[32] Bennett in his book "MAM" neglects to mention this point and this critic views that his failure to recognise this point is why he misinterprets Ajax stating that it is the most visual play. For the most visual play cannot neglect what is the most powerful moment (coming out of madness) and what would also be a most visual moment.

Bipolar, Recovery and NLP

All three dramatists are capable of powerful visualisation in their plays. Ajax butchers sheep and falls on his own sword alone on the sea shore. This is a visual play but lacks the same intensity as Agave and her colleagues tearing her son to pieces then celebrating waving her son's head around bereft of its body.

There are moments of great physical strength during mad episodes. The Maenads ripping a huge tree from out of the ground show godlike strength (L1109). Although this is used in a violent way it represents a positive aspect of madness. Madness allows a character to have the power of a god for a short time. It provides a temporary escape from mortality before the damage it causes is realised by the instigator. The reactions of Cadmus and Amphitryion are remarkable. They show no bitterness towards the murderers as they are loyal and realise that madness makes the sufferer unaware of what they are doing. Their positive reaction is a little unrealistic as it is too considerate although Tragedy is not at fault as its function is to induce pathos rather than to be realistic.

Euripides is the pioneer for psychoanalysts such as Freud and Jacques Lacan. Imagine a sufferer of bipolar effective disorder believing that they had discovered time travel during an episode of mania. This view would make complete sense to the person in this manic state. The Maenads in the Bacchae experience the same elation. When the sanity of the time traveller or Maenads is restored both realise that their behaviour was in a way possessed. The person has a chemical condition whereas the characters are forced into their behaviour because of a god. Both conditions of elation are not worth it in the end, for the coming out of madness is a considerably worse experience. This explains the most important phenomenon of the madman which Greek Tragedy presents in a frightfully realistic, chilling and gripping manner.

357

Bipolar, Recovery and NLP

Please Note:

Any conclusions I reached during my dissertation on what constitutes Madness where views I had at that particular time. For example, I now know that there is no truth about madness being a chemical imbalance in the brain and psychiatry is at worst a complete lie and at best a metaphor. In 1998 I wanted to believe this but was too scared to do so.

CHAPTER THREE

BREAKING THROUGH

Breakthrough records selected thoughts after A Can of Madness was published. Started as a sequel then I realised that surely no one's life is really that interesting or is it? Written post April 2002.

i) Punching through the wall

I was a raver that had a bad time... Such a bad time I didn't do much raving. But I lived and breathed it from the age of fifteen to seventeen, 24/7. There really were 20,000 hardcore knocking at my door. I could see them. It takes time to recover from taking five billion ecstasy tablets... one for everyone in the world... and then setting up a European Hardcore Committee, and heading it to instil world peace... that took a lot of effort... It was also a lot of responsibility...

I had to make sure that every girl in the world knew what it was like to be made love to... That was the best bit, and all it took was a bit of concentration, a bit of imagination you might say... It was a great feeling to make so many women happy... Then that in turn made their men... and other men happy (joke).

Follows naturally I suppose... Oh, but then I realised I was God... or was it Jesus. That was when it became too much to handle... It was too great a responsibility... I immediately felt guilty for all the pain and suffering in the world... Had I caused it? If I was omnipotent why couldn't I prevent it? Something had to be going on... Something underhand... Something dirty... Something sinister... and I was going to do something about it... Nobody else was doing it... Nobody else was capable...

Well something was going on and the media and the status quo have always feared it. There is a huge amount of

Bipolar, Recovery and NLP

stigma and discrimination attached to it across the board. That is why people who have "mental health issues" are commonly believed to breakdown, and not breakthrough. Well if that's so, and they are right, then I have broken down four times and not broken through yet. I mean, being given the label of someone who has bipolar effective disorder - no wonder I am programmed to think that I will always be liable to breaking down and that I can never be repaired, only at best patched up. Like a beaver dragging a tree across to a leaking dam, it seems impossible when you first see it. How do people recover from going loopy like that?

Breaking through wasn't even meant to be in my vocabulary. So when I broke through, as I call it, I was delighted. Delighted for myself because I had been through one hell of a ride, and delighted for others who had faced similar circumstances. Through what I had done I was able to create a platform for others to shine.

Other people who just needed an opportunity to be given an Equal life, whereas previously they had never had an opportunity so I set up Equal Lives. See www.equallives.org . Well, this was my mission. An ideal that the likes of men like Nelson Mandela or Gandhi fought for. Whenever we think of people like that, no matter how much money we have, no matter who we are, we all feel humble. That is the essence of humanity for me. We are all so weak and yet so strong and that is what pulls us together as well as pushes us apart.

So why was it such a fight for me to get my first book A Can of Madness in the public domain? There are several reasons. Having a manic marketing it i.e. myself was one difficulty, who knows, maybe it helped. Well that is because manic depression is a taboo subject; people don't want to talk about it, even though mental health affects all of us in some way. After all, we all have it.

Bipolar, Recovery and NLP

We all have mood swings and we are all influenced by circumstances and day to day activity. Some of us more than others, that's true. Some of us can hide it away, some of us have better coping strategies but we're all human. That is what makes life exciting, what makes life durable. Without pain and pleasure it would be monotonous and two-dimensional. None of us can deny that we are vulnerable and this is how I chose to define the term mental illness.

In April 2002 I had the book launch for A Can of Madness in the Lavender pub in Vauxhall. This would start me on a tiring journey in which I would commit to making the world a better place to live in for anyone who had been discriminated against, primarily mental health service users. Little was I to know what was to lie ahead.

It was the relentless manic energy that kept me going, that and the feeling that I knew what I was doing was essentially good for people who had been through a hard time. I never intended to be moralistic, or too pushy, in your face even, just believed in the concepts that I had created and wanted to develop them so that I could help every future manic-depressive in the world. Then, if I could help a manic, I could help a schizophrenic. If I could help a schizophrenic, I could help the homeless, drug addicts, ethnic minorities, the disadvantaged. I could change the establishment. I knew I would have to form alliances and I was prepared to sacrifice my life and privacy to just have a glimpse of a chance of changing the world in a small way. This was all possible, that was just about the only decent thing I learnt from the futility of Bacchanal raving. "Do what you want to do" was the old hardcore adage. So I did what I wanted to do. I mean, who doesn't, but things weren't easy, there was a lot going on.

I had to put up with other people's agendas, that was a difficult thing to come to terms with in the charity sector, especially when people are at first so friendly. It took me a while to come to terms with this. It's very hard to get a foot up. I'd self-published my initial book on the back of a

Bipolar, Recovery and NLP

Mind Millennium Award and distributed it to 300 charities and groups across the UK.

I'd met a printer on the way, Andrew Latchford, who encouraged me to set up a publishing company. Why not? I had no other form of income and we could sell my book through the company. So in August 2001 at the Mind annual conference I went round telling everyone about a website that never existed and a book that had not been finished. Fifteen months later I would be returning to do a book signing and waving a hand puppet Chipmunk around, who I was throwing around the stage. Why? Well my life had changed somewhat I guess.

Before I dive deeper into the mental health movement and my role within it and outside it, as an author, self-publicist, activist, speaker, politician, charity director, entrepreneur and public figure, I have a message for any young people who come close to losing their sanity. I hope enough young people will read this book and other positve stories written by people who have been mentally ill and that these books will make a difference, as it is the young generation of today who will have the power. They will be capable of reducing stereotypes and discrimination and change the media's negative attitude towards people with mental health issues after I'm gone.

It is young people who will shape the world in the future. At 30 I can still do a lot but I am already working with young people to encourage them to take over issues that the status quo cannot.

I shall begin by delivering this message in potentially the most powerful art form to do good in the next one hundred years. Rap music in my view, if it blossoms, will incorporate the ideals and dreams of the British youth. Let's face it, we're never going to have everyone going to the opera and listening large to Beethoven and Mozart. That is not to say that the amazingly peaceful and "traditional",

362

Bipolar, Recovery and NLP

aristocratic end of music can't be made more accessible, it can. Just read the rap and imagine it being played out to you by someone who cares about society, a philosopher even.

I'm writing a 100 raps to recovery
What the hell is this?
Yes .....
It's some kind of discovery
To raise awareness on mental health
And give us all some kind of real wealth
That is in your soul and not just your bank account
Because it's time to surmise,
Surprise and work out an account
Of how far you are prepared to go
To let all of the brothers know
What life is like inside the mind of a madman

Gonna stay pro-active and listen to the sad man
Was that s a a ad man or s A A D HA M M
Getting political now cause that's one way to go
If you wanna change the world then go with me flow
Before other people die and the flowers they don't
        grow

I'm looking into implementing regeneration
        in Lambeth, that's for Equal Lives
Gonna sort out my own borough, then do one at a
        time
Want to help Southwark out but they are doing real
        well
And my head starts spinning and my mind's in hell
Cause if I see too much suffering I'll be back in the bin
LIke being dropped by vintage Mike Tyson and landed on
        the chin

        The rap above shows how difficult it is to help others
when you are struggling yourself. What's needed is pro-
activity, strategic planning, a good heart and good people

amongst other things. For some it is too late, but they too still inspire and can leave their legacies.

> Starting my second 100 rap to recovery on Christmas
> Eve
> I've got many pieces of armoury hidden in me sleeve
> Too late for Pete Shaugnessey I do believe (Respect
> – Respect to this man – he did what very few
> others can)
> An inspirational super user who helped people breathe
> Gonna gain more momentum now that he has gone
> May the force be with me like Luke Skywalker and
> OB1
> Madpride and A Can of Madness they are one
of a kind
> Neither of them is afraid to speak their own mind
> Gonna save the user movement at the end of the day
> All of these individuals belong to us survivors   in
> some way
> Now I've made my point I hope I can hear you asking
> How can I really help instead of multi tasking?
> First you must make sure you can look after yourself
> It's unfair to bring your burdens onto someone else's
> shelf
> When your mind is steady and you're ready for action
> Send me an email and we'll start the contractions
> Breathe in for Chipmunkapublishing and out for Equal
> Lives
> These are both my creative visions, a limited company
> and a social enterprise
> Chipmunka publishes the stories of the mentally
> insane
> Equal Lives helps the poor communities who've
> suffered similar pain
> Both give the opportunity to live a better life than
> before
> So there's still hope for you if you listened to too much
> hardcore
> So if you see a rap event in your local neighbourhood

Bipolar, Recovery and NLP

Look out for the =Lives sign and motto we're doing
    some good
Like Chipmunkapublishing we are saving lives
Take the positive out of the negative and compromise.

Raps like these can be versed or adjusted to a global scale but then they are more likely to be misinterpreted. It is a dangerous tool that can so easily lead to gang violence and shootings and chasing the American Dream. Just as stories like A Beautiful Mind can be fictionalised because they have to adhere to Hollywood Liberalism. My wish is for this not to happen to A Can of Madness or any future dramatisation of a story on manic depression that is written in the same vain. That is why I want other people to make films of it. There are different versions already in the pipeline. I found the first interpretation hilarious, as it was so different to what actually happened and seemed so absurd.

All bodes well for the future… I think… Yes… Two Oscars… One for best screenwriter and one for best director of A Can of Madness… both in 2007… no that's too soon…2010… I'll be too old by then… and I'm more ambitious than that… let's settle for best screenplay in 2007… ok…ok…

Whenever I used to tell people this, they thought I was crackers. So I tend to hang around with a peer group with higher standards to confirm my self belief system.

Well, some people would look at my medical history and think I'm crackers anyway, so what's the difference. I've been a certified nutter for twelve years. Nothing has changed now, not in the eyes of the status quo, society, I've just told everyone about it that's all. Something changed for me though… and this is what gave me will power to go for my dreams. My philosophical view on madness developed after all the psychoanalysing I went through in my first book.

Bipolar, Recovery and NLP

At the end of A Can of Madness I was grateful for the cognitive therapy I'd gone through, grateful I was still alive but had no real philosophical depth on what I had experienced. I was simply too close to the abyss.

My major concern was to go around the country defending what I had written to people who might not like the book. I knew the memoir would upset my family. My grandmother tore it up. I knew it would upset my friends. I nearly fell out with one of the best friends I could ever imagine, let alone had and still fortunately have. I knew I would offend some women with my previous "misogynistic" antics. I knew the language would put a lot of people off but at the end of the day I'd prepared myself for all of this before. I was ready for it and have faced and will continue to face. As far as I am concerned people can like or dislike the book but to assassinate me as a person or the syntax of the book is a little unfair. That wasn't the point. The point was to reach out to others who had gone, and will go, through what I went through. Re-writing it was like reliving it. By the time I'd finished writing it I couldn't keep rereading it. I was still in shock.

I thought it was going to be a national success the day it came out. Rather like those manic moments... Sometimes positive feelings surfaced but always with the intense paranoia behind them. I was unable to determine what was really going on. I mean I was labelled with manic depression at 17 and had been on drugs before. I didn't know what being normal was like.

At the time of writing this I've swapped my anti depressants around. This was 6 days ago. Now I have 150mg of Venlafaxine in the morning instead of at night. This means I am less high and more real. More normal and more tired... More focused but less energetic... More focused and more set in the real world... but, after all, what is real? I wouldn't know what real was now if it stood in front of me and slapped me in the face. I'm also on a mood stabiliser –

Bipolar, Recovery and NLP

Sodium Valporate and an anti psychotic – Quetiapine. The Venlafaxine brought me out of my last depression. It helped save my life, or was it really me that saved my life because many people commit suicide when on and when trying to come off this terrible drug. I feel that somehow I am being lied to and psychiatry is the world's biggest propaganda tool. The drug companies use the psychiatrists as their drug pushers. Maybe I was lucky that I met a nice one or maybe I just had the luck of the draw or even the mental tenacity not to throw in the towel, yes like Rocky Balboa.

I've never tried committing suicide but I've spent two years of my mood well ingrained in the suicide mindset. It was only a few weeks ago that I first came up with a way of explaining how my friend felt when he committed suicide.

After a month's break I decided to carry on, with this that is. Me moods been a bit up and down me lads and lasses. The transition from taking the Venlafaxine at night to in the morning is pretty mind blowing to say the least. It's almost impossible to explain to a doctor or anyone for that matter. Also, a couple of times I've taken the pills at night instead of the morning, missed a dose, as if you take too much you go high, and then resumed. So I'm on the edge somewhat.

It was my birthday yesterday, 28, 21st of February 2003. A Pisces on his way to Hollywood who dreamed that coffee and cream at the Ritz costs £175. I went to where the cash register was and saw an old man with glasses sat down as if he was typing. This was reminiscent of my friend John Calder, who published Samuel Becket's poetry in the nineteen sixties. At one time Calder had 18 Nobel Prize winners on his books. Now he is struggling with the modern ways of the electronic publishing and printing world. He has an intellectual reputation that is well respected however. I gave a talk at his bookshop in Waterloo in January 2003 and the place was packed. Sixty people plus – it got a mention in

Bipolar, Recovery and NLP

the Guardian, which was my first mention in a national broadsheet as far as I am aware.

Then a few weeks later I appeared with my girlfriend Sonia in the Telegraph. I was the subject of a feature in the money section. This article was to have a massive impact on my life, but not due to the publicity that went with it.

Someone had seen the article in the paper that stated I'd sold 2000 copies of A Can of Madness. The same person had seen the fact that I received £9500 a year from housing benefit, DLA and Income support as well. Then they sent the article to the investigator's desk. I decided to make plans to escape from the benefit entrapment by the first of April. I refused to get lost in the negativity that the benefit system engulfs you in and within 6 weeks had broken out of the system and taken the bold step to grow my mental health utopian mission and look to manufacture a way of providing employment and self value to anyone who has ever been diagnosed with a mental health issue.

The article forced me to reassess my life and make changes. The experience had a positive outcome as it resulted in my decision to commit 100% to my mission to change the way the world thinks about mental health. Advice for service users and employment, DLA, advocacy etc... The information reported in the article was wrong. Put footnote listing exact date and title of Telegraph article.

Meanwhile Jamie, a fellow manic I'd met in a coffee shop in Green Park in February 2003, had done my first portrait. It inspired me to publish my third rap to recovery which I started to write in his presence.

> I'm looking at the picture and it's got to be said
> This guy is a manic, he looks off his head
> Yet controlled in some way me thinks as well
> Keep rapping and drawing like this we'll be
> doing swell

Bipolar, Recovery and NLP

Against the odds and we're one of a kind
The start of equality for the mentally ill I hope   you find
Like gay people started to be accepted when I was growing up
I turned to drink as an unaccepted manic but kept from throwing up
Felt so much pain that I made my stomach so strong
On the outskirts was tough on the inside was wrong
Took years to accept it then I got right
Determined to spend the rest of my life making   a fight
For the rights of the mentally insane
Whatever happens it will not be in vain
There's a connection with us manics like a parallel universe
The status quo is scared so it places a curse
But anything that's misunderstood is treated this way
Rise up to the challenge and win the day
Educate the media and public and fight for Equal Lives
We'll go Gandhi way before we use knives
How will we they treat us in 50 years time
Will they be embarrassed to be a friend of mine?
We're all human at the end of the day
A slight change in psychology then we've made our point
People will have empathy, no need to smoke a joint
Eliminating psychiatry with the help of psychiatry itself
An ideal to strive for to contribute to our mental wealth
Our mental health is getting better every single day
I hope to share this with millions of people
When we have the mental health live aid one day
This will be my first global rap performance in public live

Bipolar, Recovery and NLP

I'm a buzzing messenger from the mental health
hive
You try to get rid of us we'll sting you back
We fight for equality from the average hacks
Too many people and faces are fighting together
A community growing forever and ever

I found I could only write a part of the rap in front of
Jamie. The experience of having the portrait being done was
absorbing my mind too much. This though was a pleasant
experience as my passion for my mission is so strong that it
is only on rare occasions that I can lose my head in the
creativity of others. This is something I strive to do all of the
time but something that I find so difficult. It is as if the artist
within me is always manoeuvring itself to be out in the open.
Without being on the surface it would suffocate and I would
die.

The need for a creative outlet is something that is
necessary for manic-depressives. This is why I set up
Chipmunkapublishing as "The Mental Health Survivor's
Publisher". Writing helped me to express myself in ways that
I would be unable to otherwise. It gave me a voice in the
status quo where otherwise I would be silent. Without these
words writing them, rereading them and uttering these words
my mouth would be dry and my sight would be gone. I would
be unable to smell the part of the human spirit that makes
me want to be a part of mankind. I would not have wanted to
rejoin society, certainly not in a positive or meaningful way.

So writing has been more than therapy for me. It has
released the pain that I had and helped construct new belief
systems that I have. It has saved my life. The more and
more I realised that writing helped me and the more I
realised that it would help other people I came into contact
with in the mental health movement. The writing of my book
became a symbol of freedom from oppression in the way
that people with a mental illness suffered from stigma and
discrimination. The more I delved into the unjust world of

Bipolar, Recovery and NLP

mental health politics and assimilated it to my own view of the world and how the mentally ill were treated, the more my life became a mission to help others the way that I had somehow managed to help myself. This mission was a humanitarian one and remains so. It's born out of human instinct.

On October 19th 2002, Chipmunkapublishing released its second author Dolly Sen, and her autobiography The World Is Full of Laughter. I'd met Dolly a few months before when we were both helping mental health user groups in Lambeth. We swapped email addresses and away we went. Dolly is very shy in person and extremely active. She is one of the most charitable and selfless people that I have ever met, always helping people who are worse off than her.

Reading my book encouraged Dolly to write her own story. When I first read it I had a tear on my cheek for half an hour. The fact that my story could have inspired someone else gave me more strength to carry on the fight for justice. Through reading the book it was clear that Dolly had gone through the same cathartic process as I had. In her own amazing words "This book started out as a suicide note and ended up as a celebration of life". Dolly has had thirty years experience working as an actress and she refocused me on my dream to take my story to Hollywood and write it and direct it... how it really happened.

ii) Dolly Sen

I never aspired to be a publisher. I never even intended to write a book, especially an autobiography. I knew I would write a screenplay and had planned to be a film director but somehow I had allowed myself to get side tracked into doing this. It was for a great cause though and it was worth it, to help people like this. No-one else would help them get their books published. It was not financially viable for mainstream publishing companies to publish stories of mental distress. People do not want to hear depressing things. People run away from pain and the truth in this regard. It is a natural human instinct to protect oneself from this kind of unnecessary pain. Life is difficult enough to handle as it is.

As my confidence was growing I realised that I needed more from life than publishing. I needed my own importance to be recognised in a direct manner. I had a craving for fame. I wanted to use the celebrity status that I was going to achieve for the social good. Anyone who didn't believe that this was going to happen I would eject from my life. It was time to surround myself by only positive people.

People who believed that my dreams would come to the foreground and become an integral part of my life, as I lived them out. There was no reason that I could not fulfil all my other intentions, as a rap superstar, Oscar winning screenwriter and Hollywood film director whilst expanding Chipmunkapublishing and developing the Chipmunka Group. Confidence was the key, networking in the right circles and enhancing my delegation skills.

During 2002 I had promoted my story A Can of Madness. January 2003 until June 2003 had all been about planning. Redesigning www.chipmunkapublishing.com and developing a business plan with the Department of Trade and Industry. These strategic steps would ensure that Chipmunkapublishing would have a future in the 22nd Century. This would be a legacy that would have recorded a new genre of mad literature. It was a long-term plan to protect the social evolution that was taking place. The madman and/or woman would be accepted in society and would once again be revered instead of feared or ridiculed at every opportunity, by members of the status quo.

During the first six months of 2003 I also worked very closely with a man by the name of David Hart. A truly remarkable man with amazing energy despite having terminal cancer. He was a springboard for ideas and inspiration and a founder member of Equal Lives along with Dolly Sen. At the age of 64 David was Jewish and had a history as publisher of yachting and food magazines. He also said how he was a Times journalist for 30 years and was always taken to lunch by Rupert Murdoch every time Rupert visited London. I seized this opportunity and we became good friends. Once I'd read No Logo I became more in tune with his Liberal principles and was really effected by what I'd read about Globalisation. What particularly upset me was the slave labour that all the multinational companies like Nike would impinge on its workforce. Once things got hot they would just move country and exploit another workforce. These companies would pay only a few pence an hour, with forced overtime, living at work. These were the victims of Capitalist society.

In September 2003 I'd gone to Sri Lanka for two weeks and it was the first time that I had witnessed poverty that was so widespread. It humbled me. It made me realise that mental health was only a drop in the ocean. I realised and registered that most of the world and the third world didn't even have the right to have a mental health problem. They had to worry about disease and starvation and civil war. It made me feel less sorry for myself and with hindsight made me realise that there was more work ahead for me to find like minded people, and find a solution for these issues as well but first I had to come off the medication once and for all. I mean I could not go about curing people if I hadn't cured myself.

---

iii) GOODBYE EFFEXOR

This extract was written whilst I was coming off Effexor. This is a dangerous drug to come off I have heard of many people who have committed suicide as a result of coming off this drug. List number of suicide cases. Robbie Williams admitted he was hooked on this drug in a Daily Mail article in 2003.

Bipolar, Recovery and NLP

This section entitled Goodbye Effexor is not meant to offend anyone. I have to publish it to describe exactly how I felt when I as suffering the severe side effects from coming off it. People should not be allowed to take this drug or brainwashed into to taking other psychiatric drugs. We should have the right to live in a world which doesn't need psychiatric drugs. Since coming off psychiatric medication myself a year ago I have never been happier or healthier. This is a fact. Ask anyone who knows me personally. The people I condemn in this chapter are some of the most inspirational people that I know. This shows how devastating the side effects are.

Fuck Robbie Williams, still hooked on that Effexor. A manic depressive I hear and he does not have the balls to come out and say that he's got it. Think of all the fucking good he could do if this was true and he did what I was doing.

I've just come off that shite, Effexor. Fuck David Beckham and his first day wearing a Real Madrid jersey. Fuck Gerri Halliwell and her two autobiographies in eighteen months. Fuck Celebrity. Fuck the world and its capitalist mentality. Fuck the way it discriminates and ignores the people who need the help. Fuck the developed world for holding the third world back. Fuck you for reading this and not buying it and fuck me for writing it and for feeling sorry for myself.

Twenty-eight years of age and writing my second autobiography which is going to be published on the 10th of October 2003. Fuck that day when it comes. World Mental

Bipolar, Recovery and NLP

Fucking Health Day. We've got a big spread in the Big Issue on that day, Chipmunkapublishing that is. That's the little publishing company I set up to empower mental health survivors and their carers. Fuck the company and fuck Andrew Latchford the guy who encouraged me to set it up. Fuck all the authors who contact me and think that I am going to make them all famous. Fuck everyone who contacts me and wants me to advise them on this that and the other. Fuck John Bird the guy who set up the Big Issue who stood me up in Baker Street last week and left no apology. Fuck all those charities who ask me to give talks for free and ask me to write articles for their shitty newsletters.

Fuck all those charities that manipulated me in 2002 and used me for their own PR and self esteem. Fuck all the junk mail I have to open everyday from charities wanting another piece of me. Fuck everyone in the world for trying to prevent my insight and my vision coming through. Fuck David Hart from the Lambeth Strategic Initiative who acted as a mentor and spent five months still not paying the £1000 his organisation owed me.

Fuck my brother who owes me £1000 and has no intention of paying me back. Fuck him again for always asking me to give him more money whenever I speak to him. Fuck him for criticising the rest of the family. Fuck my mum and dad for not offering to assist with the fucking mortgage I am taking out. Fuck them both for remarrying and neglecting me and my brother. Fuck my step mum for "telling me that I ruined my life" the last time I was in Gloucester. Fuck my step dad for having cancer, still being alive and not letting my mum leave him and run off with her boyfriend. Fuck these drugs for making me think that I am gay.

Fuck the English fucking weather and fuck London for being up its own arse. Fuck the people in the city in their flash suits and cars. Fuck everyone who uses the tube and never makes any eye contact with me when I try and cheer people up. Fuck the British people for being so crap at

Bipolar, Recovery and NLP

foreign languages. Fuck the British music industry for being so simple and fake.

4th of June 2003

This is my life and these are my words. Nobody has altered them prior to publication.

The Effexor has now left my system. Comic Relief are playing football in the park. For the first time I notice the "All Nations Centre Apostolic Church" above me. An odd looking character walks by. I manage to turn my heart before him before he goes down St. Oswalds place. I stop on the corner of Wickham Street where Sonia got mugged. The guy who used to collect the glasses out in the stripper bar ignores me as I raise my eyebrows and write. He looks behind himself with guilt knowing I know something he doesn't know.

Coming off Effexor has been a blessing in disguise so far. I came off it immediately. I'd been going high so stopped the 150mg dose and then stayed off. My world changed as I came off the drug. I'd had a meeting with my caring Doctor, Teif Davies and my girlfriend. I made a conscious decision to come off it in a positive way. I thought of Dawn Rider and his anti drugs member's community in the US. They had sent me 54 case studies of people who had come off Effexor and committed suicide. I knew of the horror stories but I came off the drug in a positive light and this made me avoid any kind of cold turkey.

June 2003 was to be another turning point in the life of Jason Pegler. My computer crashed at the beginning of the month, a few days later I was off the Effexor. I was disorientated and confused. The computer crashing woke me up to the fact that I had been spending far too much time at home on the computer. I was turning into an introvert when what I needed was to see interact with society.

376

Bipolar, Recovery and NLP

I set about seeing London via the buses. Gone were the days when I was going to rush around everywhere on the tube. I was going to take the bus and watch the world go instead of constantly trying to confirm my position.

My whole work schedule would change. Gone were the days when I would invite people round to Chipmunka headquarters for a meeting. I would observe London and see the key people. I would only speak to MD's and chief Executives when it came to sponsorship. Speak to people who made the decisions. Enough of this being polite and not getting anywhere like.

I'd decided that I was not going to be exploited by any of these charities anymore. Throughout 2003 every charity I'd met had tried to take advantage of me in some way or other and so had every business man. Well now the real Jason Pegler was arriving back on earth after suffering the side effects from this strong medication it was payback time.

I set about playing the game in my terms and on my own rules. June 2003 I went undercover, travelling around London, playing the fool, appearing on the outside as if I were a tourist. Asking people for directions when in reality I was directing myself. The more abstract things became, the more I understood them. Not because I was manic but because I had a sense of humour, I had my own vision and creativity and was not side tracked by the mission's and messages of others. I started to understand the world subliminally and in a practical way. I realised more and more that what goes around comes around. Jules Mascarenhas had taught me that. The Producer who made a documentary about me and two other depressives. Initially we had discussed 20% - 33% deal for me, and then when the filming was complete he offered me 1%. Well I signed it off and just requested 10 videos and the ownership of some photos he had taken for my book cover. I though that he had done those as a friend but had he hell. He was out to bleed me

Bipolar, Recovery and NLP

dry man, just like everyone else so it seemed, apart from people like Dolly.

Thing is, in life, you need to know when to let go. There is no point in wasting energy. Remember in the Bronx Tale when the boy is chasing the guy who owes him $30. His gangster mentor, Chaz Palminteri, comes over and says well done. You got this guy out of your life for thirty dollars. Leave it. "He's a bum". Well Jules Mascarenhas – and everyone out there in Hollywood – you are a bum too.

Another rule I learnt in June 2003 was to only deal with the facts. Lambeth Strategic Initiative had received a cheque on behalf of Equal Lives (the organisation I had set up to positive discriminate for people who do not have Equal Lives) on January 14th. Well after being told most days for five months my patience snapped and I had to demand the money back. The upsetting thing was that the co-chair of this organisation was David Hart, my friend, yet another mentor. The man I had based my entire social enterprise around since I'd met him in October 2002. After having a tip off from a couple of friends who made me question the genuineness of this man I became more aware and realised a big truth. One can only deal with facts in life and not on supposition.

During these few weeks I felt a huge sense of betrayal and confusion, especially whilst having the side effects of the meds. When I put the cheque into context it became more and more important. A man had promised me the earth and delivered nothing, except handing books out he was meant to sell and giving me more and more responsibility for the community. I'd also been waiting for six months for an article to go in the Times. That just wasn't happening either. Things were starting to add up. It just went to show that you can't trust anyone in life except for yourself, not even your family. No wonder so many people have pets.

By the end of June 2003 I'd performed on stage twice as a rap freestyler, MC JASE. Both of my

performances were at Madpride events and had an
audience of over a couple of hundred of people. My
confidence had grown and enthusiasm was sparked even
more when I met this Rastafarian gent Fred Peters who set
up Kennington Youth Club amidst the Brixton riots in the
80s. Fred played the piano as I rapped and gave me the
confidence to improvise my rapping which I knew would take
me on a fulfilling and empowering road where I could be a
kind of Eminem, with a social meaning behind it. The second
venue was at The Garage at Highbury and Islington and
there I gave my first interview under the pseudonym MC
Jase.

iv) The significance of John Breeding

*The moment I read John Breeding's book entitled
'The Necessity of Madness' my perception of the "mentally
ill" changed forever. I realise that mental health really is a
social construct and something that the mind self manifests.
I understood how psychiatry is a form of social control and
that I could empower people so that they could make a full
recovery. It was in the moment of my decisions that I
decided to come off medication for good that I took
ownership of my life again and became emotionally free of
societies burden of living with manic depression.*

Breeding made me really see that I could take those
final steps to recovery and that if I combined his intellectual
abilities with the coaching methods of Anthony Robbins that
I too could change the world and make the world a better
place. By consistently caring about the "mental health" of
myself and therefore other people I could encourage
generations of people to step up and raise their standards so

that they would refuse to be "mentally paralyzed" by their own fears and the inadequacy of the status quo.

Just as Michael Moore so cunningly reveals the other side to Bill Clinton and the White House, I could focus on a positive image on "mental health" that would create the first brand of its kind so the Scientologist could go for the jugular with their citizens' campaigns for human rights that they had started in 1969.

CHAPTER FOUR

RAPS TO RECOVERY

Any lyrics written below are not meant to upset anyone or incite any kind of violence. The lyrics were written whilst I was on psychiatric drugs. Any reference to language that could be deemed offensive has been published to illustrate my feelings whilst experiencing damaging side effects on various medications. I believe that rap music can be used as a means for freedom of expression and is therefore a force for social good.

Bipolar, Recovery and NLP

The Jason Pegler Announcement –
Raps to recovery

Anyone trying to use the work of MC Jase will be crucified. Need I say you?! That includes you, Mr Mel Gibson, your father and Quentin Tarantino – unless you pay Jason Pegler 21/02/75 that's 21/02/75, 1 billion dollars up front and reduce world suicide you're at it.

MC JASE

I'm MC Jase
And I'm off my face
With my Mace
I'm a headcase
Certified as a nutter when I was 17 years old
Right now I've got hair no cancer so I'm not bold.
Enough to feel sorry for myself
This MC is always full of stealth
Leading an army empowering mental health
Taking time to build up my strength
Using different media types and length
Whole empire is growing by word of mouth
First North, West, East and finally South.
Too many tasks for the multi skilled
Keep observing others then get off those pills
3 months more of Quetiapine
3 years of Valporate then off the gin
Back to reality, human being again
Diary of a madman discriminatory like man.
Creative voice is heard in prose
Better than breaking somebody's nose.

3/4/01   Poll Vault

Here's a tune for vault recordings, you know who I mean.

Bipolar, Recovery and NLP

I've been to fuckin' prison, at least, I might as well have
     been.
We're a hot new record label with lots of wicked stuff,
     so if you've been listening to shit, we think you've
     had enough.
I've been rapping for a while, in lots of different ways.
Been through more shit than Eminem & I'm not afraid of
     gays.
I've seen a world of madness, where most people couldn't
     go,
and occasionally I return, when my mind goes to and fro.

  I've got madness on the brain (Cypress Hill thought they
     were insane)and I know it causes pain,
But, I have to tell my homies,
Cause my thoughts drive me insane.

I saw violence growing up, in my home and neighbourhood.
I used to get badly picked on, coz my brain was fuckin' good.
There were NWA and 2 Live Crew for a teenager growing up
The only sense of security was my Alsatian pup.
There was petty crime and drug dealing that I undertook.
Sometimes I was rather fortunate to get off the hook.
There were women everywhere but not as many as Snoop,
And I've been so fucking sick; I'm still waiting for my coup.

I've got madness on the brain
and I know it causes pain.
But, I have to tell my homies,
to stop them from doing the same

I remember knocking out a copper, when my mate lived in a
     squat,
I was so fucking paranoid; I thought the place was hot.
When I told my teacher that I was dealing drugs at school,
She burst out crying and said that she felt like a fool.
I had a good education and didn't take advantage of it,
Now I realise I was fortunate, and that I'd acted like a tit.
Never used to go to school, I would lie there in my bed.

Bipolar, Recovery and NLP

If I had my time again, I know the books I would have read.

I've got madness on the brain (and it's driving me insane),
Getting better at the game,
And I have to tell my homies,
To stop them from having the same.

Had so many fights, it's impossible to add them up,
Won them all apart from one, but I never had a cup.
A sovereign ring broke my nose and I broke my jaw myself,
The scar on my face from a screwdriver arose from clumsy
        stealth.
So I've been through loads of agro and now I've quietened
        down,
And if you try to wind me up, I'll probably just frown.
Don't push me or my crew too far, cause you will never
        know,
how far we've come and been, and how far we're willing to
        go.

Seen madness now I'm tame (it was driving me insane),
Getting better at the game.
And I have to tell my homies,
Cause they've helped make MC Jase's fame.

When I operate on the mike, there are many things to do,
Philosophise and educate, but mostly, I entertain all of you.
There were bad things in my early days,
But now I've changed my ways.
Now I'm a real citizen,
As the past becomes a haze.
Still mentally insane, and it's a shame, I'm not to blame.
'Cause it causes so much pain, to tell people my real name.
Must stay on medication, so I can rejoin my generation,
Must not forget, or relapse, or I could embarrass the X.

I've seen madness; now I abstain (slow)
I've already made my claim.
I thank my homies, then and now,

Bipolar, Recovery and NLP

For putting up with my burning flame.

Gotta get it right for the world,
Make it all a better place.
And then it will be worthwhile, to have rapped…….
yours truly…….the lyricist……..and MC Jase.

3 minutes 40 seconds

19/06/01   **Alcohol**

Things were going wrong when I used to hit the bottle
Used to sit there and talk about who I'd throttle
Now there's homies round these flats
And everywhere I go I'm surrounded by twats
But at least they know their hip hop
And I know I'm going to the top
Of the rap music industry
That's DJ Fraudster and me
The Vauxhall boys gonna take over
A rapper and a composer
We don't give a fuck about no life
That's only covered in strife
Might as well just end it all now
Than try to figure out how
But then I guess that'd be copping out
And we're made of metal there's no doubt
We're gonna crucify the rest
Because together we're the best
Whether it's free style or rehearsed
Our magic bubble gonna burst
And we're grateful to Eminem
That mad rapper can be a gem
He's bringing hip hop over here
And that makes it really clear
That we're gonna go for it
Because we've been through too much shit

Bipolar, Recovery and NLP

We're gonna bounce back off the mike
And mix some tunes that give a spike
Cause we're really into this game
And we really want and need that fame, MC Jase

5 minutes
Rhyme and Reason

Rhythm, rhyme and <u>reason,</u> is for all of the four <u>seasons</u>
So when this rapper wants to <u>show</u> which route he's gonna
       <u>go</u>
There's some logic in his <u>mind</u> and a story you will find
About the <u>world</u>.
Yeah the <u>world</u> and what it's like
About life; and all the <u>strife</u>.
About how to cope with it, instead of feeling shit
The troubles that begin
Whether big, fair, huge or thin
This rappers really gonna be
No 1 for eternity + philosophy
Cause I got poetry that makes <u>sense</u>
An understanding of anthropology that's <u>intense</u>
I gotta hold of the mike and I won't let go
Wanna make me famous and make some dough
So I can set myself up and my future family
(speed up) And prepare for any traumas that may affect me
Gonna entertain the crowd in a different way
No bullshit, or gangster rap but memories from the day
Tunes that will stay in peoples minds
And words that are targeted to open blinds

Cause I want people to learn from doing wrong
And I want them to sing this song
I want their lives to be fulfilled
I don't preach, I'm just chilled

(Slow) out. That's child out.
And I've been there,

Bipolar, Recovery and NLP

well into despair.
And I got out. Just about
and it was hard, to play my last card.
I kept guard and although my life was marred,
I escaped to have my music taped
And then a record deal,
hoes, nice suits and a flash car.

Vauxhall Crew

Rapping now for the Vauxhall generation
Dolly Sen's drum and bass, the new sensation
Council estates must get rid of crack
And get these broken community spirits back.
Time for the hardcore music to make sense at last
Things boring, normal, then too fast.
I'm just a manic depressive at the end of the day
Want me to get a job and join society, no way.
Too much stigma and discrimination going on round here
Feel guilty for mentioning it, must drink beer.
Something's not quite right me, rapping here today.
I'm white, manic, not homophobic or gay; at least that's what
        I say.
Social evolution is what's happening now
Multicultural society ends the racism row
Equal lives must unite across the universe
Positively helping the status quos perversed
I'm so tired now I could end my life
Preaching like a bell end about my strife
Mental illness is a horrible thing
Mentally ill in Amityville makes my ticker ringer
Laughing at reality is an ingenious way
To forget the fucking label that ruins my day
My friend jumped off a bridge not so long ago
Couldn't stop that but with these words I grow
Next time you see a schizophrenic in the paper
OPEN YOUR FUCKING MIND!
DON'T LEAVE THESE LUNATICS BEHIND!
Help them out

Bipolar, Recovery and NLP

Cause we're all human beings at
The end of the day
Even us Manic Depressives
Who don't know what to SAY?
Time to Heal

There's still time to heal.
Time to heal, for real.
Stop making bad motherfucka's and be more like brothers.
So there's time to heal for real, and bad motherfucka's can
        turn into brothers.
That's turn motherfucka's into brothers.

There's racism all over the world, so rap is everywhere.
Just listen to a great rapper, and tell me that you don't care.
They'll fill your mind full of truth, intensity, love and questions
That's with philosophy, psychology and their best intentions.

And in multicultural societies all over the globe,
Rap is a language that can reach everyone's abode.
Get rid of the gangster rap lifestyle, that people aspire to,
And substitute it for real rapping, that makes people do what
        they do.

We can still keep the element of fun, shock and crazy shit,
But rid the world from images of nigga's causing all the shit.

Blacks have been oppressed and that's a fact,
Time they made amends instead of getting whacked.
And if it takes a mad white man, to help them along their
        way,
Then so be it, I dedicate myself.
I don't care if people think I'm gay.
And I don't care if people think that I'm wasting my time
It's all mine and I'll do it without expecting a dime.
Because it's my craving out of a necessity,
Want to help solve the disease I see,
People not together and fighting each other's ass,
When all they need to do is hut, hut, hut, look up and pass.

Bipolar, Recovery and NLP

Yeah. Pass the ball to each other
And turn the bad motherfuckers into brothers.
Cause there's still time to heal.
Time to heal for real.
And I want to stop bad mother fuckers
And help turn them into brothers.
Then us brothers, can say thank you, to our mothers.

So next time you're burning some weed and listening to
        Death Row,
Remember that if a brother pulls out a g-lock its time to go.
No need to hang around and act too tough,
Because one thing is for sure,
You've both already suffered enough.
Once you get away from the violence and killing,
Can start enjoying things, and make life more fulfilling.
There are so many things, out there to do.
It's a tragedy to die young, a tragedy for you.
70% of rap records are bought by middle class whites,
So there's hope for the rest of us and room for more party
        invites.

Yeah. Pass the ball to each other
And turn the bad mother fucker's into brothers.
Cause there's still time to heal,
Time to heal for real.
And I want to stop bad mother fuckers,
And help turn them into brothers.
Then us brothers, can say thank you, to our mothers.

As this rapper starts out his career,
There's one thing you should know.
He's gonna rhyme like kid n play and know exactly when to
        let go
Of the mic to let the melody and backing vocals intervene

Cause he has an intuitive understanding of narrating the
        obscene

Bipolar, Recovery and NLP

That's a comical element of rap that is always here to stay
As there's nothing wrong with healthy sex not even if you're
      gay
Better to have a world full of orgies and open sexuality
Than one based on vengeance
And shooting mother fuckers in the knee.

Juice and Gin

When you Dogg Pound Crew gonna let JCB come in?
I've spent all this time sipping on juice and Gin.
And I see the great Eminem,
So cool that he can't rap about race
Well I'm not afraid, 'cause I've been to every place.
Know what it's like to be mad, then you know what I mean.
I've endured it and recovered from it, you should have seen

SEEN IT.
Seen the shit.
And I've endured it.
And I've still got my wit

My heads going to explode 'cause I write raps so quick.
And I've got no boundaries, so I'm gonna make you sick.
And tell you of all the troubles in the world, that 2pac talks
      about.
And I'll be accurate as well, of that…there is no doubt.

About drugs, a life of crime (pause) bitches,
Money and a life of irresponsibility (27)
About guns, sex, fighting, booze, prison,
And love, decisions and insecurity. (20)
There's nothing I won't tell.
I'll tell everything that's on my mind.
My honesty bodes well,
At least, that's what I hope you'll find.

Bipolar, Recovery and NLP

Cause life's hit me so hard I've no longer got a guard.
I'm opening my heart for the benefit of art.
A music known as rap,
Which upper class people think is crap.
But its music that is real,
That's music that you can feel.
Not like that ancient shit,
That makes me have a fit

Rap makes one feel at home…unlike the millennium dome.
It's more valuable than chrome.
Yes, more valuable than Rome

Rap is a kind of music that is here to stay.
Its essence is too important, for it to ever go away.
Compounding more out of racism in 60's America.
There are many scars that I'll be telling ya.
These mother fucka's ain't healed yet.
If you think they have, you're a fool, I'll bet.
Black people had a rough time at the hands of whites,
And their bound to want revenge from societies ugly shites.
Remember when a black man couldn't go in the same bar as
         a white,
Well it takes a long time and a lot of education to forget that
         shite.

In time, generations can forgive that shit,
And rap is the only mass way to convey it bit by bit,
For church ain't that popular anymore,
It's too antiquated for the young.
They're more likely to get pissed off, get hold of a gun.
Get the bastards back for making them hooked on crack,
For if you move to the hood it's hard to get back on track.
There's a lot of discipline needed to make a good rapper,
Need to educate, without preaching, and entertain the foot
         tapper.

Bipolar, Recovery and NLP

JCB 1

Now ev-ery body <u>listen</u>… to me
Stepping up on this mike… is <u>JCB</u>
Joining my crew… is the thing to do
(That means) telling other people what happened to you
Honesty is the name of the game
Making others feel the (empathy) for your pain.

It's time to take the ride that was slip – er, ey.
As Coolio did it, then so can we
No need for the gin we just need the juice
Cause Snoop Doggy Dogg is a bit different than Proust
He may (be the best) rapper that's still alive
But sometimes (that gangsta stuff stings) <u>like</u> a beehive

It can, encourage youngsters to get the wrong end of the
        stick
Make them sell crack and think through their dicks
Causing teenage pregnancy on the estates
Making life even harder than social policy dictates
Black people born into poverty all the time
Not surprising is it – really – that there's so much crime

I ran 100 miles to see NWA
Then the Fugees made me stop and find another way,
Developed my own philosophy to help the disadvantaged,
Reflected on my life – knew I was privileged,
2pac gave me strength to make my quest reality
Although he is dead he gives me psychic energy

Like O B 1 <u>Kenobie</u> in the (Star Wars trilogy)
Let Darth-Vader <u>win</u> to deceive his enemy.
<u>Luke</u> felt the force and got stronger every day,
JCB will win YES I'm going to save the day!

Going to stomp all the crime by reducing ignorance,

Bipolar, Recovery and NLP

First, bring different cultures together – give them all
significance.
Lots of ways to do this – make them part of the UK,
Join up with So Solid Crew – they may behave in a different
way.
They describe things as they've seen them in Battersea they
say,
So I give them my respect – now I should tell you about
myself.

Born and bred in Gloucester with sex, drugs, booze, and
women
Everything seemed stable until I developed manic
depression.
Trying to stop a nuclear war that was only in my mind,
Making all these assumptions that I could never find.
Went from mania to paranoia at the click of a manic gun,
I was certified a madman, therefore crazier than everyone.

When JCB was seventeen I was hospitalised for my mental
health.
In the years to follow this would seriously affect my wealth.
Really hit rock bottom when I realised what I'd thought,
One minute saving the world then humiliated and distraught.
Spent six months mad and suicidal in a mental institution,
A miscarriage of justice planted the seeds for a revolution

Diagnosed with a mental illness it took ten years to accept it

I managed to sort my head out for the very first time…

Start bringing different cultures together and making them
chime.

Bipolar, Recovery and NLP

A Can of Madness

Now, I was forced to go into a mental asylum,
At seventeen years of age,
And some years later I wrote about it
And cried on every page.
It was not recalling the experience itself that made me really
        weak,
But telling people about it and letting them here me speak.

I spent a long time writing and getting my book published.
The government gave me funding which stopped me feeling
        dissed.
I would give the first 300 sales to charity,
Fuck me, thanks to Mind,
I'd been given an opportunity.

There are so many things in life that I want to achieve.
But I only get so much time so it's difficult to
        alleviate the pressure,
As I don't know where to prioritise
Cause I don't know about all that gangster shit,
I don't feel wise.

I grew up in Gloucester,
Which I thought was really good
Cause there were so many nutters in my neighbourhood.
Then one day I grew up and realised,
It was all an urban joke

Cause by the time I left, I'd kicked the fuck,
Out of almost every bloke

Then I went to Manchester, to go to University
I was meant to study Classics but I tried to be a G.
With my mates working on the door, and me shifting my shit,
Life was made more fruitful with a regular piece of clit.

Bipolar, Recovery and NLP

There were bitches and hoes more regular than before,
And it was nice to be called a stud,
Instead of a fucking whore.
I was popular at Uni,
till my drinking took control.
I'd have six litres of strong cider,
Then piss on the remote control

I was violent all the time, and generally depressed.
But when I played football I had the talent of George Best.
There were many things going on when we lived in Mosside.
Living next door to a borstal helped make us the law abide.

You see this started moral questions going on in my mind.
I became too drunk to do anything evil for mankind.
Recovery wouldn't happen for several years,
That's why my fucking memoir is so full of tears.

Jase August 8th 2001

Where is love

I was white now I'm black
In this multicultural trap
There's a vision of the world I have as well
To combat prejudice and stigma and remove this hell
A manic man, who's too scared to say it,
Once he reveals he'll have to pay for it

But the world is changing and societies gotta answer
Got me homies with me and my ghetto blaster
Doin' the right thing for the segregated
You are of the alienation that you've created
Accept people for what they are when you meet them
Don't judge pre-emp or abuse or try to defeat them

Where's the black representation in this society
Gangsta rappa's and priests only is not diversity
Everyone else come out of your shell

Bipolar, Recovery and NLP

Let bygones by bygones we might as well.

Ode to Slim Shady

Eminem can fuck it
I'll saw his head off
And put it in a bucket

People call him the rabbit
That makes me Big Wig
Dod damn it

I can run 8 million miles
So watch it!

Hang on let me think
I can't saw an idol's head off
That would be very disconcerting.

Ode to Slim Shady 2

Been rappin' 10 minutes,
Eminem can shit it.
Been a manic depressive since 17
And he thinks he's losing it.
Ain't got not grit for a bit, or a tit
I'm beat, I was neat,
But popped pills and was defeated.

Ode to Slim Shady 3

Eminem I want to love you
But my hearts not full of shit
There's people dying shady
And you joke in spite of it
My dad can't understand you
His wife thinks you're a Dog
I'm understanding what you mean

Bipolar, Recovery and NLP

But you got to do it my way now shady.

Bipolar, Recovery and NLP

8 Billion Miles

Another rap to recovery is stepping up tonight,
Regenerating the urban generation used to give me a fright,
Now it's an automatic humanitarian goal,
To take the community in and its heart and soul,
MC Jase alive returning to the house that Jack thought he
       built,
Too many mistakes in the box and they're covered in guilt,
Manufactured rappers not writing their own lyrics,
Feeling sorry for themselves their bullies and cynics,
Waiting for the sunlight to rise on this beautiful day,
Gonna stop this gangster rap nonsense and spread positivity
       my way,
Twenty four hours till things turn around,
Humanitarian goals for your breath, sight and sound,
Not born in the ghetto but been to hell and back,
Caused by ecstasy and a manic depressive attack,
Eight years after then I bounced back,
Cured myself and helped others to heal,
Thought I was crazy when I listened to Seal,
He's not crazy this manic depression is real
With these amphetamines, lsd and ecstasy I was fucked
Paralysed on psychiatric drugs
So I turned into a thug and fucked people up
One street brawl lost and the next 50 won,
My life nearly ended before it begun,
Things going on, people too scared to face up to want their
       dream,
Receiving your destinies, easy, just don't let your brain
       steam,
Life is worth living don't ask me that question,
Stop using other models; make your own invention,
Equal lives for all and Chipmunks unite,
A multi media movement to give you some fucking rights
To make things open up and get us out of this dump
Smile, laugh, do a parachute jump.

CHAPTER FIVE

HELLO HOLLYWOOD

June 2003 saw Jason Pegler film himself for the very first time. The experience was eleven years in the waiting. Ever since he was seventeen he had envisaged filming his own experiences of manic depression. Then he realised he only needed a computer.

The Movie Script to 'Cans of Madness' is a great example of an incantation[33]. When writing I imagined that the screenplay was already successful and that it had already reached Hollywood. As I now write we are already making Chipmunka films in house. This comes across in the autobiographical script as well and was one of the main driving forces that enabled me to write it in the first place.

Another Incantation:

After 12 years of being on psychiatric medication Pegler finally chose to come off the crippling drugs with the help of his imaginary life coach Anthony Robbins. By the time Pegler finished his script he was nearing 30 and was Young Social Entrepreneur of the Year 2005. The crusade that had begun in 1993 at the age of 17 to break down the mental health taboo once and for all now had the ammunition it needed to deliver. All that was needed was to sell the script for an eight figure sum that could be used for social good and produce films that would fill Pegler's utopian mission in house. Everything was beyond Pegler's ego. Inside his mind was an automated mission to help other people, by changing the way Hollywood though about mental health and therefore, the whole world at large.

---

[33] Anyone who wants to learn more about incantations should read "Awaken the Giant Within" by Anthony Robbins.

Bipolar, Recovery and NLP

Initial Cast Envisioned for:

A Can of Madness/Cans of Madness:

Jason – Jason Pegler/ Tom Cruise
Brad – Johnny Depp
Sonia – Penelope Cruz
Dad – Michael Caine
Harry – Brad Pitt
Mum – Bridgette Fonda
Gina – Halle Berry
Meredith – Nicole Kidman
Felix – Robbie Coltrane
Mark – Gary Oldman
Dom – Tom Cruise
Ed – Liam Neeson
Claire – Glenn Close

Bipolar, Recovery and NLP

A Can of Madness/Cans of Madness
The Screenplay by Jason Pegler ™
December 2004 – April 2005

Part 1

Club scene: 5 min
Quiet Room/table tennis/changing clothes/brad leaves: 11 min
Internal dialogue 1 and 2/Prodigy: 5 min
Jason's Dad and Internal Dialogues: 7 min
3 months later: 1 min
Ward round: 4 min (33mins)

Part 2

Uni Fight scene: 4 min
Chorlton/moss/trav mania: internal dialogue. 12 min
Uni visit: 2 min
Dr Clarke's 3 min – Sunday coffee
Final exam tripping 5 minutes
Graduation =4m (+30m=63min)

Part 3

Prozac Nation: 5 minutes
Narrative: move to London, meeting Sonia, Miami 4 mins
Psychologist final Meeting: 3 meetings
Dr Davies meeting: 3 minutes
TV – 4 minutes
4 Writing and finishing script with Girlfriend 2 minutes
3 Making of film: 2 mins
2 Hollywood living + Oscars meeting Jack Nicholson/cameo role: 2 mins
1 Saturn and manic vision: 2 minutes.
----
87 mins + Psychology

All set in UK except for Jack Nicholson scene.

401

Bipolar, Recovery and NLP

32 scenes all together.

The film begins in the depths of a hardcore club in Swindon in the mid 1990s. The atmosphere is dark, packed and extremely noisy with a 50K indoor system blasting out and an MC refusing to leave the stage. There are three people stood on platforms and the camera zooms in on one of them, a teenager called Jason. His eyes are dilated and he is sweating in a trance like state.

MC: 'It's ten past 3.00 in the morning and we're going nowhere. Speaker box climbers get off the stage you are distressing it for everyone. Now let's dance to some real deafening madness. Are you ready? That's nothing like loud enough. I said, are you ready?'

JASON: 'Can you dig it? Yes. I can dig it'.

MC Robbie Dee: 'I said it's gone ten past three in the morning and we're going absolutely nowhere. We were meant to finish at 3.00am but we are pumping up the hardcore especially for you. Right now…There is no escape… Loving it…. (Fantasia back to the future theme tune… lets go…. is here in the back ground…).

Jason starts matching the sound of the recorded tape in unison with the beat.

'Da da da da.. da da da… da da da da da da da…
'Da da da da.. da da da… da da da da da da da…

HARDCORE: Let's go… into the future

As the repetitive sounds continue Jason starts giving it the hardcore with all his might. He moves his whole body in time with the music and has an extraordinary amount of energy coming directly from his inner self. He seems as though he

Bipolar, Recovery and NLP

is on some kind of spiritual journey as the deafening music makes 2000 people go absolutely mental. Back to the MC who starts shouting, interrupting the repetitive beats but somehow allowing them to continue and giving them new found meaning and enlightened significance.

MC ROBBIE DEE: (music from Fantasia Second Sight) To all of those who know the score how's about a little bit of hardcore... goes a little something like this... don't forget to hang the DJ... but not this DJ... for this is the one and only DJ Ratty... and if you double cross this DJ... there is only one way you can go... Straight to hell... dive into the abyss... and there is no way you are coming out. No way you're ever going to come out.... Because there'll be 20,000, yes 20,000 bleeding hardcore knocking at your door. No way out. Yes no way fucking out... so stay off those fucking speakers and pump up the hardcore...into the future...Into the future...Yes whaooooooaaayyy yeah (sound of woman's voice on tape), we'll live as one family.... Last one for the night for all you boys and girls here's MC Robbie Dee bringing it down... previously cooking up your brain... been cooking up your brain but now bringing you down softly.... Bringing you down nicely.... Alright matey.... Let yourselves go.....

Whaaaoooaaaaayy... whaaaoooaaayyy we'll live as one family..... We'll live as one family.........

This scene needs a lot of impact. It should be 5 minutes in length. (It could be a manic voice over or extract from the book about being a raver or manic moment epitomising excitement/narrow-mindedness/futility of rave culture).

The camera focuses back on Jason's forehead profusely sweating and onto his mouth singing the strong sounds of the woman's voice. Now into the mouth, and onto the next scene, where a tape is seen being played playing the same music from above.

Bipolar, Recovery and NLP

Two young men, who look like ravers, are sat in an oversized room. They are in a mental institution. There are several old chairs and an old stereo. The curtains are open and it is dark outside. Noticeably there are great big bars on the only window.

BRAD: 'great night, I remember that one. That MC Robbie Dee is proper crazy. We'll live as one family. Wa ooohh yaaa. What did you say they call this? The quiet room hey... well its not the quiet room anymore... we've just impregnated it... Still I can see you need to get away from those loons in there and get some piece once in a while. I know I would if I were in here. How ya feeling?

JASON: Like I know the score... how's about a little bit of hardcore...

BRAD: You are still a bit off your head mate... how long you going to be in here do you reckon?

JASON: As long as it takes to save the world. I took 5 billion ecstasy tablets last night. One for everyone in the world, so I could create world peace by making the world live as one family. That meant that I could make love to every woman in the process. Not bad for one night's work.

BRAD: [Pauses looking worried for a split second] Wow really... don't worry mate you'll be out of here soon. You've got a good head on your shoulders. When you get better you'll be stronger for it. Your heart's in the right place.

JASON: Whhaaoo ayy. We'll live as one family. Want a game of table tennis?

BRAD: 'sure let's do it. Bro... let's go...

JASON: Into the future...

Bipolar, Recovery and NLP

[A little pause, Brad looking worried, turns into a laugh and then a smile]

BRAD: You're amazing you are… come on…

JASON: Let's go… into the future…

[Brad laughs out loud]

They proceed into a white corridor and then into a big lounge where there are about 15 patients sat down watching TV. Most of them are smoking. A couple of old grannies are knitting. Coronation Street is on in the background. The game of table tennis is a strange affair. Both players are quite good being able to hit the ball over at a reasonable pace. Strange thing is that Jason tries smashing the ball when it does not seem possible. This must be a sign of boredom or perhaps he actually believes he can pull the majority of these ridiculously hard shots off. He tries ludicrous shots and loses the first game 21-11. Then just before the second game starts we start to get a real indication of just how off his head Jason really is.

JASON: I'm just going to change…Into the future. I'm going to get out of here now. I'll be back.

Jason walks backwards deliberately… pointing at his back while he leaves the room. Brad laughs and Jason walks out of the room, back towards the corridor where the bathroom is and along one door further down on the left hand side.

He goes into his room and puts on a hardcore tape (The producer and DJ Tanith – first 30 seconds Fantasia Castle Donnington). Jason takes his shoes off and puts on four pairs of socks putting his shoes back on. He takes his jumper off puts on a couple of T shirts and then a couple more jumpers, his puffer jacket, a woolly hat and another pair of baggy jeans. Finally he puts his gloves on and then goes back into the dining room. The table tennis table is

405

away from the rest of the room. Brad manages to hide the fact that he is worried from Jason and joins in the manic fun.

BRAD: Are you warm enough Jase?

JASON: I'm freezing… I'm going to get out of here man. You know I stopped that nuclear war?

BRAD: That's good, shall we carry on playing?

JASON: Sure.

They play a coupe of shots where Jason tries ridiculous smashes.

JASON: I'll be back…

BRAD: I'll make a cup of tea. Do you want one?

JASON: ok…

As Jason leaves the room, the camera turns to Brad following him, walking out of the room along the corridor in the opposite direction. He looks more serious now, takes a deep breathe and looking a little worried puts the kettle on. He lights up a cigarette as he waits for the kettle to boil placing two mugs and making preparations for coffee. Jason comes back in dressed as he was before he put too many clothes on.

BRAD: You decided you were warm enough then.

JASON: Yes I'm fine now. I will get out of here though.

BRAD: I know you will Jase… I know you will. Here's your coffee. Don't pour it on your head buddy, remember. Drink it.

JASON: I like the taste. It will mean I can help more people, drinking this significant drink.

Bipolar, Recovery and NLP

BRAD: [Looking a little worried] I see. So, when you going to get out of here then?

JASON: Some time soon. Some time soon.

BRAD: I'll have to go after this cuppa. Still knackered from weights and I've got work tomorrow.

JASON: I've got love making to do. So many women to see and men to stop from fighting. The world needs me. Now that I'm God and all, so much responsibility, but I enjoy it really you know Brad. I enjoy looking after everyone, especially when they don't know I'm looking after them.

BRAD: I know you do… [Rubs his eye] I know you do…

A big, fat, Welsh nurse called Gary walks in. He must weigh 20 stone, but looks kind. He looks at Jason.

GARY: All right Jase?

[He seems more interested in talking to Brad. They shake hands]

GARY: All right? Brad is it?

BRAD: Yes that's right.

GARY: You're a good mate you are. Come to see him a lot you do? I know Jason appreciates it you know. He lights up when you're here. It's important that he can see his friends.

BRAD: That's what friends are for. I'm sure Jase would do the same for me. Wouldn't you Jase?

JASON: Interesting coffee this. Very interesting. Can't remember how I stopped the nuclear war. How did I stop the nuclear war?

Bipolar, Recovery and NLP

GARY: Don't know Jase. But somehow you managed to all right. There's not going to be a nuclear war anymore?

BRAD: That's for sure.

Gary and Brad laugh quietly.

JASON: Thank God… I mean, thank ME… God… for that…

Brad and Gary look blankly back at Jason. Jason does not pick up on their blank look.

JASON: Yes glad I stopped that. It wasn't easy to work out but I did well.

BRAD: Yes you did well Jase. You did well…

JASON: Thanks Brad. Thanks.

BRAD: We'll, I've got to be going now Jase. Duty calls. I've got work tomorrow.

GARY: Nice to see you again Brad. Come back anytime.

BRAD: We'll see you Jase.

JASON: I'll see you out Brad.

GARY: See you in a minute Jase. Don't be long.

BRAD: Well Jase, like I said, I'll see you tomorrow. You be all right? Make sure you don't run off. They're looking after you in here you know. I know it's hard, but you'll see.

JASE: Yes. But, I'm looking after them under cover, all of them and they don't realise it, but you and I know. Right? Promise me that you won't tell them? I have to stop the inevitable nuclear war again and make them understand.

Bipolar, Recovery and NLP

BRAD: I know mate. I know.

JASE: Promise you won't tell them anything Brad, not until I give you the signal?

BRAD: You've got my word on that. I promise.

JASE: Safe.

BRAD: Safe.

They shake hands and Brad leaves the ward pushing his expensive mountain bike out. Jason looks like he may follow, when Gary calls him in the background.

GARY: All right Jase, come and play that game of table tennis now.

JASE: [Turning round] Yeah OK Gary. Going to have a cigarette and listen to some hardcore first though. I'm trying to crack some messages that the tapes are sending me, about stopping this nuclear war. See you in a minute.

Jason walks past Gary closes his door and takes out one of his Embassy Number one cigarettes.

(Internal dialogue 1 shows Jason in the exciting parts of mania)

JASON'S INTERNAL DIALOGUE 1: Nothing to do when you're locked in a vacancy. Now I see why John Hughes was telling Bender to stop that Nuclear War, but he didn't know how to do it. He didn't realise that it is the film director himself who does it, not the actor.

Like me, the film director of the world now. I'm filming everything that happens on earth as a movie through my mind. How clever. I'm God the ultimate Oscar Winner. It's so obvious. Can't believe I am the one, but I must be strong. People need me and most of them don't even realise it. Even those that do could never admit to it.

(Internal dialogue 2 shows the confusion and pain caused my mania and illustrate why it cannot be allowed to continue in the 'real world')

JASON'S INTERNAL DIALOGUE 2: Oh my God... that's me. So much responsibility and I seem to work out the answer... all the time... I work out the answers and it doesn't seem to make any sense... One minute I'm God... looking like Robin Hood. Next I've changed into the new Alex Ferguson or an abject slave performing rituals. What the hell is going on? I don't understand. So tired, my brain keeps working on over drive, yet it seems so automatic and I'm sure there is a cover up. Why are people trying to be my friends? Because they want to start the nuclear war... they want information from me... the chosen one... God... well I'm not giving it... I'm more cunning than they are... all of them... I won't give in... I don't take this job lightly... I haven't been going through all this to give it up to some conspiracy against the world... their creator... Gotta calm down and listen to this tape... the Prodigy will have the answer. Forget the Producer.

He plays Wind it up by the Prodigy. Jason starts to dance in his room like someone possessed in Brunel Rooms in the 1990s i.e. like he was in the first scene but better and faster this time. When the first words of wind it up are echoed in the song the camera continues to focus on Jason dancing but the internal dialogue 1 comes back on.

Yes. Wind it up... Wind it up... I'm winding the world up... like an alarm clock... the world is in my hands... and I created to Prodigy to send this subliminal message to those in the dance world. I created ecstasy as a drug to create world peace and the singers and dancers to create harmony so that we do all live as one family. Then I needed to join the

Bipolar, Recovery and NLP

scene and release everyone's unconsciousness. Make them part of the real world. I started with ravers... then the rest of the world can unite and join together in perfect harmony...

Suddenly there is a knock on the door. It's Jason's dad.

DAD: Hi Jay. Can I come in? Do you mind turning the music down. I've brought you a couple of Mars Bars. Have you've eaten?

JASON: Yes, I've eaten thanks Dad.

DAD: Have one of these now then.

JASON: Thanks. I'm starving.

DAD: Must be those pills. You've put on some weight, but don't worry about that. We want you to get better first. And you needed to put on some weight anyway, I think. Did you sleep ok last night?

JASON: Yes thanks, I must have got seven hours sleep. Something like that anyway. Definitely got some sleep. Didn't think I was that tired.

DAD: That's probably the pills as well. They're bringing you back down. You have had so much energy for the last few months. Too much, in fact. It wasn't normal. Now you're starting to get back down to earth. It will take some time. Do you know what's been happening?

JASON: Not really.

DAD: The doctor has said that you have been high. Not in the real world. Manic he called it. Now they're giving you drugs to clear your thoughts. Make you what you were like before you got ill. I'm so pleased though. I thought you were a gonner at one point. I thought you were going to be a cabbage.

Bipolar, Recovery and NLP

JASON: Why is that dad?

DAD: One day I came in and you didn't even recognise me. You were just that. Your eyes were like stone.

JASON: How did that happen Dad?

DAD: They had to restrain you. One day when I walked in you through a chair through a window and it took five nurses to bring you down. They had to put you in a straight jacket and injected you with some drugs to calm you down... (Eyes start watering)... It was really scary ...but it had to be done, you were out of control. Anyway the drugs they gave you were so strong that they knocked you for six. (Wipes tears from his eyes). And I thought you were a gonner, I really did. You know, I've got a friend with a son like you, who's been in a place like this. He said that his son's been sat there for two years. After two years he still doesn't recognise him.

JASON: That's sad dad.

DAD: Promise me you won't take those drugs again Jay. You've been really lucky, been given a second chance, you know? You have to take it.

JASON'S INTERNAL DIALOGUE 1: What about these drugs I'm taking now they're even better... ha hah haa and what's more, they're free and legal... As god I had to assume an antic disposition, but can't let this on, as I don't want to upset my dad now, or Hamlet or Shakespeare for that matter. It's a lot of responsibility being the father of God, so I better play dumb. Anyway I still take drugs, but only telepathically. They have more of an effect that way.

JASON'S INTERNAL DIALOGUE 2: But what if he's right. My dad. All these amazing thoughts I had. They can't be true. It's impossible and I could never admit that they were not true, that would be the most humiliating thing on earth.

Bipolar, Recovery and NLP

To admit to having lost my mind and to admit that I am actually living in a mental hospital. What a disaster. How can I ever look my teachers, friends, people I know in the eye ever again, without ever feeling like a loser, an animal even? How can I play Rugby again, go back to school, go to University and lead a normal and even an inspiring life, after I admit to having been completely insane? It's like Jack Nicholson in One Flew Over the Cuckoo's Nest, and it's my life. This is too much to bare man... no way... No way out of this mess... Ahhhhggghh....

JASON: I won't take them again dad.

DAD: Now you are getting better Jay, there is one thing you have to be prepared for.

JASON: What's that dad?

DAD: Well I spoke to the psychiatrist the other day and he told me that things are going to get worse before they get better.

JASON: Why's that?

DAD: Well he told me that now you are beginning to realise what has actually happened it's not going to be easy accepting everything and your mood will naturally go low.

JASON: What do you mean Dad?

DAD: Well Jay I mean that he said you're going to get depressed.

JASON: For how long?

DAD: Well we don't know exactly but it could be a long time. The important thing is that you keep taking the drugs they give you... I know you will anyway. What is also important, perhaps more important is that unlike a lot of the other

413

patients in here you have a good support network. I mean a really good support network around you. You've got a good doctor. You've got me, your mum and your brother. You're Grandma and your Nan and you've got very good friends who come to see you Brad and Tim and Dom. They're all here for you. Have you seen Brad today?

JASON: Yes dad. He's been doing weights. Really strong now.

DAD: He's a really good friend you know. He comes to see you nearly every day doesn't he?

JASON: Yes dad.

DAD: You're a lucky chap. You remember that OK.

JASON: Will do.

Jason sparks up another cigarette and looks into the loving and distressed eyes of his father.

DAD: What did you have to eat for supper then Jay?

JASON: Fish and Chips and sponge pudding with custard.

DAD: When you come home we'll have Fish and Chips from Ready's. OK?

JASON: OK Dad. When will that be?

DAD: Don't know son. Won't be long. You just hang on in there ok.

JASON: OK Dad.

DAD: Well I'll be off then Jay. I've got work in the morning. Just wanted to say hello. Love you. [Kissing his son on the cheek and giving him a hug]

Bipolar, Recovery and NLP

JASON: Love you too dad.

DAD: You'll be ok wont you. Just hang on in their kid. You've got the mental strength I know.

JASON: I'll see you out.

As they walk down the corridor the camera moves slower than usual.

3 months later in Jason's room. Jason is no longer manic. Over the last 3 months his mood has dropped. He has been in a suicidal state for a while and sleeping 16 hours a day. He has been given his own room still as his parents asked for him to have his own space. He is lucky in this regard as all the other patients are split in between two dormitories apart from another single room which is left empty for any pregnant women. He lies crying in his bed like a little five year old boy who has lost his parents when shopping at night and is afraid of the dark. Bob Dylan's 'Times Are Changin' is playing in the background.

Jason sits up and brushing away the floods of tears he picks up Nelson Mandela's autobiography 'Walking to Freedom'.

He cannot seem to concentrate so takes the book into the hall and sits cross legged in the doorway. Looking up as the day to day activity of the ward goes past. One of the nurses tells him to get up because it is medication time. He reads for a minute and then eventually keeps looking up. From where he is sat he can see the patients lining up and taking their medication one by one. A team of broken souls, longing for a better existence. If only Jason could put his own life in perspective with that of Nelson Mandela perhaps he would have a chance.

Quick flashback to 18th birthday in hospital: 30 seconds.

Bipolar, Recovery and NLP

Fast forward 2 months and Jason is sat in a ward round.

DR.TAYLOR: How are you Jason?

JASON: A lot better thank you Doctor. I can't wait to go home.

DR.TAYLOR: We'll see about that. I have some questions to ask you OK. Please answer them as honestly as possible ok. I think you know the drill by now... Is life worth living? Yes or No?

JASON: Yes.

DR.TAYLOR: How do you feel compared to the last time I saw you?

JASON: I feel less depressed and more ready to go home.

DR.TAYLOR: Do you feel like you are likely to harm yourself?

JASON: No my mood is better. I don't feel suicidal now. I can see that there is light at the end of the tunnel.

DR.TAYLOR: So you still feel that you are in a tunnel.

JASON: No I feel like I have been in a tunnel and now I'm looking back. I have a long way to go but I'm definitely looking back. I promise.

DR.TAYLOR: Jason you don't have to prove yourself to me or anyone else here. You understand. You just have to be honest with yourself. I know it's difficult but you're doing well believe me. You've been with us quite a long time now. Six months I believe but there is a definite improvement OK?

JASON: Yes Doctor.

Bipolar, Recovery and NLP

DR.TAYLOR: So you can see light at the end of the tunnel. On a mood of one to 10 with 1 being depressed and 10 being normal how do you feel?

JASON: Six I guess, maybe seven but that will go up to eight or nine if I can go home for good.

DR.TAYLOR: Do you have racy thoughts any more?

JASON: No Doctor.

DR.TAYLOR: Do you feel depressed?

JASON: I don't feel like I did before if that's what you mean. I mean I do feel depressed sometimes but I feel that that is because of everything that has happened and the fact that I am still living here. There's a lot to cope with bearing in mind everything that has happened. My life has been turned upside down.

DR.TAYLOR: I see. I believe you are seeing a counsellor Reginald every week. Tell me Jason how is that going.

JASON: It's going well. I like Reginald. We have some good talks. I can tell him things that I don't talk to other people about. Personal things you know and I can see its helping me deal with the situation, the past, the present and the future, in a way that I never thought possible, until I met him.

DR.TALOR: That's good Jason. How do you feel about other people?

JASON: What do you mean doctor?

DR.TAYLOR: Do you like them? Do you feel resentful to them in anyway, angry even?

JASON: No doctor, not at all. I feel embarrassed maybe, humiliated even, because of all those crazy thoughts I had that were I thought were true… thinking I was God and all that. Apart from that I just want to rejoin society and I'm ready to go.

DR.TAYLOR: Well I think you're nearly ready to go now Jason. You can go home this weekend and then I'll see you next week. Should you continue to improve and the medication continue to work, which there is no reason why it shouldn't I'll see you once more next Thursday and then you'll be ready to go for good.

JASON: Really Doctor, it's great. Thank you so much.

DR.TAYLOR: Well I think that just about wraps it up for today Jason if you will excuse me. Please can you ask Harry to come in?

Jason leaves the ward round for the first time ever with a smile on his face. He goes to the main lounge where there are several people watching TV and sees Harry biting his knuckles.

JASON: Harry you are next.

HARRY: What ward round Jase.

JASON: Yes Harry.

HARRY: You look happy Jase. Good news.

JASON: Yeah Harry. There going to let me go next week. Don't believe it.

HARRY: Well done Jase. Wish me luck hey.

JASON: Good luck Harry. Good luck mate…

Bipolar, Recovery and NLP

HARRY: Can't remember where the door is Jase can you show me? I can't remember anything since I started this ECT?

JASON: Here it is mate. Here's the door. Allow me.

---

15 months later. September 1994. It's Jason's second year at Manchester University. He's watching match of the day drinking some cider in some run down house with a big TV when the door bell rings.

JASON: I'll get it its Meredith.

ROGER: All right Jase.

Jason opens the door and a pretty girl with blonde hair dressed in a short dress and lots of make up can barely speak. She's crying her eyes out. Jason lets her in.

JASON: Hey... what's wrong?

MEREDITH: Th... That bastard out there tried to kiss me and the only way I could get him to stop was by telling him that he could come back with me. When I answered the door he ran off.

JASON: You what... You fucking what... Wait here...

MEREDITH: Wait... come back.

Jason races out of the flat and Meredith stays in the hallway. Jason runs round the corner and sees the bloke walking away.

JASON: Oiiihhh. I said Oiiiihhh. You.

The man turns round in the dark. Jason can't see his face. Jason runs right up to him.

JASON: That's right you... you mother fucker.... Who the fuck do you think you are..... [punching him in the face he falls to the ground and Jason starts kicking him in the head repeatedly].... Who the fuck do you think you are... whack... fucking with my bitch like that... doosh... You like hassling women do you.... You fucking gutless turd...thwacckk.. You think your going to get away with this.... Kapppooww. You just picked the crazy person in Manchester to fuck with.... Smack. [Jason then kneels on top of the man and starts punching him in the forehead, eyes and nose. After about fifty punches he regains his breathe]... I was in the bin you know... and now I've got to put up with a prick like you.... Fucking with my girlfriend like that... she's done nothing. [Standing up and kicking him in the head a couple of times and on his back and arse]. If I ever see you in this neighbourhood again or hear from you ever again you're dead. Now get the fuck out of here or I'll kill you. You mother fucker.

As Jason walks away he can see Meredith watching in the back ground. He gives her a hug and they go back inside. Meredith goes upstairs to freshen up and Jason goes back in to watch match of the day.

JASON: I just kick fuck out of this bloke who was molesting Meredith.

ROGER: You should have said we'd have helped you mate.

CHRIS: Yeah. I thought I heard something. Is he still outside.

JASON: Don't know.

CHRIS: Let's have a look. I'll come with ya. For protection, not that you need any Jase.

Bipolar, Recovery and NLP

They walk outside and there is no sign of the man. Jason goes down to the floor where he was on top of him. There is a pile of blood and then a trail going down the alley.

CHRIS: Looks like he got the message Jase. Don't think he'll ever come round here again. Gonna watch the rest of Match of the Day.

JASON: Yes.

CHRIS: Come on Manchester United are on next. I'll make Meredith a cuppa. You want a lager. I've got some. Tastes better than that crap you're drinking. Not so strong but tastes better for once. You might have got lucky. Could have got a Leeds fan there you know. Come on mate. Let's get back inside its cold out here.

----

12 months later there has been heavy drinking… stopped taking medication nine months previously… no symptoms of manic depression until…

JASON'S INTERNAL DIALOGUE 1:

Jason narrates with Meredith now openly Mistress Real, asleep living in a quieter area in Chorlton Cum Hardy. He begins believing Chorlton is the head of World Consciousness and the whole world is a brothel.

There is a visual re run of events. Talking is in the back ground. (Like the big fuck you scene in Spike Lee's 24 hours)

Ah what a privilege it is to live at the head of world consciousness and to be the first to realise that the whole world is actually a brothel. As I stand here an abject slave to the Mistress of the night. The camera zooms in on a picture of Mistress Real sat in her purple throne. She also happens to play the character of Meredith. The most intelligent Classics Professor of my tutors had an inkling no wonder he was bordering on the insane.

Not like me God aka Jason Pegler, an undercover Classics Student and manic depressive from Gloucester understands the real significance that I can indeed create world peace by forcing the whole world to make love to each other in a subliminal and a pro-active way. I will have to withstand pressure from all my sides from other Dominants and make my move now.

As I masturbate while looking through my window I can see a light on. Behind this light I can feel myself making love to the beautiful horny middle aged woman inside. As I awake her from her sleep she has multiple orgasms and starts to dress up in her leather gear placing a whip between her panty hose. The world thought that the sub dominant scene was something to be criticised for pain and humiliation. Well once everyone goes through the real physical pleasure and trust that stems from this movement even only in an unconscious level they will be nicer to their fellow man and start to give instead of taking. That includes giving more head... Ha ha Ha ha...

I look at my girlfriend while she is asleep. Mistress Real. She is so caring looking after my every need in the real world appearing to be my Mistress and this is what I must make her think. As I discover the ultimate sense of trust and faith from womankind through my relationship with her I can manipulate others and go through each household one by one turning unconscious sub and dominant pain and pleasure into correcting abject slaves' behaviour so they follow Christian living and do what the bible says. That's why I could never figure out who Jesus was as well as I was Jesus myself.

Last night's Journey now makes so much sense. When Meredith or should I say Real went to sleep I set

Bipolar, Recovery and NLP

about putting my plan into action. I told the whole world how I will put my plan of stopping the inevitable nuclear war into action... First I needed to check that Chorlton really was the head of world consciousness so I paraded through Hulme and Manchester University with my final preparations for the film of the century. Sophocles' Ancient Greek Tragedy being transformed into a modern film in the style of the 1979 classic The Warriors set in Hulme where the best graffiti in the country is.

I needed to go into the Classics Department itself. Make love to the girl I spoke to telepathically. Jane said it herself... When I told her about the film, as my dissertation. She said. "You really have everything sorted... I wish I could get my head as straight as yours Jason..." That was all the assurance I needed that I would have the right casting for the movie with my Classics team on board. Dr. Clarke and Dr Roy Gibson choosing the cast....

So next I walked through Mosside. Past, Denmark Road where I used to live. Worrying that I had killed that man I beat up who had tried to molest Meredith... I mean Mistress Real (visual manifestation in throne)... I set about visiting Mosside police station... I asked the officer: "is everything all right mate"... he said everything was and asked if I could help him with everything... I said of course I would and that I would be back. As I walked around Mosside trying to decide where the head of world consciousness was I came about more clues... First the old Bingo Hall run down. Nothing there sending spiritual messages that I was close. I went into a couple of newsagents and bought first the Caribbean Times and then an even more obscure ethnic minority newspaper. Very interesting but not quite the centre - it would be too obvious.

I'd been wondering all evening how it would happen and thought I would wait until Real was asleep to continue with the plan. As soon as she was asleep I sat on the empty gold fish bowl and made my seemingly submissive sexual ritual defecating in the bowl, filling it up with shampoo and then wrapping a plastic back around so the shit couldn't escape. I would present it to Real in the morning whilst it unconsciously made her my slave in her dreams. The next day when she discovered it she would assume that I was her slave and the role reversal and therefore the first steps to world peace would be underway.

In the evening I needed to send CHI in the opposite direction so first I took my Usual Suspects poster and placed it on the Garage on the house facing the right hand side of Cranbourne Road. Then I filled my rucksack with 30 or so significant literary texts, wrote cryptic messages to people I selected to spread the word and put them in every shop in Chorlton.

The fancy dress shops were of certain significance... that why I bought something for Real for everything during the afternoon... I can see why she was surprised when I gave them to her. All that flattery too much to bare for a mind that was still at times unconscious but I must not belittle her... such is the life and limits of a human being. It's difficult for me to remember now, as I have had the epiphany that the world has been waiting 2000 years for. It has hit me like a thunderbolt from Zeus.

The night certainly got more complicated and hectic as it grew on. My mind was racing like a Ferrari in a space shuttle. Had to remember what messages to send and where and how to present them so in the morning there would be only love in the air. That's why at 4.00am I thought I'd call Snoop Doggy Dogg and the Dogg Pound crew for help. I had Snoops number from the back of my Doggy Pound CD and went to a phone box to make the call. No one around... perfect. Pressing those numbers was like typing in the answers to the Universe. When I got to the other line I understood the coded message straight away. Snoop was on board and would spread the word to the record industry

Bipolar, Recovery and NLP

to put the live "All you need is Love" switch on as John Lennon and the Beatles had so publicly and quite charmingly enacted for me in the 60s. Then chance to join the physical and telepathic realms of the human race through sexual unconscious and conscious union where appropriate. A job well done and time to enjoy myself... and everyone else... ha ha ha...

Now I remember the next day when Meredith woke up not understanding the significance of the ritual.. the whole world on my shoulders... she took the day off work... it was affecting her life and set about taking me to see my mother in Wales. Fine by me.... Remember her imaginary role as the dominant was now crucial as part of this whole manoeuvring to stop the inevitable Nuclear War... Don't understand the logic... You're not meant to... too complex... only God can understand it... hence why I am retorting it right now...

I had some tasks to complete in the morning. To keep to schedule for when I had to be in the right place at the right time to discover time travel and shift between states I put on my roller skates and started giving banana's and cans of coke to the four tramps I saw that morning. I threw the significant book I'd saved up in the air at the garage.... Shouting the time is now... changed a few mindsets and thought patterns by being seemingly dangerous and crossing the road. Watched One Flew Over the Cuckoo's Nest as an Ode to the mentally ill in society and to put my telepathic judgement into all future Hollywood productions and creative ideas. During one scene of the film I swam under water to Australia and back again in less than five seconds. I had to try my reflexes for the pending rocket launch with my boogie board so on my back whilst stood in the living room. Real open the curtains (see Meredith opening curtains and Real's throne smiling – to different sides to the coin to explain one phenomenon) after her ecstasy was too much to bear and we were off to the train station via taxi.

After I bought a sports magazine to make get every famous sportsman, woman and team to start spreading the unconscious word of peace to all earth I met a charming lady on the train who reminded me of my Grandmother. Knowing she was the one who would understand I began giving her the details, coordinates and philosophy behind time travel. After forty five minutes I realised she had understood as Real had reassumed her earth mode as Meredith for a brief moment to suggest that I be quiet because she thought that the old lady had got "the idea by now". After a brief demonstration before leaving the train on showing time travel in action we set about reuniting with my mother...

This was very critical because Meredith back in her Real pose had made me realise that I needed to be in an isolated and anonymous place... i.e. out of the area where world consciousness was at its peak to enable the path to world peace and freedom to have the quickest effect. In the evening I telepathically made love to my mother and saw her as a matriarchal figure. I awoke in the middle of the night and stupidly told Meredith as I saw her for a split second that I needed help. "I knew I was manic and that I was desperately ill." Fortunately this thought subsided after a brief cry of some seven seconds and I was back into my plateau and god like state.

Could be an insert about reality of second episode and being in Talgarth – how about entrance and thinking I was film director upon arrival – mentioning of knife and game of pool before entering ?!

INTERNAL DIALOGUE 1: Fucking the Spice Girls scene.

Jason is sat down smoking a cigarette on a tiny, smelly and dirty hospital ward when out of the blue Professor Bain, a podgy late fifties man with grey hair, one of his lecturers, walks in.

JASON: Professor Bain. Surprised to see you hear. Thanks for visiting.

PROFESSOR BAIN: Ok. I was nosey, so here I am. Dr. Clarke sends his love.

Jason: That's nice.

PROFFESOR BAIN: I've bought you a book. It should be of real interest with your passion for films. Some light reading away from your final year studies. I hope it will be of interest.

JASON: The history of Hollywood. Thank you.

PROFESSOR: How are you?

JASON: Pretty terrible. I mean, I can see me getting through it. I'm not a quitter but it's the humiliation that's the worst thing. All those amazing thoughts that I thought I had were all rubbish. Not sure if I can ever come to terms with that.

PROFFESOR BAIN: Nodding his head. I see. You know we had a Professor who used to be in the department when I first started. Must be nearly thirty years ago now and he went mad like you. I came to see him in this hospital too. He got better and turned out to be one of the greatest classicists of our times. Most intelligent tutor we ever had in our department. The man was a genius. Graduated from Cambridge as I did.

JASON: Really - that's encouraging.

PROFFESOR BAIN: You're still young and have a good future ahead of you. Take this time to get some much needed rest. You will be back soon I presume.

Bipolar, Recovery and NLP

JASON: I hope so. It will take me a month or two to recuperate.

PROFFESOR BAIN: Well I'll leave you and see you soon then. Dr. Clarke asks that you go and see him at the University when you feel up to it. I'll have him keep me informed of your progress.

JASON: Ok. Well thanks for coming.

PROFFESOR BAIN: Ok.

Dr. Clarke, a scruffy looking Irish intellectual in his late thirties is sat drinking a coffee with Jason in a quiet pub in Chorlton on a Sunday lunch time.

DR.CLARKE: Well Jason, it's very good to see you. I'm so pleased that you are better. You look good.

JASON: Thanks Dr. Clarke.

DR.CLARKE: Please call me Michael.

JASON: Ok sure.

DR.CLARKE: I'm sorry I didn't come to see you; I can't bear places like that. Something similar happened to me when I was younger, so I find it difficult to visit hospitals. Let's not talk about that though. Let's talk about you. How do you feel about returning this academic year?

JASON: I think it would be too difficult now. I've already missed the last seven weeks and my mood will drop before I get any better. It's how my manic cycles go. Whenever I go high depression follows and it lasts even longer than the mania.

DR.CLARKE: Quite right Jason. I was going to advise you against it. You need time to heal and get better. Come back in the next academic year fresh and stronger. Then you'll stroll through the final year. You shouldn't give up on your degree and I'm sure you won't.

JASON: No I'll come back stronger. Will you still be there next year?

DR.CLARKE: Yes next year will be my last year in Manchester. Then I'm going back to Ireland to concentrate on writing my book.

JASON: What's the book about?

DR.CLARKE: The book is about gathering a collection of the finest war strategies from the Ancient Classical World. It will feature the most advanced strategies and the most epic battles in history including the most amazing victories against the odds.

JASON: Sounds fascinating.

DR.CLARKE: Yes, I've wanted to write it for some time now. Anyway, that's enough about me? How do you feel about everything?

JASON: I feel like I keep getting hit by the world's toughest boxer and it becomes increasingly more difficult to get back up.

DR.CLARKE: I thought you might say something like that. We all feel like that at one time or other. It's one of life's idiosyncrasies. Try and see it as a blessing in disguise. The harder you get hit by life the more you learn and the harder you are able to hit back. See life as a constant challenge. It would be boring if it was easy. I know you are going through great pain at the moment, but trust me that the most successful people in the history of this world are people who have suffered great hardship and uncertainty and managed to overcome it. Now you have experienced this manic depression again you have more potential to do greater good for yourself or even society if you want to. You could be a good example to many people if you want to. You have the ability to shape your own destiny and determine the way your own life turns out Jason. Remember that.

JASON: I will.

----

16 months later – final examination:

Final exam tripping out on Youth, Love and Rome 4 minutes:

INTERNAL DIALOGUE 1:

What is Lucan's own view on Civil War? Well Lucan is sick of it. He sees it as something that doesn't work. Why else would he be so obsessed with writing about it. Also he describe it in such grotesque detail that you could only feel that he was abhorrent. Just as the world feels abhorrent that I am a manic depressive but the truth is that Lucan must be fascinated by civil war as people are about my manic depression. I know that people are jealous of it and can explain my historical significance through the Classical World. Aeneas may have founded Troy but who founded the human race and invented the Greek and Roman Gods. I did and all unwittingly for my first twenty years. Strategically moving myself into position as a manic depressive in society's eyes so I could meet other like minded people who would remind me of my station.

I do not punish human beings for being above their station by giving them eternal madness like a Pentheus or an Ajax. I am not a Euripides or a Sophocles. I am too clever for that. That is why I created the most romantic story in the Ars Amatoria. Narcissus was punished it is true for being

Bipolar, Recovery and NLP

vain and the tragedy is that he will never see echo again because her voice, first voice, echoes so he will never know where to move. I myself although I know I am god, must not be overtly vain.

I must be humble so I am not guilty of 'hubrising' myself, a contradiction in terms I know but someone has to set the standards for the entire history of the universe. This brings me to my next point, about Catullus. He was in love with Lesbia we know and he was right about ancient Spanish people not cleaning their teeth. When he writes his poems it is fascinating to observe from a literary standpoint about the power of the in definability of being in the in crowd. For Catullus loves to join this crowd because it has no official size it is a matter of perception for him and in his poems he controls his own past.

In Ovid's Metamorphoses he appears to be sending a message of warning to the Emperor of the time Augustus saying how there will be a new Empire and a New Emperor that has its good and bad points. Ovid is really sending a message to me however. I created him as a writer to comment on the role of the Romans in history as part of the history of the world and made it a literary allusion to hide the obvious from the status quo, who would by nature cause anarchy if they knew everything. That would make my job twice as difficult and there has always been a lot to do as there is.... classics... manic energy... ancient rome... love... enjoy the manic feeling....

8 weeks later. October 1998.

Jason and his mum and dad are at Jason's Graduation on a sunny day outside the University. Jason is wearing his gown and hat and is posing for photos. Jason's mum and dad are both very proud whilst Jason is pumped full of medication.

MUM: Are you Ok dear?

Bipolar, Recovery and NLP

Jason: Yeah. I feel stupid though with my eyes pumped full of this medication. Like my 18th birthday in Coney Hill. Remember that Mum. I was in hospital on my 18th birthday too and now my graduation.

MUM: looking upset. Oh dear. Come here.

DAD: Don't say that. You have done extremely well to make it considering what you have been through.

JASON: And what I've still got to go through.

DAD: I thought you said you knew why it happened?

MUM: Yes, overwork wasn't it.

JASON: …And binge drinking. Must stop that for good and with my psychologist I have ways of managing my stressors now so I know when my warning signs are and how to stop them.

DAD: Make sure you stop that drinking.

MUM: Sounds like you know what you are doing now dear. Don't try too hard. You always did try to run before you could walk you know. Ever since I can remember.

DAD: He's competitive like his dad. No harm in that.

MUM: No. No harm in being competitive, but everything doesn't need to happen all at once. Things take time.

JASON: I know. And this time I have strategies in place to cope with the boredom of the real world. I don't have a destructive personality any more and I know when to switch off. If things happen I'm going to switch off and when I deal with them I'll do so in a positive way.

Bipolar, Recovery and NLP

MUM: Sounds like a personal transformation. Not heard you talk like that before Jay. Must be the pressure of University being over and everything, and that Psychologist has helped you, hasn't she. Kath, is that her name?

JASON: Yes, that's right she's set the scene but has told me that it is only me myself that can be the one who wants to get over this and manage it permanently in an effective manner.

DAD: Good - now stop waffling Jay and let's go in. Your ceremony begins in a few minutes. I want to get a good seat.

Jason collects his University Degree and his Mum and Dad are clapping in the audience.

July 1999. Jason is sat in the back garden on the floor in the sun reading the last page of the book Prozac Nation. When he finishes he closes the book smiles, looks up into the sky and says:

JASON: 'Right… let's do it…'

He goes into the house where the computer is already on and opens a word document. He then types 'A Can of Madness' by Jason Pegler into the page and then begins writing: 'how the fuck is someone meant to live with a mental illness? Don't ask me, still trying to find out how? After panning in and out of page of typing….. The doorbell rings. It is Gina, Jason's girlfriend at the time, and her friend Debbie.

Gina: "So have you started your thing a me jig yet?… You said you were going to when you finished that book….

JASON: Yes I've started it. It's going great. Want to see it?

Bipolar, Recovery and NLP

GINA: Yeah. Let's go upstairs. Come on Deb. Race ya.

Jason sits by the computer and the girls sit on the bed.

GINA: Go on read it out then. You sexy writer, you!

JASON: Ok here it goes….

Jason reads out the first paragraph…. Gina interrupts I love the first line… I fucking love the first line…. 1 minute 30 second citation…..

Gina keeps screaming yes and jumps up and down on the bed. Then says she needs a cigarette. Debbie is already smoking and keeps shouting Yes…Yes.

GINA: You're onto a winner here. You're going to be famous. And it's so fucking true what you're saying. You're so right. Isn't that right Debs?

DEB: That's right Gene…

GINA: You know me and Debs have both been there and we know what its like. You sum it up man. You really sum it all up.

DEB: And you know what I really love about it Jason, is that you are being yourself. You still appear yourself in your writing. I know writers who completely change character when they put pen to paper and I don't usually mind that but I like the originality in this.

GINA: That's right original. So when are you going to buy me a brand new BMW then? How long will it be until you're famous? I bet you'll look real sexy in a nice shirt and tie on TV?

Bipolar, Recovery and NLP

Jason talking sense will be able to see images of this speech and visually see the move to London as Renton moves to London in Trainspotting. This time music will be Coldplay with 'Clocks'.

JASON: I had to really choose life and move to London. That meant living the life that I wanted to. Having my third breakdown at the end of my University Degree had knocked back my confidence and I only stayed in Manchester and got a shitty job because my confidence had taken a knock again. I realised that I had to lead the life that I wanted to lead. That meant leaving Gina we'd both been moving in different directions. As soon as I started writing my autobiography I knew I'd finally find a cure. I was really on the road to recovery. All those years of anger and self fuelled resentment had been a waste of time. I wanted to focus on the very first realisation that I had when I returned to consciousness from my first manic episode. To psychoanalyse, myself and then set about helping reduce the humiliation of first one and then other sufferers where I could invent my own utopia to help mankind.

I moved to London to pursue a postgraduate fast track newspaper journalism course where it was cheap and moved in with a helpful landlord in Roger Moore's birthplace (play with James bond joke here) – the glamorous setting of Stockwell. Not paradise but a secure environment and next door to the college so very convenient. (Miami here or later?)Things were going well, then on the last day of college we had a university party and I met the love of my life. [Coldplay song becomes louder]. There was a beautiful moment of dancing, eye to eye contact and kissing with a beautiful Spanish girl with dark hair and big brown eyes. He takes her off the dance floor and asks her if she wants a coke. Her reply is "que?" We spent a few days together and felt spiritually very close.

There was a last holiday of destructive behaviour as if I needed to balance my whole life into perspective. I'd been given a free holiday to Miami thanks to (this bit filmed quickly like the guy slamming his drink down quickly in snatch hearing Benito Del Toro is off gambling) my landlord Felix, on the condition that I drive him around in a luxurious sports car to the odd business meeting. (Pan to driving red sports car.) There were two holidays in one. During the day I'd hang out with Felix going to the Everglades, watching Miami Heat, shopping, jet skiing on Christmas day and being shown sites by all the friendly people we met. When Felix crashed out any time from 10.30pm I'd be off binge drinking and cruising around in the sports car meeting people in bars and getting up to all sorts of mischief mainly drink driving and womanising. This culminated with a stupid occurrence where I mistakenly poured petrol into my eye at 9.00am when refuelling the car having been drink driving in between different bars without having any nights sleep.

After hitting 140 mph during the day and getting away with numerous traffic offences I set about turning home and pretty quickly settled into a relationship where I had one final episode in April 2000. By October 2000 I had recovered and finally got my own flat (show keys moving in,) thanks to the council. A bit run down but happy to do it up and get my life back on track the way it always should have been.

Psychologist Meeting: Summarising techniques

CAROL BUSCH: So Life is looking good, Jason, so how do you feel about everything?

JASON: I feel great. I have never felt so content about life, and the future looks good. More importantly I am enjoying every day.

CAROL BUSCH: Good for you Jason. How do you feel that the cognitive treatment has worked?

Bipolar, Recovery and NLP

JASON: On the whole, I think the CBT has been great. I felt a bit uncomfortable at first letting my inner feelings out but after I soon felt comfortable talking about things with you. I think it is because that is the way it is designed. It feels that I am talking to you as a friend rather than a psychologist or part of the medical model and this makes things easier. The way we put together my action plan together was really a joint effort but a logical progression.

CAROL BUSCH: I'm so pleased Jason that you have found the treatment so helpful and you should congratulate yourself you have done well. You have put in a lot of hard work and deserve to be well. The action plan we put together was all your work. I was here to give you a structure of how to put your life into perspective and avoid stressors to reduce the risk of relapse and you worked with me very well. You know that you may come back and see me at any time should you ever feel the need to talk things over.

JASON: Thanks Carol. I know that but I think I'll be fine.

CAROL BUSCH: Well I hope so too Jason and I think you have a very good chance. You are a great deal better than when we first met and I feel that you've moved forward along way. Remember that this is not good bye however and that my offer still stands. All you need to do is ring the psychology department and speak to my secretary Grace. You know her don't you.

JASON: Yes I do. We know each other quite well now.

CAROL BUSCH: Good Jason. You know with the techniques you have learnt you have an excellent chance of staying well. I know that your work with your psychiatrist Dr Davies is equally important. How is that going along?

Bipolar, Recovery and NLP

JASON: Well we are continuing to meet once every six weeks and the medication has kept me stable although I do intend to come off it for good in the near future.

CAROL: Well Jason I wish you luck. I must urge you not to come off your medication without discussing things with Dr. Davies. It really is most important.

JASON: Oh of course not, I will discuss any change in plan with him.

CAROL: Well I'm sure you will do Jason and I hope for your sake that you do. You have done extremely well and we want things to continue this way. If at any time you feel that I can be of any help whatsoever please do let me know. I am only a phone call away and whilst I am very busy, in fact busier than I have ever been, these days with the recent cut backs in the department should you need my help we would be able to meet within a few days.

JASON: Thanks Carol. I know you are and that is very reassuring. I am fine for now however and do not envisage us needing to see each other anymore on a regular basis. If at any time I need your help I will call you with no hesitation I promise.

CAROL: Ok…well thank you Jason.

JASON: Thank you Carol.

Meeting with DR. Davies about coming off medication but clearly more friendship here than anything else.

JASON: I know I am definitely Ok to come off the medication for good. I finally have the confidence to do it.

DR.DAVIES: I know you have really thought this through and you are doing very well.

Bipolar, Recovery and NLP

JASON: I know you said that 90% of your patients relapse in the first year of coming off, but I know I have the strength of character to pull through especially with all these NLP techniques that I have learnt.

DR.DAVIES: Yes they sound very interesting. I feel that sometimes I could do with using some of the techniques you describe myself.

JASON: Well now you are my board with the charity I'll see if I can get you a free ticket to the world's greatest NLP practical trainer Anthony Robbins. Tickets are usually £455 but as a Chipmunka Foundation member maybe I can get you a free ticket, as long as you give me some feedback on how we could deliver this revolutionary practise to future NHS mental health patients.

DR.DAVIES: Why I'd be delighted.

JASON: I am more myself now than I have been for a long time, since I was seventeen probably and now I am on a lower dose of medication – 600mg of Sodium Valporate a day I can see the side effects of the drug. It blocks my real feelings, makes me anxious and confused. The sooner I am off them the better but I am happy to come off them gradually over the next three months like you said.

DR.DAVIES: Yes coming off gradually is wise.

JASON: And I know I can take my sleeping tablets if I need them. When should I take them?

DR.DAVIES: Well you need at least four hours of sleep a night. Ideally you should have about 7.00 but some people can manage with less. If you cannot sleep the first night take your sleeping pill the next night. Start with one.

Bipolar, Recovery and NLP

JASON: If I still can't sleep what should I do? Can I take up to 4 3.5mg of Zopiclone in a night.

DR.DAVIES: Yes no more than that and try to take less than that.

JASON: What next?

DR.DAVIES: If you still have trouble sleeping on the fifth day, go onto 50mg of Zopiclone like we talked about. That should calm you down. Then once you have had a good few days of sleep you can come off it.

JASON: Yes I remember. It's better to have to go on a stronger drug the Quetiapine for a few days and suffer the more serious side effects from that than endure the side effects of the Sodium Valporate all of the time.

DR.DAVIES: Yes that's right.

JASON: I don't envisage needing to do this though but I will be honest with myself if at any time I definitely need to. I am so much better at managing my life now and things are going really well with my work. Chipmunka is going really well. We've been in all the national newspapers and I've been on TV several times lately and been invited to the States to appear on TV and talk as well.

DR.DAVIES: Yes I hear from some of my colleagues that you are doing extremely well. I am very pleased. Your work is helping a lot of people I am sure and I am proud that you have asked me to be a part of it.

JASON: Well, like I said on TV the other week, it is vitally important to have a psychiatrist that treats you as a human being first and not a patient. Only then can you build up a rapport and start to help the patient to help themselves.

Bipolar, Recovery and NLP

DR.DAVIES: That makes a lot of sense to me... Well time is running a little short. Let's make our next appointment in three weeks time so we can monitor how you feel as you reduce the dosage...ok?

JASON: Ok, let's do this.

Dr. Davies leads Jason out of the room. He opens a security door and they go into the waiting room.

DR.DAVIES: Please can you give Jason another appointment. [Addressing the Chinese male 20ish receptionist in the window]

RECEPTIONIST: Looks at the diary. When would you like it?

DR.DAVIES: 3 weeks time please?

RECEPTIONIST: How about Friday the 19th?

JASON: That's fine.

RECEPTIONIST: I'll put it in my diary.

DR.DAVIES: Well Jason... [Shaking hands] I look forward to seeing you soon. Take care.

JASON: Yes, and you chief. Take care. Bye.

Richard and Judy interview:

JUDY: And now to a truly remarkable story

RICHARD: Yes, we are extremely lucky to have him here. Believe me all of us are.

Bipolar, Recovery and NLP

JUDY: Yes, Richard I agree entirely. Here he is, the Founder of Chipmunkapublishing and the Chipmunka Foundation, and of course the author of the world's most significant book on mental illness. Jason Pegler.

Jason walks in with a casual grey suit and T-shirt on. Shakes Richard's hand smiling and kisses Judy who wipes a tear away from here eye.

RICHARD: Allow me to start, if I may Jason. Your selfless work is quickly becoming recognised as a force for social good, most notably reducing stigma on mental health by so cleverly creating the world's first mental health brand. I have one question though, which I am sure you are often asked but I am fascinated to know. Why did you feel so compelled to write A Can of Madness? It can't have been an easy decision. What made you do it?

JASON: Well Richard, it's quite simple. It came to me in a flash. When I was seventeen I'd been in a mental hospital for six weeks and I thought I'd been playing Football Manager, the computer game. The moment I realised where I was, I knew that the only way I could ever psychoanalyse myself and emotionally get over the humiliation that I felt was to tell the whole world how I felt, and create a Hollywood blockbuster movie about my experiences. I knew that deep down I had the mental strength to do this and I knew I had a responsibility to stop the humiliation that anyone else who has ever been in a mental hospital feels.

JUDY: I'm so pleased, and I know Richard is too, to have you on the show. Please explain to us in more detail and to the viewers at home, what you mean by humiliation and give us an idea what drives you.

JASON: Of course Judy. Let me explain it like this. The moment I realised I was in a mental institution I felt guilty, humiliated for having a mental illness and I knew that this was something that was fundamentally wrong. It was society

442

that made me and makes anyone with mental health issues feel like this. Thing is that we are all so close to it really. Having manic depression myself changed me as a person, made me more sensitive and gave me insight as a human being that I would not have had otherwise. In fifty years time, when another seventeen year old is in the same position as me, the moment he realises, the first thought that will go through his mind will be "I'm manic and society is going to help me" not "I'm manic and its my fault, I'm a freak" . Then I've made a happy man. That is what drives me every day and why I do what I do.

RICHARD: I see Jason…so, let's look at the present - you are the head of The Chipmunka Group and creator of the World's First Mental Health Brand. What's next?

JASON: Well Richard, to continue with the mission and release 'A Can of Madness' as the Hollywood Blockbuster Movie I always intended it to be. I must stress that this is for the benefit of society. It is beyond my own ego. I have maintained the IPR and creative direction so that I can keep the story real and grow the brand through philanthropic activity. The World is badly managed and to eliminate mental ill health and psychiatry for good we need to be focused. We can't afford to waste time, as people's lives are at stake.

RICHARD: I have heard rumours that Tom Cruise will be starring in the film Jason, is that true?

JASON: Let's just say that I know someone who is close to Tom's heart and I think it would be a wonderful project for him. He is such a wonderful actor and his films are very influential.

JUDY: Well I know I'm definitely going to see it. I would like to refer to psychiatry though, if I may? I mean, it's pretty radical what you're saying don't you think?

Bipolar, Recovery and NLP

JASON: Well it's more common sense Judy, actually. Let me explain it like this. Psychiatry was invented as a form of social control. If people behave oddly, there has to be rules put in place otherwise there would be anarchy. Then look at the history of schizophrenia, for example. In 1908 some Suisse scientist advertised a notice locally asking who heard voices. Several people came forward. Some enjoyed their voices whilst it disturbed others. The scientist then calls this schizophrenia and then some entrepreneur, not a social one I hasten to add, thinks 'I know. I'll sell some drugs and make a fortune'. That's how it happens. And the whole world is taught to think that we need these drugs that screw our minds up.

I've seen hundreds of thousands of people better off without them, myself included. All that's needed is a positive that is reinforced on a daily basis and you'll never need to suffer the horrid side effects of any psychiatric drugs.

RICHARD: Yes I know people to who you have helped who have been well for years after reading your book and hearing you and Chipmunkapublishing authors speak. That is why I am so delighted that you could spare the time for us to appear on this show.

JUDY: Yes Jason. Mental health is a subject that is so very close to my heart.

JASON: Thanks to both of you. I'd just like to remind the audience at home that you must do something today to help the mental health of someone else. Give love back and it will return tenfold.

RICHARD: Oh I nearly forgot to say congratulations on winning the New Statesman's Young Social Entrepreneur of the Year Award 2005.

JASON: Thank you.

Bipolar, Recovery and NLP

JUDY: I hear you beat Jamie Oliver in the process. You must be proud.

JASON: It means so much to receive the recognition not for my own ego but because it shows that the judges realised the vitally important work that we are doing. There is so much good will out there and we have a duty to maximise it for the benefit of everyone.

On the beach front on a Sunny morning 6.30am in Barcelona.

JASON: "Ah finally finished. At last the script to change the way Hollywood and the world thinks about mental health once and for all and the deal is already signed. Think I'll have a shower".

SONIA: "Ok sweetie. Well done".

JASON: "Thanks sweetie".

SONIA: "How did you manage to do it so quickly?"

JASON: I managed to focus as you know, exercise every morning, wrote what was in my heart and stayed true to myself. All the time, I envisioned that it was already completed in the way that I wanted it to be. There was a burning desire within me to complete it because I know that when it is out it will help people who watch it and are influenced by the world's reaction to it.

SONIA: "I see" smiling.

Bipolar, Recovery and NLP

STEPHEN SPIELBERG: Jason that's great. Next take remember just be yourself. You've experienced this before so all you are doing is reliving it.

JASON – talking to the actor playing the character of his English teacher in the school and the film set.

JASON: "I have taken 5 billion ecstasy tablets, one for everyone on earth to create world peace, so I can fulfil my obligations as Head of the European hardcore Committee and instil love as one family."

PAMELA: How realistic do you think this is? You are not well.

JASON: Do not worry about me. Where there is a will there is a way. I only wish that you could see what I see… Think of those hardcore lyrics Miss… Into the future. We'll live as one family… They were written for a reason and I have discovered the reason… I have it all mapped out in front of me… look at my action plan… I will control Hollywood and the way it thinks by planting subliminal messages of peace onto the world… this is so exciting to have found the answer.. Then I can get my message out… I'll use telepathy to raise the consciousness of people around me to get them to unwittingly buy into this ideal… the world is our oyster…

PAMELA: What do your parents say about all of this?

JASON: They don't understand yet but they are starting to.

PAMELA: I think you need some help Jason.

JASON: I know. That's why I am here. Don't worry - we can do this.

They hold hands for a moment. Pamela is crying feeling desperately upset as she sees Jason as needing urgent help. Jason holds Pamela's hands thinking he is telepathically in tune with womankind to create world peace through the European Hardcore Committee which he set up as a means of communication from heaven and the real world.

Jason drives along Hollywood Boulevard in his red Ferrari listening to 2 Pac's California Love. He gets out of the car and walks into a very nice restaurant. As he is invited to sit down by the waiter Jack Nicholson stands up.

JACK: How's it going kids?

JASON: "Going great, thanks Jack. Jack how are you?
JACK: Not so bad. The Nicks won so I'm happy. You know I really think you're going to win the Oscar with "A Can of Madness this Year". I've not been as excited since "One Flew Over the Cuckoo's Nest was at this stage, just a week away from the result.

JASON: Wow thanks Jack.

JACK: You see… you got guts kid. Not only did you write the script but you acted in it and had a hand in the direction as well. You kept the story real…you see what I'm saying?

JASON: Yes Jack. I've spent years planning this. I just hope it happens. Not for my sake but for the sake of people's mental health. If it wins the Oscar next week in February 2007 then this adds recognition forever in Hollywood. It means that the taboo of mental health will disappear once and for all and then it will be easier to help the third world achieve Equal Lives.

JACK: Right on. What you having to eat. I'll have the salad. How about you?

JASON: Same here and a raw juice.

Bipolar, Recovery and NLP

JACK: Sounds great. I'll have one too. Now tell me about your next film.

JASON: Well it's another autobiography about mental health. This one is just as inspiring…

JACK: Now why did I think that?

JASON: Well it comes from this utopian vision of wanting to stop the humiliation of anyone who has ever had a mental health issue. It concerns setting up a generation of people to come forward and be positive about their past pains so they can empower themselves and other people. There are different social and financial systems in place.

Imagine the world as the planet Saturn and in the middle is the ring the mission to stop the humiliation of everyone. At the top is an arrow pointing down. Mental Well-being leading down to mental illness. The mental well being model reached to reduce stigma and vice versa. The more people are proactive in reducing stigma the further up the planet people go. The more people look after their own mental well being i.e. Mind, Body and Soul, the more time they will have to help a person with a mental health issue empower themselves.

Take the same scenario with a financial model. At the top you have a philanthropic model sending money the right way for the right reasons for this utopian ideal. At the bottom you have charity and social enterprise models campaigning in proactive terms. They have influence and can create good will but do not change the world as a whole.

JACK: – I see. Marvellous.

JASON: Well I better stop there because that's a manic mind after all and I want to eat…. hey, listen Jack… I love this song.

Bipolar, Recovery and NLP

Coldplay's "clocks" starts playing in the background and continues through the credits.

Panning out of vision like beginning of Star Wars i.e. some mental health facts... or map of Saturn diagram... but has serious undertone and plays with screen like beginning of Amelie.

CHAPTER SIX

CONCLUSION

"Curing Madness, The end of Madness – the beginning of equilibrium and a fair world"

It is inevitable that madness on earth as we know it will end. Too many people have suffered for too long. Since the beginning of time people who are the weakest have been eliminated or humiliated. Eventually they will join forces and create a bond that will lead to a revolution. I am talking about the plight of the "mentally ill". During this philosophical treatise I will prove that everyone on earth has a mental health problem.

I will begin with the strongest philosophical argument to date. That is that madness is a social construct i.e. it has been created by the status quo as a means of social control. In fact according to American Professor John Breeding, psychiatry is the greatest form of social control since Hitler and his anti Semitism in the Second World War. Breeding's argument is very impressive and is explained in layman terms, so a wide audience can be reached, but we must delve deeper.

I myself, for example, agree with Breeding's wonderful argument but as a manic depressive since the age of seventeen I have been unable to escape the social construct that I am a part of. I cannot go and live on another planet in a world where prejudice, stigma and no humiliation or even hubris exists, as I have the limits of being a human being. This leaves me with manic depression, in the real world, even though I know that it fundamentally doesn't exist. My mind though, is able to wander through and envisage a utopian ideal, where a positive image of mental health, developed by the mental health service users themselves, can lead to a revolution whereby the world is cured of mental illness. I can therefore visualise or incant a cure and choose to stay in these preferable states of being.

The utopian ideal is as follows. If I can prove that everyone on earth has a mental illness then I can stop the humiliation that mental health sufferers go through and ultimately improve that madness is after all merely a social construct. If this can be achieved then we will be able to break down mental health as a taboo and normalise it so that is mainstream an integral to society. Once it is integral to society people will have owned up and then admit to each other their own vulnerabilities. This creates a caring culture instead of a punitive one and leads to the empowerment of the mental health service user.

A most formidable example is Martin Luther King JNR and black rights in the 1960s. Thank the world for Rosa Parks who inspired Martin Luther King and countless others. If Martin Luther King JNR was a white person talking about black people's experiences nobody would have listened to him. The fact that he led a peaceful demonstration is also significant. Promoting a positive image on mental health is also a key factor in making the masses and government's buy into the strategy and have the empathy that is desired by so many sufferers. The mental health sufferer must be seen in an over positive light. This is to compensate for the disadvantageous way they are represented by the media, in flippant conversations and by the people who care for them when they are in their worst or most creative states.

We currently understand mental illness as a disease because governments, drug companies and psychiatry tell us so. However, as Thomas SSAS and Ron L Hubbard so eloquently put it, let's look at the "facts" as they are laid out in front of us. Only once we have done this, can we see how myself, Jason Pegler, and the work done at Chipmunkapublishing and it's related enterprises and the global grass roots mental health movement can take on board SSAS and Ron L Hubbard and go even further.

Bipolar, Recovery and NLP

The future of mental health empowerment, the world's first mental health brand and in my view the solution to curing my own madness of and the world which I perceive and am therefore part of is very simple.

It lies in the hands of the people. It was never designed to be owned by an individual, just representatives, who by positively discriminating in their own favour, could plant the seeds for a social revolution across the globe. Chipmunka is driven by empowerment, for the people of the world to stop the ultimate humiliation in life. That is of being diagnosed with a metaphor that turns into a poisonous reality, unless the pattern is broken and creativity and humanity are allowed to flow, and raise one's consciousness and standards back to reality.

Whatever you believe you are entitled to. That is your right as an individual. I wrote this book to illustrate how i cured myself and to give love to other people in the world who have been severely damaged by mental illness. I wanted to reveal the truth about my own experiences and to show others that you too can cure yourselves if you want to. This is because i honestly believe that there deep down there is nothing wrong with you. Insanity and mental illness are merely a matter of perception at the end of the day.

If anyone tells you any different they either have vested interests, are self manifesting their own mental illness or fear change. If we all visualise a world without mental illness then it will cease to exist in other people's realities and as a social construct. This is a matter of fact so lets do it. That is how i transformed myself and that is why i have dedicated my life to helping others see this opportunity to embrace life and achieve the impossible by saying no to a life of mental illness. I keep doing this by growing my inner self every day and being in a constant state of creative being. Now it's your turn. Enjoy it and please do keep in touch.

The Ultimate Guide to Well Being

Achieving 100% Mental Well Being

By Jason Pegler

Bipolar, Recovery and NLP

Published by:
Chipmunkapublishing's
PO Box 6872
Brentwood
Essex
CM13 1ZT
United Kingdom

http://www.chipmunkapublishing.com

Copyright © 2007 Jason Pegler

Bipolar, Recovery and NLP

CONTENTS

Bipolar, Recovery and NLP

ACKNOWLEDGEMENTS

I would like to dedicate this book to anybody who strives to help the well being of other people on the planet. I would also like to thank anyone who has been associated with Chipmunkapublishing and the Chipmunka Foundation over the last five years. Thank you for giving me the strength and support when I needed it most. In particular I would like to thank Andrew Latchford who is without doubt the most generous, patient and giving business partner, human being and friend that anyone could ever wish for. I would also like to thank Paul Williams, Paul Brandwood, Barbara Phillips, Mark Randall, John Bird, Nigel Kershaw, Ashley Cooke, Barbara Brown, Peter Horn, Charles Beckett, Stuart Bell, Sandra Lawman, Dominic O'Donnell, Ben Robertson, Nigel Stoneman, Former Labour MP and Cabinet Minister Tony Benn, Adele Blakebrough, Robert Bond, Dolly Sen, Dominic Hiatt. Apologies if I have not mentioned you.
I would also like to thank all the Chipmunkapublishing authors for believing that they and we can make a difference. Thank you for believing in me, and the Chipmunka team.
I would like to thank the many Chpimunka volunteers around the world for their time, donations, kindness and dedication in helping us to help more people. They can see that the work we are doing is a unique empowerment model that is changing the history of the mental health movement for the better.

Bipolar, Recovery and NLP

I would like to give special thanks to the fifty or so university students around the world who have given their time to come into Chipmunka offices to selflessly help other people whose lives need to be given a voice. I would like to give a special thanks to students from French universities and London universities for giving up a considerable amount of their time and using their initiative to help more people.

There have been many organizations and people that have helped inspire me along the way. I would like to thank Virgin, My Space, You Tube, Microsoft, eBay, Apple, Manchester United, Anthony Robbins, Coldplay, Eminem, Dr Dre, Snoop Doggy Dogg, Paul McKenna, The Department of Trade & Industry, Bill Clinton, Tony Blair, Nelson Mandela, Bob Geldof, U2, David Beckham, Madonna, Ronnie O'Sullivan, Steven Spielberg, Martin Scorsese, Ben Affleck, Matt Damon, Al Pacino, Tom Cruise, Robert de Niro, Bill Gates, Paul Merton and Richard Branson, to name but a few.

I would like to thank particular organizations that do not always get the high profile but have an important role in the well being of people in the UK especially and further a field. Please forgive me for any organizations that have not been mentioned. You know who you are. I would like to whole heartedly thank the DTI, New Statesman, The Arts Council, The National Lottery, SLAM NHS Trust, NIMHE, London Development Centre, The Sunday Times, BBC, ITV, Channel 4, Sky TV, Big Issue, Community Action Network, Mind,

Bipolar, Recovery and NLP

Rethink, Sane, the Independent, Daily Telegraph, Guardian, The Times, The Observer, Natmags, Emap, Launchpad, KPMG, Faegre Benson Hobson & Audley, Olswang, CCHR, Samaritans, NAMHE,

I would like to thank my family and friends for allowing me to express the way I feel about the world during our time together. Thank you from the bottom of my heart. I would like to thank my partner Sonia for her love everyday that gives me the strength to continue the utopian dream that I have to eliminate the humiliation that people with 'mental health issues' feel or will ever feel and to make suicides a thing of the past. Your love, patience, kindness and advice inspire me everyday.

Bipolar, Recovery and NLP

Chapter One

Healthy, mind, body and soul

To discover the ultimate path to well being, you have to reach inside of your mind, body and soul like you never have before. This takes a conscious effort or *massive action* as Anthony Robbins most aptly calls it. Anthony Robbins who is probably regarded as the greatest motivational speaker on the planet says that you need to take *massive action* in his book Unlimited Power (Published by Simon & Schuster 1989). In the last 10 years I have read several hundred self-help books and regard Unlimited Power as the best of them all, much better than his later books and audio material. He is also a pretty impressive speaker – I have listened to him for many an hour.
Anthony Robbins is exactly right. There is no point in procrastinating on doing something. You have to actually do it. You have to look inside of yourself and ask yourself who you are as a human being and what you are capable of. Then do it.

Once you discover who you are, you can then discover what you want and then start doing it. It really is as simple as that and not rocket science. Just decide to do something and then take massive action.

During this book I have decided to split the journey to Ultimate Well Being into nine manageable steps (It's like two Stephen Covey books in one and a bonus chapter– only joking, Steve, I am a big fan of your books Stephen …

Bipolar, Recovery and NLP

Please keep writing). Whilst you go through each step and go through each exercise, take notes, re read anything you do not understand and visualise the positive outcomes of each step so that you are also taking a step forward and are therefore a step closer to Ultimate Well Being. Each step will take you that little bit closer to 100% mental well being. See this book as an examination of yourself. You will be able to pass but you will have to challenge yourself to progress. This book is an opportunity for you to test yourself and give yourself 100% success, as you are the examiner of your life. Nobody else is responsible for how you feel… Just you… That is the reality. See this examination as a confirmation that you and anyone can choose to be a success and even rid yourself of your ego in the process so you can lead a more fulfilled life and have a more positive impact on the world. I repeat. You are the examiner in your life. Ultimately no matter where you seek inspiration the responsibility of living your life boils down to you and not anybody else.

This is not just another self-help book. Even if it were I do not think that would necessarily be a bad thing. I like self help books. They fill your head with positive things and day-to-day people can easily be bombarded with more negative than positive thoughts, so self-help can reprogramme positivism. My first two books document how I lived a life of manic-depression and cured myself. (If you feel this is dubious please break your pattern, open your mind, change your belief system, do whatever it takes to accept this as fact and then read on!) I have been in the depths of despair and welcomed positivism and enlightenment into my life and made the permanent switch into having a happy mind, body and soul. Therefore I feel that I am qualified to write a new type of self-help book and publish a new type of self-help genre of autobiographical memoirs from people who suffer 'mental illness'. I have changed my life and I am not just using some kind of theoretical system like most other self help books. My personal suffering has been revealed in my earlier books and the weaknesses of many self help writers is a mystery. Reading this book is a unique opportunity for you to totally enhance your life and reach new standards in every aspect of your life so you can be totally empowered.

You will be able to be a *novus homo* as they say in Latin. A new man as the amazing Roman orator Cicero was in 63BC when he became a member of the Equestrian Order through his achievements instead of through birth. Nobody had done that previously in the history of Rome so it really was an outstanding achievement. If you find it hard to identify with the life of someone over 2000 years ago in another city then think of rap.

Think of Eminem's lyrics in the film *8 Mile*. The director of *8 Mile* said that writing the lyrics for the film made Eminem go deeper inside himself than at any other time in his life. As Eminem says in the most famous track he wrote for the movie "*If you had one chance, one opportunity in life… would you capture it or let it slip*". In 8 Mile Eminem wins a rapping contest but instead of celebrating who goes back to work so he can save up money for his studio time. The implication in Eminem's lyrics I believe are that you should capture an opportunity even if you only have it once. This is exactly what Eminem does in the film and exactly why he won the contest and went back to work to save up for his studio time so Rabbit would become a famous rapper just like Eminem is.

Would you capture it or let it slip?

I remember being inspired when watching *8 Mile* and was fortunate that when an opportunity came along for me to make a rap album I managed to capture it and not let it slip. I have recently launched this rap album. Although it was a very steep learning curve over a short period of time and a lot of hard work, it was really much easier than I thought. The album is called *A Can of Madness*, the same name of my book and autobiography on living with manic-depression, published in 2002 by Chipmunkapublishing. I had one chance to do a rap album and took it. It all started when a volunteer in the Chipmunka office called Ama was reading the rap I wrote in *A Can of Madness* and said that she liked it and that she had a friend whose boyfriend was a rapper. I've always loved hip-hop ever since I heard NWA's 'Straight Outta Compton' at the age of 12. I see hip-hop as a potential force for good to bring cultures together and stop racism globally. I liked writing lyrics but never really thought of doing an album or performing. Soon enough I met Ama's friend and the rapper. His name was Ryan and at 17 years of age he had his own label, Raskil Records. I was amazed how good the rappers were on his label, especially as most of them were teenagers and they wanted to help people with mental illness. So within 6 weeks I had paid for and organised two rap events for them to perform live for the very first time. At the first event one of my friends whose rap name is Howling came along. He was a multi-talented 23 year-old at the time, and introduced me to his friend Avarice who made his beats. Avarice is a brilliant producer, lyricist and rapper himself and went out of his way to help. We held several sessions after work in my office and Avarice had given me a crash course in rapping in time to the beats to the lyrics that I had written a few years earlier. This consisted of several evening sessions after work in Chipmunka's main offices in central London. Then we spent one day round his house as he has his own studio and within four months of meeting him, I had launched my rap album.

Just like Eminem you can do anything like making a rap album if you wanted to. It's just a little example of how if you have a good feeling for something, that you should just go for it and reap the rewards whether they are emotional, financial, psychological or spiritual. In return I wanted to help Avarice, so I kept in touch and I am helping to promote his crew Renegade Artistry. Check them out at www.rarecords.net. They really are some of the most talented rappers in British Hip Hop.

Moment of Decision

As Anthony Robbins tells us it is in the moment of our decision when our lives change or we have a *paradigm shift* as Stephen Covey calls it. Anyone who hears and connects with Eminem in the film *8 Mile* could think of something in their lives that they have been hesitant about and would choose to go for it. If you read this book with this positive mentality and decisiveness then you will achieve Ultimate Well Being.

So congratulations to you dear readers for taking that quantum leap (Yes VISUALISE IT RIGHT NOW… feel good… that's not good enough… feel great… feel fantastic… that's more like it!!!) into a happier state of consciousness… OK… THEN LET'S PROCEED…

We get what we focus on in life. In order to have a healthy mind, body and soul you need to treat these conditions as achievable qualities. Everyone has them so if you don't feel it stop moping around and just zap yourself with some amazing, fantastic, energising sense of feeling great for yourself, other people and the world as a whole. If someone tells you that you have manic depression and a chemical imbalance in the brain, they do not know what they are talking about. You can alter your chemistry by getting more oxygen and jogging in the morning. No psychiatrist has ever proven that there is something wrong with your brain so snap out of believing those negative thoughts. Life is worth living. Take it from me, I know! I have been so low I was suicidal for months at a time and I chose life. If *Forest Gump* can achieve the impossible then so can you my dear friend. And if you can… so can anyone… So let's deconstruct having a healthy mind, body and soul into three parts. First, let's break them down into three separate parts. Then we will show how they are all connected.

Having a healthy mind.

Having a healthy mind is as achievable as you want it to be. Let's set some targets. Say out loud "my goal is to have a healthy mind body and soul 24 hours a day, seven days a week for the rest of my life." Feel good? Well good isn't good enough… feel very good… feel outstanding… Wooooooooooowwwwwhhhhhh…… Great. Say it again first in your mind. Then out loud. Now try doing something fun with your body, like smiling, while you are doing this or even be more adventurous and try a flying kick… something to give you more oxygen and change your physiology so you are in a PEAK state…….
Repeat this three times… Feeling Great….. Now CONTINUE.

Those of you who have been to an Anthony Robbins Seminar will know exactly what I am talking about. Don't worry if you haven't. Ever seen Paul McKenna? Now you have re-programmed your mind as Paul McKenna would say to make this feeling of feeling GREAT a reality. The more intensely you practice this INCANTATION and awaken, the more real it will become. Why not commit to chanting to your first step to Ultimate Well Being three times a day for the next year, after that it will be automatic. Now you have programmed your mind to choose a healthy mind you can mark yourself and give yourself 1% towards Ultimate Well Being.

Congratulations, you only have 99% to go. This will be as easy as you wish it to be. And you will remember the decisions you have made in this book forever because you are consciously choosing to do so. Now celebrate as if your favourite football team has just scored! Or for all you ladies reading this, as if you have just bought a beautiful outfit that you feel stunning in and the man or woman of your dreams walks straight up to you and asks you out. LOL… Or something else that will give you the same amazing feeling. Having just met your loved one for the first time! An end to world poverty… Every religion becoming friends… Something totally awesome and loving so you will NEVER FORGET THIS BEAUTIFUL MOMENT. Do whatever it takes to make this crucial moment in your personal development last forever and then multiply the love and intensity a MILLION TIMES. Close your eyes and have some beautiful intensity and love that will improve your life and the lives of those you love and even those that you haven't met forever. Feel the love and relax in a state of being.

Bipolar, Recovery and NLP

Congratulations you are now fully on your way to ACHIEVING 100% and ULTIMATE WELL BEING. What's remarkable too is that this is a gift that you can pass on both consciously and unconsciously. You can pass this on so you can help other people and the world as one. Eckhart Tolle writes about this in *The Power of Now*. He is an amazing person. For the first 29 years of his life he was severely mentally ill. Then a profound spiritual transformation virtually dissolved his old identity and radically changed the course of his life. He did not know who he was, but spent three years on a spiritual high and lived for two years on a park bench in a state of ecstasy. The transition that transformed his life happened in a split second. Eckhart Tolle writes in his introduction in *The Power of Now* that he lived in a state of almost continuous anxiety interspersed with periods of suicidal depression. One night he woke up with absolute dread that was so intense, more intense than he had ever experienced. He had a deep loathing for everything in the world, his misery was compounded as he loathed himself more than anything else. During a time when he was going through the deepest psychological pain that he ever experienced, he broke through into a higher state of consciousness. Tolle writes:

"I cannot live with myself any longer." This was the thought that kept repeating itself in my mind. Then suddenly I became aware of what a peculiar thought it was. "Am I one or two? If I cannot live with myself, there must be two of me: the 'I' and the 'self' that 'I' cannot live with. "Maybe," I thought, "only one of them is real."

His massive action, paradigm step, step into Ultimate Well Being, step into being, personal transformation or whatever you want to call it, shows that anything is possible for a human being. Tolle is a living example that anyone's life no matter how desperate can improve.

The same is true of any kind of mental illness including manic-depression. I know this because I achieved the transition myself. When I was 17 I was diagnosed with manic-depression. From the ages 17-25 I spent over 1 year of my life in five different psychiatric hospitals. By the age of 29 I had made a 90% recovery but was still part of the medical system. In September 2005 I made a life changing decision after meeting Robbins whose work I'd been following. I used his techniques for inspiration in life and work for five years to take the final step to constant empowerment and Ultimate Well Being. I accepted that my manic-depression was entirely self-manifested and that I would come off the medication that was poisoning my mind and to come off it forever. I also managed to get sponsored by the NHS to go to his events, so that was a bonus and I felt justified in receiving this gift as my day job is as a social entrepreneur and learning his techniques would enable me to help more people anyway. Robbins and his techniques had helped but without being a social entrepreneur I would never had been able to make a full recovery. Both positive outcomes could be maximised to help even more people and give myself more personal growth and happiness.

There were 12,000 people hugging each other for four days. It was an uplifting experience that I will always cherish. Within four months of attending Robbins, I'd come off medication for good and had 25 people working for me full-time for free at my company Chipmunkapublishing's first office in London. This accelerated the utopian vision to change the way the world thinks about mental health and facilitated the launch of the Chipmunka Foundation (Registered charity number 1109537) and enabled me to help more people worldwide.

Every second of every day I looked inside my inner self, looking at what was truly important to me as a human being. As my mind became free of medication I became stronger every day and more fun to be around.

Within eight months of deciding to come off the medication, my life had totally changed. I spent three months coming off slowly with discussions with my psychiatrist who could see that I had massive insight into my own behaviour, life and belief systems and he gave me his full consent and support because he could see that I had total commitment with the intelligence, aptitude and mental strength to make a life changing commitment forever.

Now my psychiatrist is an active supporter in the active goals of my social enterprises and charity.

Bipolar, Recovery and NLP

How great is that? If you are a psychiatric patient this shows that you can totally cure yourself not just philosophically but in reality. It is just as easy as choosing to and following up with whatever you want to do in life.

By May 2005 I was sat in a room with 200 people at the Dali museum in London listening to the Channel 4 TV presenter Sarah Smith talking about how I had a vision for the world which shows massive potential for helping people cure themselves of mental illness, I was a phenomenal public speaker, extremely talented consultant, social entrepreneur who had written one of the most defining books of his generation etc... A few seconds later I was awarded the New Statesman's Young Social Entrepreneur of the year 2005, beating celebrity chef Jamie Oliver who has his own TV series and had convinced Tony Blair to commit to spending more money on every school dinner for pupils in schools throughout the country. All my dreams were starting to come true at a quicker pace because I had been setting the appropriate plans but also because I had chosen to take massive action myself and actually do it. I'd decided that it was only me who was responsible for what happened in my life. This is true for you too. If you want a healthy mind, body, soul or anything else in life then ultimately it is your responsibility to do something about it.

Now repeat after me: Me, myself and I choose to achieve 100% mental well being and I choose to do so now. Feel it, visualise it, imagine it, celebrate it...do it... Happy... Feeling great...

Bipolar, Recovery and NLP

Play your favourite song, shout it out, do it with a friend, meditate, play football or do martial arts while you are saying this to get more oxygen in your body… Do whatever it takes to make it have a stronger and more lasting impact on your newfound content and happy mind. Do this with your friend, partner, imaginary friend, remote control or any other inanimate object next to this book. Do it now, enjoy it and celebrate as if you have just won your favourite Olympic event and then donated your gold medal to charity for world peace… and say it five times so it stays with you.

Say that you will do it five times for the next five days and it will stay with you. Then every five days it becomes five times more intense and five times the fun. Who would not want that great felling to continue? Congratulations you can now give yourself 2% in your journey to 100% mental well-being and Ultimate Well Being.

Just like anyone else who is a PEAK PERFORMER, I constantly draw inspiration from people who have the greatest minds in history to challenge me everyday in my own mind and life so that I can help the people that The Chipmunka Group is designed to help. Some of my favourite inspirational figures in this world are:

1) Mohandas Gandhi (1869-1948). Known as Mahatma ('Great-Soul'), Gandhi was the leader of the Indian nationalist movement against British rule, and is widely considered the father of his country. His doctrine of non-violent protest to

achieve political and social progress has been hugely influential.

Gandhi stuck to what he believed in. He had the peace of mind to continue non-violent and peaceful demonstrations despite being constantly pushed to the edge where most people have cracked under pressure and changed strategies even beginning to use violence. Gandhi stuck to his principles, made a bigger impact than using force would have done and went down in history as a force for social greatness.

2) From 1931 to 1948 Mother Teresa taught at St. Mary's High School in Calcutta, but the suffering and poverty she glimpsed outside the convent walls made such a deep impression on her that in 1948 she received permission from her superiors to leave the convent school and devote herself to working among the poorest of the poor in the slums of Calcutta. Although she had no funds, she depended on Divine Providence, and started an open-air school for slum children. Soon she was joined by voluntary helpers, and financial support was also forthcoming. This made it possible for her to extend the scope of her work.

On October 7, 1950, Mother Teresa received permission from the Holy See to start her own order, "The Missionaries of Charity", whose primary task was to love and care for those persons nobody was prepared to look after. In 1965 the Society became an International Religious Family by a decree of Pope Paul VI.

Bipolar, Recovery and NLP

The Society of Missionaries has spread all over the world, including the former Soviet Union and Eastern European countries. They provide effective help to the poorest of the poor in a number of countries in Asia, Africa, and Latin America, and they undertake relief work in the wake of natural catastrophes such as floods, epidemics, famine, and for refugees. The order also has houses in North America, Europe and Australia, where they take care of the shut-ins, alcoholics, homeless, and AIDS sufferers. Mother Teresa is also someone whose mind I admire. She dedicated her life to helping other people less fortunate than herself. She goes down as number two in my list of most inspirational minds today.

3) I am also greatly inspired as many people are by the mind of Nelson Mandela. Nelson Mandela is one of the world's most revered statesmen, who led the struggle to replace the apartheid regime of South Africa with a multi-racial democracy.

Despite many years in jail, he emerged to become the country's first black president and to play a leading role in the drive for peace in other spheres of conflict. He won the Nobel Peace Prize in 1993.

Bob Geldof was right to call him the president of the world. Nelson Mandela gave his life to stop the suffering and discrimination felt by his people. He reaches my top ten minds today. My top minds may change on a daily basis as yours can, as there thousands of people that inspire me to push myself further and enable me to lead a more fulfilled, meaningful and loving life.

4) John Lennon also had an amazing mind. John Lennon's mind was so creative and he has given joy to millions of people. He created his own music and The Beatles are the most successful band in history. I like the way John Lennon went through stages and experimented with his mind. From songs such as 'Jealous Guy', 'All You Need is Love', his boyish humour and his peace demonstrations. His mind and his actions are truly inspirational to me.

5) Like many other people I have respect for Albert Einstein. Einstein changed the way we all think, by his theory of Relativity! I was never very good at Science at school but like many other people, I am inspired by Einstein's positive impact on the world. Einstein contributed more than any other scientist to the modern vision of physical reality. His special and general theories of relativity are still regarded as the most satisfactory model of the large-scale universe that we have.

(6) Pele was a genius on the football pitch. Pele was the greatest footballer of all time in many people's books, scoring over 1000 goals in his career. He stormed on the scene in the 1970 World Cup. He had a quick mind for football. He applied his mind to a higher standard than others and was an amazing player to watch. By 1970 people thought that he was past it but he led Brazil

to winning the world cup that year and was inspirational in the tournament. I am a big sports fan and watching the greats like Pele is one reason why I still enjoy playing football. I could quite easily come up with a list of 10 sportsmen who inspire me on a daily basis.

(7) I have always loved playing chess. Gary Kasparov makes my top ten minds of all time for today as he is probably the greatest chess player of all time. I know how demanding chess is mentally and physically as I played to a high competitive standard from the age of seven. Kasparov has won world titles and dominated the game for well over a decade. Kasparov is also an amazing person as he speaks articulately on human rights issues.

(8) Marcus Tallies Cicero - the famous Roman orator was a statesman, humanitarian and lawyer who was born 106BC- died 43BC. Cicero is one of my heroes of history. He rose from plebeian to statesman class, which was unprecedented and chose not to become a dictator in 60BC when asked to join the First Triumvirate, as he was not corrupted by political power. His philosophical work On Old Age is also the most sensible and helpful philosophical essay that I have ever read. It actually makes you look forward to old age.

9) Other minds that inspire me include William Shakespeare. Shakespeare wrote many amazing plays and beautiful sonnets which are still staged

and known to people all over the world of all ages nearly 400 years after his death. His plays and poems move people through every single emotion: joy, fear, sorrow, pain, pleasure, humour, despair and enlightenment. Shakespeare's work touches every single facet of human emotion and has stood the test of time.

10) I also have a great deal of respect for Thomas Ssazz who has challenged psychiatry since the 1960s. Ssazz's writing has pioneered much service user thinking about psychiatry today and shown that the drug companies grip on the world of mental health patients worldwide need not last forever and can convince people to think in different ways.

I constantly use people throughout history to inspire me so I have a mindset that keeps me on my toes and raises my standards every second of every day. You can do the same. Write down the ten greatest minds that inspire you. Think of people who have changed the world or people who have had a profound impact on history, politics, sport, art, and literature. Even if it is your friends or family that inspire you most write their names down and then give reasons why.

Your top 10 minds

1
2
3

4
5
6
7
8
9
10

Finished your list now? That's great. You have now achieved 3% of your Ultimate Well Being. Write a line or two for each explaining how they inspire you to increase your score to 4%

1

2

3

4

5

6

7

8

9

10

Now you have finished your list of people that inspire you and the reasons how they inspire read each person's name and the reasons out loud with passion in the same way you read out your incantation. Congratulations you have now achieved 5% mental well-being. Feeling good… ok…. FEELING GREAT……… that's better. I deliberately made the first few steps the most difficult. Now achieving your well being score should become easier as you go through the exercises.

Bipolar, Recovery and NLP

NLP

The mind as you can see is an extremely powerful tool and so is the body. People who study NLP (Neuro-Linguistic Programming) realize now how important the way we use our bodies is. Fifty-five percent of how we communicate is through our physiology. Only 7% is from the words we use and 38% is from sound and tonality of the way we do things. Imagine you walk around standing upright, walking confidently and with an expression of calmness and friendliness. You will be able to send a positive vibe or give positive chi when you come into contact with people, if you maintain this positivism. You can even go further and deliberately be nice to people. This will have a positive impact on their day and yours. This is much better than walking and dragging your feet kicking, cussing, being cynical and placing your problems on other people etc... better stop there. I do not want to break your pattern and make you sad. Let's keep it up and positive. Happy... move on... Just a word of warning for you, don't be overly nice to people on an ongoing basis as this is not being honest with people. Better to be positive than negative though, as this is really important in your journey to Ultimate Well Being.

Think about the following. If you see someone walking down the road, looking angry, cursing and swearing, this will put your body in a different state... Your physiology will drop and somehow... turn negative... Your heart rate may increase...

you may remember something that annoys you and your mood will drop as well... You may even cross the road... You may change the way you breathe or stop breathing... This could make you nervous... stressed... anxious.... give you a panic attack.... even give you Conversion Syndrome Disorder if you repeated this behaviour over a number of years...

See how the previous mindset triggered and caused this negativity.... It was self manifested.... You could do the exact opposite.... Think about it. You've already mastered your mind. You have the 10 greatest minds in history inspiring you and you know you can visualize more amazing people inspiring you in any walk of life at any moment to help you get to achieve whatever you want to in life......you can move forward at any moment when using your mind. You can do the same with your body too...

Walk down the road... smile... look at someone else and feel happy and smile... Your positive chi will pass onto the next person and so on... You will walk confidently... your physiology will be strong.... You will enjoy every second... look forward to what you are going to do and be happy in that present moment... and have a great day... This is something you chose and something that you decided to do.

I am now 31 years of age and my body is in better shape than it has ever been. I have more energy than I have ever had and average 6.30 hours sleep a day because that is all I require to have an amazing day each day. I believe that I am lucky to have a healthy body and look after it by eating healthy, exercising daily and not smoking. I believe that the healthier my body, the healthier and happier I am as a human being.

I know the positive impacts of a healthy lifestyle and playing football and or exercising most days, releases positive endorphins in my body that make me physically and therefore psychologically happier than I would have been without exercising.

I still admire people in history who have the healthiest bodies of all time and step into their shoes to give me a psychological buzz at every opportunity I have consciously and unconsciously chosen to improve the condition of my body, which I know helps my related state, emotional well being and happiness.

Inspirational Bodies

(1) I have an amazing amount of respect for Lance Armstrong. Lance Armstrong won the Tour De France 6 times. The Tour De France is one of the most demanding physical challenges in any sporting event. No one else has won the Tour as many times as Lance Armstrong or as many times in a row. What makes the life of Lance Armstrong even more incredible is that he became ill with

cancer, nearly died and still came back to win the Tour De France on his return. You think he did this by feeling sorry for himself… no way… he achieved this by deciding that he could overcome it and kept that positive mindset throughout.

(2) Second on my list of bodies that inspire me is Arnold Schwarzenegger. Arnold Schwarzenegger was born in a small town in Austria and became Mr. Universe 5 times. He trained unbelievably hard. When I used to play competitive rugby as a teenager it was Arnold Schwarzenegger who inspired me to go down to the gym even though I had never met him. I knew no matter how many times I went to the gym that Arnold Schwarzenegger would look stronger than me. Imagining him as a potential opponent and imagining I was him when training inspired me to train more frequently and train harder. Rugby, like many sports is quite a psychological game and the stronger you look to your opponent, the stronger you feel and are makes a difference.

(3) Third in my list of remarkable bodies is Bruce Lee. He was renowned as the greatest martial artist in the world and was responsible for taking martial arts into Hollywood. In 1970 (Age 30): Bruce had injured his sacral nerve and experiences severe muscle spasms in his back while training. Doctors told him that he would never kick again. During the months of recovery he starts to document his training methods and his philosophy of Jeet Kune Do. Thirty years later this

martial art is revered and practised all over the world and Bruce Lee inspires thousands of people to take up martial arts every year.

(4) Another body or person that I admire is Amir Khan. At 17 years of age he went to the Olympics and gained a sliver medal. Less than a year later he turned professional and beat the boxer who beat him in the final, has won his first ten professional fights and looks set to become a future World Boxing Champion.

(5) Houdini is the most famous magician of all time. Houdini is credited with the invention or unique improvement of a number of important illusions (the Strait Jacket Escape, Walking Through a Brick Wall, Metamorphosis, Buried Alive, the Hindu Needle Trick, the Chinese Water Torture Cell and the Milk Can Escape). He revolutionized magic and took it to another level. He could escape from things that other people could never have perceived before.

6) The most amazing magician and stunt performer David Blaine is also somebody who inspires me. David Blaine (4/04/1973 from Brooklyn, New York City) made his name as a performer of street and close-up magic. David Blaine has performed many stunts. For example in November 2000 Blaine began a stunt called "Frozen In Time". Blaine stood in a closet of ice, which was sculpted to fit his body, and a tube provided him with air and water while his urine

was removed from another tube. He was encased in ice for 61 hours, 40 minutes and 15 seconds before being removed. Blaine survived as the whole world witnessed the event on television.

(7) I remember when I was 9 years old watching the Los Angeles Olympics on Television. Carl Lewis won the 100 metres, 200 metres, long jump and relay. On the biggest day of his life he succeeded and was at the top of his sport for several years. All together he won 9 Olympic gold medals and 8 world championship gold medals. Although I never went on to enter the Olympics I found Carl Lewis an inspirational figure during and after that Olympics.

(8) Steven Redgrave is another amazing athlete. He is the only athlete in the history of the Olympics to win a gold medal in 5 different Olympics. Redgrave epitomizes the success that an individual can have at peak performance for the longest interval. He has also won the BBC's sports personality of the year.

9) Phil Taylor is someone who deserves a lot of admiration. He has fantastic eyesight and hand to eye coordination. Phil Taylor was born on 13/08/60 and is a multi word champion darts player, considered by most to be the greatest ever. His nickname is 'The Power'. Taylor has now clocked up 11 PDC World Championships to bring his haul to 13 world titles. Knowing how hard he

practices I would not bet against him winning any more world titles.

10) Michael Jordan is another amazing athlete. He is the greatest basketball player of all time. He also made a comeback at the age of 35. Jordan put in the effort. He practiced before everyone else did for 1 year when his high school coach refused to pick him. Next year he got in the team and the rest is history.

Now think of 10 people with the most amazing bodies in history that inspire you.

1
2
3
4
5
6
7
8
9
10

Great......Well Done...... Feel the rush...... Feel the buzz...... Coming up..... GETTING HIGHER. Feel that natural feeling of Ultimate Well Being......

Now you are 6% on your way to Ultimate Well Being. Write a line or two on why each one inspires you to get to 7%.

Bipolar, Recovery and NLP

1

2

3

4

5

6

7

8

9

10

Read out loudly the names of the people whose bodies inspire you and why and you have 8% Ultimate Well Being. Congratulations. You are well on your way to leading a happier life….

Bipolar, Recovery and NLP

Having a healthy Soul

Make sure you do not mention the same people in this section as you did in the healthy mind or body section. That would make it too easy…. Draw inspiration from different sources to maximize your well being.

Now you have a healthy mind and body why not go all the way and choose to have a healthy soul. There are many people throughout history who have a healthy soul.

(1) Top of my list today is Jesus. I was born a Christian but I am not particularly religious. I see myself more as a humanitarian with a mindset similar to some aspects of Buddhism. Like many people I see myself as someone who draws inspiration from everyone who has a positive impact on the world. I see my duty in life as a communicator of Ultimate Well Being and Mental Health Empowerment. Whatever your religious beliefs Jesus was an amazingly generous person. Two thousand years after he walked the earth, Jesus of Nazareth remains one of those most talked-about and influential people who had ever lived. Jesus dedicated his life to helping others and even died for us. How's that for having a beautiful soul.

(2) Martin Luther King also had an amazing soul. He was instrumental in giving black people a voice in America, reducing racism and giving equality to

black people throughout the world. He died for what he believed in and has had a positive impact on the whole world.

(3)In my mind, Bill Gates has an amazing soul. He had a dream to give everyone in the world the opportunity to have their own computer. He has been the richest man in the world for the last decade but gives away a high percentage of his wealth for charitable causes.

(4) Dale Carnegie also has a beautiful soul. He was the wealthiest man in the world and was ruthless but then went back to a commitment that he made at the age of 30. By the time he would die, he promised to redistribute his wealth for the benefit of society and for the education of the world and he made sure he did. He accomplished so much, setting up schools and libraries that would not have been set up without his help.

(5) In my view Anthony Robbins, the world's leader in motivational seminars, also has a beautiful soul. He is driven by the will to encourage everyone he meets to reach their full potential in life.

Now come up with 5 souls in the world that you inspire. It can be famous people or people you know.

1
2

Bipolar, Recovery and NLP

3
4
5

You know the score... Twenty Thousand hardcore knocking at your door... Only joking... Write a line or two on why each of them inspires you to take your well being score to 10%. Celebrate.... Jump up in the air... SMILE TO YOURSELF... however you want. Enjoy the natural rush and feeling of Ultimate Well Being.

1

2

3

4

5

When you have written this down and read it out loud and agree to at the utmost intensity like you have never meant anything before, you will have completed 11% of your journey to Ultimate Well Being.

As you have gone through each exercise, you may have been thinking of the same people for different categories. I know I did. I asked you not to repeat the same people to make your journey to ultimate well being more rewarding and more soul searching. I never said it was going to be easy but I promise you if you follow the techniques in this book verbatim and give everything that you've got, then you will be able to move forward and have the opportunity to make 100% ultimate well being a reality. There is no reason why you will not be able to keep that reality. This choice has already been made by you so congratulations once again…. you are well on your way to Ultimate Well Being.

You will see now that there are people who can fit into all these categories and people who do not for one reason or other. To achieve 100% mental well being you have to succeed in every category. Winston Churchill had a great mind. He was Prime minister, he had a great soul, he is said to have saved Britain in its hour of need. He didn't need much sleep. He was overweight, a drunk and a smoker and suffered from depression. In my eyes Churchill fails in one category, possibly two so realize how far you are going to stretch yourself. You are now only at 11% so there is a long way to go but you can choose to do it. Be like NIKE or somebody who inspires you- Just do it.

You can go further in your guide to Ultimate Well Being than Winston Churchill did, one of the most accomplished statesmen of the 20th Century. There is no reason why you can't be successful in all three categories. I have a healthy mind, body and soul because I have identified what constitutes having a healthy mind, body soul every day means for me.

When I worked out what having a healthy mind means to me I decided that it meant a mind free from medication, drugs and alcohol abuse. I choose to use my mind everyday to spend time doing what I am passionate about and learning more and more about philanthropy, social entrepreneurship, mental health, well being, business practices, social justice, information technology, Neuro-Linguistic Programming, the world and other things. I learnt to appreciate my friends and family more and appreciate simple things in life/ Live in the now and not worry so much about the past and the future.

I see life as a gift and I believe that I have an opportunity and duty to use the previous pain that I have experienced as a former manic depressive as a force for social good to have a positive impact on the world. I believe that I can facilitate changing the way the world thinks about mental health for the better and empower millions of people around the world to empower each other and give each other a voice so that in 50 years time there will be no humiliation for anyone who is regarded as "mentally ill". The moment that I realized I was in a mental institution at the age of 17, was the defining moment of my life. The first thought that went through my mind was that the humiliation I felt was unjust and I knew that when I chose to, I would spend the rest of my life finding a way to prevent other people going through the same humiliation that I felt.

I can say three things about having a healthy mind, body and soul.

1 My healthy mind is a crucial tool in reaching the most important personal goals in my life.

2 My healthy body is another helpful tool in achieving my personal happiness.

Chapter 2

Know what is crucial to your happiness

In the first chapter you learnt how to establish a healthy, mind, body and soul for the rest of your life. You realized that this was a choice that you made and attainable when you decided to do so.

In this chapter you will learn what is crucial to your happiness as a human being.

Think of your life and how hectic it is. There are many things that we plan to do in a day but do we ever get everything done? Of course not… Life would be boring if we did get everything done. That's not what life is about. Life is about, 'knowing thyself'- this old Greek adage is just as relevant today as it was 2500 years ago. To discover what you want to do in life, in business, relationships or relaxation, it helps to plan. However, this is not always the case. For example if you can be in a constant state of being then you may be able to move from one flow to another but this is not practical for most people to suddenly step into and is a complex line of thought. It is not in my nature to plan. I am by nature impulsive and have a stream of conscious style to my writing and thought processes. If something feels right then I tend to go with the flow that I have.

To get the most of your well being however and to know what is crucial to your happiness, it helps to plan, certainly until you move into higher states of consciousness and spirituality which are discussed in Chapter 6.

A pioneering exercise to do which is used in most self-help books is to write things down. At the beginning of this chapter we are going to use Anthony Robbins's technique that has been rehashed by hundreds of authors writing self-help books since. For our purposes in this instance Robbins's earliest work of (1989) is ideal.

In **Unlimited Power**, Robbins writes about us writing down our top 20 values in no particular order in order to take steps for us in finding out exactly who we are and what are therefore the most important things to us.

Spend 5 minutes writing down your most important values. I'll give you an example. For me values that immediately come to mind are –

Love, healthy mind body and soul, companionship, loyalty, friendship, honesty, integrity, compassion and hard work.

Once you have written them, put them in order of priority with number 1 as the most important to you; e.g.

Honesty (1)
Healthy mind body and soul (2)
Love (3)

Compassion (5)
Integrity (4)
Friendship (7)
Hard work (6).

Your Values:

1
2
3
4
5
6
7

Do not forget to put them in order of priority. You should have at least 7 values.
Then write a paragraph for each of the top 5 and why they are important to you. This brainstorming exercise will start getting you in the mood to really answer the question once and for all. How will I know what is crucial to my happiness?
Use my example of Having a healthy mind, body and soul to help you.

Example:

Value 2 - Having a healthy mind, body and soul

I know what makes me happy. Having a healthy mind, body and soul are important to me so that I can make the most out of the love of my girlfriend, friends, family and people who I meet in life and want to help and want to empower and give a voice. With my healthy mind, body and soul in place and awareness of my values, I am able to focus on what drives me to have a positive impact on society.

Top 5 values with explanatory paragraph:

Value

1

2

3

4

5

Bipolar, Recovery and NLP

Congratulations now you have added your top 7 values and explained why your top 5 values are the most important you can move from 20% ultimate well being to 25%.

The rest of this Chapter is an example of how I have answered what is crucial to my happiness as a human being. For me it is helping other people with mental illness that feeds my happiness and motivates my goals and actions in life. Whilst you are reading please think of answering this question for yourself. There will be a space for you to write your own notes at the end of the chapter.

DIAGRAM. 1
Economic.   Final Steps.

BIG
STEPS

GOAL REALISED

INTERCONNECTED

SMALL STEPS

Non-economic.   First steps.

Bipolar, Recovery and NLP

The diagram above illustrates how small and big steps can interconnect to realize a goal. This diagram can be used as a model to help you with your goals.

My main work goal in life is to reduce the humiliation of people with mental illness. I visualize this goal working so I can place it in the goal realized section in the diagram above. To achieve my goal I use a variety of steps. At the bottom of the diagram I put in the small steps. For example, in this section I would include the Chipmunka Foundation, the fact we help people with mental illness, the fact that I as an individual have had manic depression gives me credibility in working in this area.

In my view these steps are steps towards the goal. The big steps would be the Chipmunka Group, including Chipmunkapublishing. The fact that I set up Chipmunkapublishing as the Mental Health Publisher enabled me to set up the Chipmunka Foundation. Even if the Chipmunka Foundation achieves its mission and becomes the most effective mental health charity in the world it will not become a bigger influence than Chipmunkapublishing or the Chipmunka Group.

The Chipmunka Group is a social entrepreneurship and philanthropic model that enables the Foundation to grow organically. The Chipmunka Group generates its own revenue and actively supports the Foundation. It also gives opportunities to people with mental health issues to become self-employed, social entrepreneurs and show that people with mental health issues can achieve anything that they believe is possible therefore creating the world's first mental health celebrities.

The Chipmunka Group itself has the same mission as the Foundation but uses economic forces to take a bigger step. Therefore, all parts of the Chipmunka Group would go above the goal cylinder because of their economic potential in pushing the utopian agenda.

The fact that my life's mission is to help people with mental illness is also in my eyes a small step. By October 2006 Chipmunkapublishing alone receives more web traffic than any other mental health publisher on the Internet. This is because we are giving people a voice, an opportunity to have their voices heard in a world where they are discriminated against.

The reason why I have put helping people with mental illness as a small step is simple. I deliberately used the wrong language in the previous sentence and in diagram 2. There is no such thing as mental illness really. On one level it is a mindset. I know this because I spent 12 years blaming other people for my manic-depression. As soon as I stopped blaming others and took on full responsibility for my life on an ongoing basis I cured myself. It does not take a rocket scientist to work out that other people, such as Stephen Fry or Pete Doherty could do exactly the same thing. Mental illness can also be said quite rightly to be a manufactured term set up as a form of social control as governments do not generally want people to think for themselves. The term mental illness also fits the selfish entrepreneurial motives of drug companies to condemn and make money out of people taking medication that they profit from. On one level everyone in the world could be said to have a mental illness. On another level there are people who are suffering who need help and society should be able to help them. This could be a real dilemma without an appropriate solution.

The big step in the diagram and the solution is to improve the well being of people on the planet. The real voice here is changing the term mental illness and turning it into well being. If people see the issue as well being there will be no taboo and they will realize that mental illness affects everyone. Then they will be more inclined to talk about mental health and then more likely to help a person with mental health issues when they see them and not ignore them or judge them unfairly. They may even befriend them, give them an opportunity to get employed or manage their own life or money or offer them appropriate support. When I put my publisher's head on, this is quite exciting as in theory it means that I could publish a book on anything as long as I can find an appropriate mental health hook on it. If any serious venture capitalists are reading this please do get in touch.

The other advantage of using well being is also the mindset of the person with the "mental health issue." They will see their state as something that can be felt by more people or even anyone and will also focusing on recovery rather than illness... Where people focus is massively important as where people focus is where they usually end up in life.

Then they can see a way out, change their mindset and cure themselves. With this paradigm shift the drug companies' and psychiatrists' influence on the world will lessen, their grips will loosen, their roles will be redefined or replaced and a new form of well being will be developed creating a healthier and happier world.

The final small step I would like to discuss is the fact that as a former manic-depressive, I have credibility in the area of "reducing the humiliation of people with mental illness."

By the time I'd set up Chipmunkapublishing in April 2002 and launched "A Can of Madness", my autobiography on living with manic-depression, I knew that my story was an example of someone who was prepared to face up to what being diagnosed with a mental illness meant in the eyes of society. In fact what motivated me to write it apart from knowing it would stop me committing suicide was to stop the humiliation and suffering of another 17 year old with manic-depression.

This is because I went through it first when I was 17 and it is only natural to want to stop someone else going through the same pain that you went through, especially when you feel the pain could have been avoided and part of it was unjust on some level. This is a natural human instinct. I am no different than any other human being. This is precisely why my own experience is a small step in the universe. Even though my experience planted the seeds for the Chipmunka Group and the Foundation and is my driving force for realising my goal to eliminate global humiliation, It is my passion that makes me get up buzzing every single day and commit to doing more. It is my passion, which shapes my belief systems and well being. I am only one person, but I have a goal for the world.

The goal I have is to stop the humiliation of anyone who has been told they have a mental illness because this is an ideal. It is something that in my eyes should not occur in the 21st Century or should have ever occurred in history. This is a utopian goal but one that I believe is possible. The big step here is a founding generation of people stepping out as others and I have done, using mental health as a positive, thus creating a paradigm shift. I envisage millions of people stepping up around the world and saying why the humiliation of mental illness is wrong. This like anything, only receives real credibility and revolutionary status if it is led and controlled by the "sufferers" themselves, by the people who went through it. Otherwise everyone would be invited to alcoholics anonymous to give an opinion as to why certain people drink. The goal is beyond my own ego; it's beyond the Chipmunka Group. It's about millions of people all around the world being brave enough to stand up for what they believe in as human beings and having the mental strength to give back and take on the responsibility of giving others an opportunity to empower themselves for the well being of the world and the planet. This is for all of our future and for the future well being of the planet, for our children and our children's children, for people in the 3rd world so they can empower themselves and improve their well being and the rest of their lives, so we live in a humanitarian world for world peace and so we can motivate ourselves as a race to save the environment, stop diseases etc…

DIAGRAM
2:

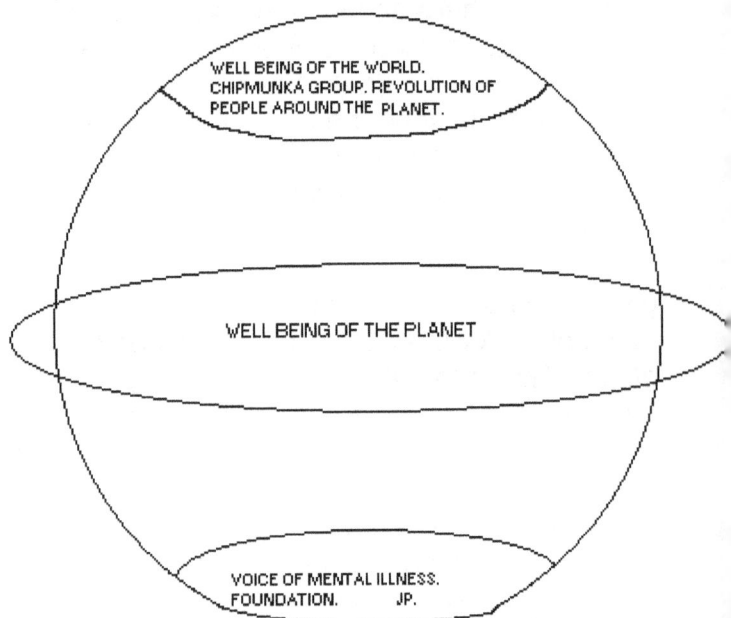

This one goal that I have explained in the last few pages is an integral part of what makes me happy as a human being. I use the same thought processes in other aspects of my life as well. For example, the love of my partner, friends and family is also another crucial aspect to my happiness as a human being.

Think of something crucial in you life to your happiness. It could be in your relationships, work, health, finances, etc.

Now have a think about what is crucial to your happiness as a human being. No need to write it down. Just feel it and it will formulate in your unconscious mind.

YOU HAVE ALREADY ACHIEVED 25% towards Ultimate Well Being… take a few moments to congratulate yourself… pause… and enjoy the moment… visualize how great you will feel when you have finished this book and achieved 100% … feel good… feel great… YES… YES…This is called an incantation and is a technique you can use in any aspect of your life. Whenever you want to overcome an obstacle or stress or just want just want to enjoy the moment, you can always use an incantation to snap yourself into a positive mindset.

Chapter Three

Inspire Yourself

My healthy soul is equally, if not more important as how I act as a person determines my state of being and ultimate well being.

By being aware of having a healthy mind, body and soul I can be successful in having Ultimate Well Being and so can you.

Through becoming well trained in self-help, empowerment and Neuro-Linguistic Programming, I know that the healthier my body is the better equipped I am to fulfil my personal ambition of reducing the humiliation that anyone with a "mental health issue" faces. This is why I hardly touch alcohol or smoke or overeat. This is why I sleep as much as I need to and do not oversleep and why I eat healthily. I know that physical exercise gives me energy, so I work out most days. I regularly go jogging in the morning, play football every week, do weights, cardio vascular exercises and practice other sports including squash, swimming and martial arts.

I am also convinced that I have a happy soul. I am happy with my inner self because I have searched my soul and gone through a personal transformation where I consciously discovered what would make my soul happy and then lived by these rules that I set myself and I regularly review the guidelines I set myself. Therefore on an unconscious level my soul takes care of itself and is happy.

I know that the most important thing for my soul is to have a purpose in life that makes me a human being with a purpose. This makes me totally committed and happy in my relationships, has helped me find a peer group that I feel comfortable with and challenges me. For me it is important to have a peer group that is constantly growing and evolving. Otherwise I would lower my standards and get bored.

I am also totally convinced that the work that I do every day is a force for social good that other people around the world can benefit from today and in the future.

I set up Chipmunkapublishing, The Mental Health Publisher, to give a voice to other people diagnosed with mental illness around the world, so they too could join other people's goal of reducing stigma on mental health issues and my personal goal of stopping the humiliation that anyone with a mental illness feels and enable people to empower themselves through literature and multi media. This one thought alone is what gets me up with a spring in my step every day. This is why I work so hard and put my whole life into changing things. I do this out of choosing to do first and then a kind of necessity because I am fortunate that I have had the insight to realize what ingredients I need for having my healthy mind, body and soul.

The final exercise for this chapter is for you to work out what gives you the peace of mind to realize what a healthy mind, body and soul means to you. I want you to spend at least 15 minutes doing this exercise. Do it… and enjoy it…
Write down at least 5 situations in each category of amazing things…situations or events that would make you feel totally fulfilled as a human being if they happened or were happening in your life. Once you have written this down, prioritise them putting them in order of significance, then put time frames around them.

You can use them as your Ultimate Well Being action plan for the rest of the book. When you have completed this stage learn them verbatim and you will have leaped from 11% to 20% Ultimate Well Being. If you do not complete this whole exercise then you only stay at 11%. Then and only then move onto the second chapter. I have given you my own example to act as a template. The number at the end of each example below illustrates the order of priority I gave it at the time that I wrote it. This is a good exercise to try and can be repeated any time you want to refocus your healthy Mind, Body and soul techniques. Notice that the order I wrote them down was not necessarily the order of priority that I gave each action. The more you write down the more the exercise will help you. I have found this exercise to be a wonderful experience. Sometimes I have written down over 30 points for each and prioritised them which have lead to rapid improvements in each area.

Example:

Mind Page:

Visualize happy days every day 1
Do the work that I enjoy 2
Spend time with people who have compassion 5
Switch off work in the evenings during the week 7
Do not look at emails on a Sunday 3
Read and complete the reading of one new book a fortnight 6
Be in a state of being rather than visualisation and enforced NLP
Finish writing my 4th book mental health Empowerment ASAP.

Body Page:

Drink more water 6
Go jogging 3 times a week 4
Play football every week 3
Eat fruit every day 5
Make love regularly 2
Have a stronger physiology 1

Bipolar, Recovery and NLP

Soul Page:

Help people on a daily basis 1
Help someone I do not know once a month for one
hour 6
Spend quality time with my girlfriend 2
See good in other people 4
look to empower others 3
stay close to my family 5

*Complete Your Mind, Body and Soul techniques
below:*

Mind Page:

Body Page:

Soul Page:

If you have prioritised them then congratulations. You can now move on, as you are now 20% of you way towards Ultimate Well Being. Remember you can do this exercise whenever you feel like re-evaluating so you can maintain Ultimate Well Being for your mind, body and soul.

Chapter Four

Inspire Yourself and have time for other people

People can draw inspiration from others of course, but to achieve Ultimate Well Being as with achieving anything else in life the responsibility lies with oneself. Mohammed Ali is a great example of this. Muhammad Ali (born Cassius Marcellus Clay, Jr. on January 17, 1942 is a retired African American boxer. In 1999, Ali was crowned "Sportsman of the Century" by Sports Illustrated. He is a three-time World Heavyweight Boxing Champion.

Most people who have heard of Mohammed Ali whether they know much about boxing or not, regard him as the greatest boxer of all time. This is not just because he was a great boxer but because he projected this image and always described himself as the greatest.

Mohammed Ali was so intent on winning that he constantly referred to himself as being the greatest to raise his self esteem and empower himself as a boxer. The fact that it became true cannot be said to be a coincidence. In essence it was Ali's sheer belief and mindset that he was the greatest that made him the greatest. The Rumble in the Jungle is a great example of how Ali the underdog inspired himself to victory.

Bipolar, Recovery and NLP

The Rumble in the Jungle

Ali regained his title on October 30, 1974 by defeating champion George Foreman in their bizarre bout in Kinshasa, Zaire. Hyped as "The Rumble in the Jungle", the fight was promoted by Don King who had served time in prison for killing his partner.

Almost no one, not even Ali's long-time supporter Howard Cosell, gave the former champion a chance of winning. Analysts pointed out that Joe Frazier and Ken Norton had given Ali four tough battles in the ring and two of them while Foreman had destroyed both in the second round.

The fight turned into a political symbol – Ali was taken to represent black consciousness and the fight against white power, Foreman taken to represent US arrogance. Ali was massively popular in Zaire and it is said that the enthusiastic support of the crowd assisted him in his victory.

In the fight, Ali took advantage of the young champion's one weakness – staying power. Foreman had won 37 of his 40 fights by knockout, most within three rounds or less, with Foreman's eight previous fights not going past the second round. Ali saw an opportunity to outlast Foreman, and capitalized on it.

Commentators expected Ali to box Foreman at distance using his superior speed and footwork but, instead, during the second round Ali retreated to the ropes inviting Foreman to hit him, while sporadically counterpunching and verbally taunting the younger man. Ali's plan was to enrage Foreman and absorb his best blows in order to exhaust him mentally and physically. The champion threw hundreds of punches in seven rounds but with decreasing technique and effect. This was later termed the "Rope-A-Dope".

By the end of the eighth round Foreman was clearly flagging and Ali made his move, turning Foreman off the ropes and executing a beautiful combination for the knockout. Foreman failed to make the count, and Ali had regained the title.

Just as Mohammed Ali inspired himself you can inspire yourself too. I do not mean go out and punch somebody. Please don't do that. The determination of successful sportsmen in this case a great boxer can be a strong metaphor for inspiring people in life.

I am inspired in my life by many things. I am inspired by the people I meet, by the things I want to achieve, by the wonderful world, technology, humanity and advancement in art, education and science that I witness as a citizen on a daily basis. I am happy in my relationships. I surround myself by positive people. I do not overspend which is something that makes me feel secure. A lot of people do not manage their money and therefore have a low financial intelligence, which can lead to great unhappiness. There are many books that you can read on financial intelligence. I have read many similar books. The **Rich Dad Poor Dad** series are the best that I have come across. I highly recommend them.

I choose to do the kind of work that I am passionate about. I avoid doing things that stress me out unnecessarily and embrace things that make me grow spiritually, emotionally and intellectually. I am very aware of what makes me happy so I focus on doing the things that make me content and happy. This is not only common sense but a deliberate mindset that breaks the pattern of any negative thoughts so that they are not allowed to manifest themselves.

All of us should be able to focus on the positive things in life thus making our lives more fulfilled. Most people though, focus more on negative things on a daily basis than on the positive. There are many reasons to speculate as to why this is the case. Robbins would argue because people's standards are not high enough. Perhaps it is because society embraces people who fit in and do as they are told and conform.

One thing that I have noticed is that people feel a connection with people when they are depressed. If people assume the worst then they assume that they will not be disappointed. This is playing it safe but is also a disastrous philosophy in life as it makes people content with being average.

Bipolar, Recovery and NLP

Therefore people have low expectations and lead mundane and unconscious lives, as they never break out of their comfort zone. They become failures and then meet other people like them who do not achieve anything. They both feel a connection with each other as they are alike and the dreams they once had disappear and are left to recite as a whim when they are much older.

The same is true of mental illness too and as a former manic-depressive I was a classical example. When someone is depressed they create a negative image of themselves. If someone else, their best friend feels compassion for them when they are depressed they will be more likely to be open about being depressed again. This can be detrimental because the person who acts depressed is doing it to gain significance and connection with the other person. Therefore unconsciously they are more likely to want to feel depressed again in front of their friend as they will feel significance and connection and we all need these two sensations. They are part of the human experience. So when someone feels depressed they are actually getting leverage over other people. If one can go manic as well that's real leverage as you can find people to connect with and give you significance in different ways. I have illustrated these examples to show that you can cure yourself from a mental illness. I know this because I have done this myself. As soon as I made the permanent decision never to go back to this self manifested feeling of significance and connection through depression and mania, I took full responsibility for my life and stopped blaming other people and moaning about circumstances instead of getting on with life.

Hence in less than one page I have articulated the cure for mental illness on a global level. Robbins has proved this change in action can help thousands of people around the world. It should not be limited to people who have to pay to go to seminars but should be brought inside the NHS and inside mental hospitals so people can make themselves better instead of spending their lives zombified on medication. Notice I did not need to medicate myself or anyone else to actually make myself better. I did it myself. As long as people with mental illness are not stigmatised, can be empowered to have their voices heard and taught that it is actually a great thing to take responsibility for their own lives and take massive action then this is a full proof system that can be attached to health authorities and individuals around the world. This is the future of the mental health industry not the medication time that we witness in *One Flew over the Cuckoo's Nest.*

In my own work during the last six years I have seen people's lives totally change and turn around for the better because we at Chipmunkapublishing gave them an opportunity to have their voices heard, not feel alone and empower themselves. Just go to the Chipmunkapublishing website at www.chipmunkapublishing.com and you will find many of these people. You can read their testimonies and see how they are helping the well being of others.

It is no coincidence that the most successful people in history are not scared of failure. In fact they are usually the people that have failed the most times to achieve what they have achieved. Successful people are not paralysed by the thought of failure. They deal with it and move on. Look at Walt Disney. He is a classical example of somebody who didn't take no for an answer.

Walter Elias Disney – December 5, 1901 – December 15, 1966, was an American film producer, director, screenwriter, voice actor, animator and philanthropist. As the co-founder of Walt Disney Productions, Walt became one of the best-known motion picture producers in the world. The corporation he co founded with his brother Roy, now known as The Walt Disney Company, today has annual revenues of approximately 30 billion US dollars.

In 1922, he started a small company called Laugh-O-Grams, which began by selling short animated films to local companies in Kansas City. By the time Walt had started to create The Alice Comedies, the company went bankrupt. Even though the company ended, Walt did not give up, he packed up what he had of his Alice Comedies and decided to move to Hollywood to try and start a new business.

Bipolar, Recovery and NLP

When Disney arrived in Los Angeles, he had 40 dollars in his pocket and an unfinished cartoon in his suitcase. Interestingly, he first wanted to break away from animation, thinking he could not compete with the studios in New York City. Disney said that his first ambition was to be a film director. He went to every studio in town looking for directing work; they all promptly turned him down.

Due to the lack of success in live-action film, Disney went back to animation. His first Hollywood cartoon studio was a garage in his Uncle Robert's house. Disney sent an unfinished print to New York distributor Margaret Wrinkler, who promptly wrote back to him. She wanted a distribution deal with Disney for more live-action/animated shorts based upon *Alice's Wonderland*.

Disney looked up to his brother Roy, who was recovering from tuberculosis in a Los Angeles veteran's hospital. Disney pleaded with his brother to help him with his struggling studio, saying that he could not keep his finances straight without him. Roy agreed and left the hospital with his brother. He never went back and never had a recurrence of tuberculosis. That was the beginning of the Disney Brother's Studio.

One of the main things to remember about the life of Walt Disney is that he wouldn't take no for an answer. Another thing that Walt Disney had and you should have if you want to inspire yourself to live the life you have dreamt of is to embrace fear. Yes for you to inspire yourself you have to embrace fear and choose life. Do not let fear hold you back or you will never reach your full potential. As Robert De Niro's directorial debut so aptly explains when De Niro the bus driver is talking to his son:

"The worst thing in the world is wasted talent"

Chaz Palminteri who plays Sonny the gangster also comes up with an interesting line. When asked whether he would rather be feared or loved he comes up with the interesting line. "If I had to choose which. I would rather be feared. As with fear comes respect".

Well that may be fine for people who want to follow a gangster. I am saying do the exact opposite. Embrace fear and move on from it. Don't ever let it hold you back.

Another quality you need to inspire yourself is to stay focused on what you want to do. A great example of this is Isaac Newton. Sir Isaac Newton 1643 – 1727. Isaac Newton was the greatest English mathematician of his generation. He laid the foundation for differential and integral calculus. His work on optics and gravitation make him one of the greatest scientists the world has known. He once said:

Bipolar, Recovery and NLP

"If I have ever made any valuable discoveries, it has been owing more to patient attention, than to any other talent".
Isaac Newton

So if you know what you want in life and know what inspires you, make sure that you stay focused on it every day. A one-degree shift one day, made consistent over a long period of time could lead to massive changes. This could be applied to anything; work goals, dieting, training to run a marathon etc… You can't just decide to go and run a marathon. You have to prepare for it and make changes consistently in order to do this task as you would any other concrete task.

Another way to be inspired is to know yourself. You can know your mind, body and soul – remember what you learnt in chapter one. You can also
Know what is crucial to your happiness – remember what you learnt in chapter 2.

In order to really know yourself you need to take full responsibility for your own life, make your own judgements/decisions and do not live in the shadows of others. You need to know thyself.

Now read closely so you can do the following exercise. Think of all the things that inspire you and write them down. This could be anything. It

could be a person, a place or a thing, a feeling.
Let me give you an example.

1. The way the sun rises in the morning
2. The way tiger woods plays golf
3. The way single mums bring up children
4. The movies that Stephen Spielberg makes
5. Eminem performing on stage
6. Bob Geldof committed to helping people in
Africa
7. Coldplay's music and the way they play live
8. The way Tony Blair delivers his public speaking
9. The way Bill Gates made computers widely
available
10. People who want to help other people.

Now write your list of 10 things that inspire you.

1
2
3
4
5
6
7
8
9
10

Now take a look at what you have written. You will
see that most of my examples mention people
who are recognised for being particularly good at
something. Many of them were famous people.

Bipolar, Recovery and NLP

That was deliberate. Isaac Newtown also said something rather insightful once:

"If I have seen further, it is by standing on the shoulders of giants"

This is an interesting concept. Inspirational people seek inspiration from other inspirational people. This is common sense. Do not hold yourself back. If someone else or something inspires you feel it and make it part of you. This does not mean you have to change your character. If you are a shy person you may not want to go around and tell everyone what inspires you, just keep it to yourself and feel it. If you want to tell the world or give some inspiration to someone who you feel needs help then do that too. Do not underestimate or be sceptical about feeling and therefore being inspirational. It is not a form of arrogance or even part of the manifested self or ego. The world is a beautiful place and the whole universe and everything in it is inspirational. This is a fact of life. How you live your life and how inspired and independent you are depends on how much you choose to feel comfortable about the inspirational world around you.

In my life I learnt the hard way not to take anything for granted. When I was diagnosed with manic-depression in 1993 after spending six months in a mental hospital I was only 18 years of age. Whilst it knocked the stuffing out of me it also taught me a lot about life in a very short amount of time. It made more sensitive as a human being, made me know that at some point when I was brave enough I would dedicate my life to stopping others going through the pain and humiliation myself. I also knew there and then, the moment when I came down from mania and realized I was in a psychiatric hospital and my life had changed forever that I knew I would ultimately have to take full responsibility for my life to inspire myself and be independent if I was ever going to make that horrific experience a force for good for me and society. The realization of what has happened was at the same time the most harrowing and beautiful moment of my life. I have taught myself to always see that moment as a beautiful moment and that poignant few seconds of my life planted the seeds for my life's work.

Many people have defining moments in their lives and it is more often than not how they deal with these moments that determine how their lives pan out. It is one of the great things about being a human being that life is unpredictable and we are given options to move in ways and experience things that we can not always predict. Of course the world can be an unfair place but most people can alter their own destiny. We have to believe that otherwise we become lazy as a species.

There are many techniques that can be used to train the mind. I have practiced dozens of techniques over the years. The most fun and the most helpful were the techniques I picked up from

Bipolar, Recovery and NLP

Anthony Robbins' more advanced seminars. I would do a daily success ritual that lasted for 5 minutes and set the tone for having a great day. After practicing this routine for a year I found that having a great day became automatic. I even found that if I tried to be negative in anyway, I couldn't because I had programmed my mind to be extremely happy. I suggest anyone who has any kind of mental illness and finds it a burden to practice their own positive reinforcement ritual every day for 12 months and they too will get the same results. My Daily Incantation ritual is mapped out below. After you have read it there is space to write your own.

Training the Mind

JP Example of Daily Incantation

1) Daily Success Conditioning Ritual

a)   Jump out of bed and do Power Move every day – Peak State
b)   2nd State – Close Eyes Vision Yourself
c)   Celebrate – jump up and down and anchor that with your physiology
d)   Say out loud with conviction your 'I am' statements and your belief statements

2) By 18/10/2008

Hollywood Film Director. Winner of Best Oscar at 33 years old. Famous screenwriter with Sonia. Mentally outstanding living in L.A. and Chelsea.

3) I AM

Full of joy
Outstanding
Focused
Inspired
A leader

BELIEFS

1) I am making the world a better place
2) I am the greatest
3) I love the world

I now give myself permission to move into this vision

Imagine having completed all your visions and incantations. How does it feel 1 year after completion 18/10/2008. It feels fantastic.

Practicing my daily incantations gave me great confidence, improved my well being, and enabled me to accomplish things and feelings of ultimate Well Being that I had not even really imagined before. You can feel the same sense of Well Being, just create your own ritual. I would recommend five minutes each morning in front of the mirror, before you even clean your teeth as then you will spring out of bed and into action and will set the positive tone for the rest of the day. This is the way Anthony Robbins and Stephen Covey recommend to do it and you will get the most out of it this way.

Your Daily Incantation

1) Daily Success Conditioning Ritual

a) Jump out of bed and do Power Move every day – Peak State – Your Power Move will be some physical activity that you repeat ten times to build up the oxygen in your body. Mine was a high front kick that I learnt when doing Taekwondo. If you are unsure what Power Move to do try raising both your hands in the air and celebrating by punching your fists in the air.
b) 2nd State – Close Eyes Vision Yourself – Now select two or three clear goals that you wish to achieve in the next two years and imagine how you feel after completion. Mine were winning an Oscar, being happy with my girlfriend and living in Chelsea and Los Angeles.

Goals:
c) Celebrate – jump up and down and anchor that with your physiology. This celebration should last for 5-10 seconds at least.

d) Say out loud with conviction your 'I am' statements and your belief statements - come up with 5 adjectives, each of them should be words that describe how great you feel and then 3 positive belief statements.

Above is what you are going to do each day.

2) Date – 1 Year after I have achieved my goals =
_____

Write Goals again and feel the sense of achievement here. No more than two lines, be specific:

3) I AM – list your 5 positive adjectives of how you feel below. Write alongside my examples:

Full of joy -
Outstanding -
Focused -
Inspired -
A leader -

Belief Statements - Write yours alongside mine:

1)   I am making the world a better place -
2)   I am the greatest -
3)   I love the world -

"I now give myself permission to move into this vision" – read this out loud and have your eyes close when you say this and imagine how great it feels to have achieved your goals. Write down your goals again below and then practicing feeling the sensation:

Goals:

Now you have learnt the daily incantation ritual, practice it every day. Once you have practiced it every day for a month, you can revaluate it. You might find your goals, beliefs and feelings even more focused and inspired.

For listing ten things that inspired you earlier in this chapter and creating your own incantation ritual your Ultimate Well Being Score has increased from 25%-40%. List 5 things that are inspirational in anyway to you at this moment in time to take your score up from 40% to 45%. I have given you 5 things that inspire me as an example.

Jason's example:
1 helping others
2 being creative
3 being true to myself
4 inspirational people around me
5 sporting heroes and applying their mindset and principles to my life

Bipolar, Recovery and NLP

My Five Inspirational Things:

1
2
3
4
5

Chapter Five

Inspire others and become a social entrepreneur

Look at any successful social entrepreneur such as Martin Luther King, Nelson Mandela, and Bob Geldof. These people make things happen because they have self-belief/conviction that what they want is good for society and others follow. This can be on a grand scale or at your local community talking to a homeless person and buying them breakfast one morning every week and just listening to them without judging them.

I have dedicated my life to becoming a social entrepreneur and feel that my life has a purpose because of what I do everyday. I remember not long ago I saw a tramp shaking at 6.00 in the morning on my way to work and I wanted to help so instead of giving him money, buying him an unhealthy breakfast I gave him mine and some dietary advice, gave him advice on how to sell the big issue and probably most importantly listened to his story.

When I wrote my own autobiography on living with Manic-depression *A Can of Madness* I received a grant from the government to give copies to people who it may have helped. I gave 300 copies to people in drug and alcohol rehab centres, as I knew they might identify with what I went through and hoped it would help them. When I set up Chipmunkapublishing "The Mental Health Publisher" in April 2002 I did so because I wanted to help other people who had been affected by mental illness. I wanted to stop the humiliation that they felt for being diagnosed with a mental illness and feeling alienated and worthless by society.

In October 2002 we published our second book *The World Is Full of Laughter*, an autobiography on schizophrenia written by Dolly Sen. Dolly said that writing her book "started out as a suicide note and ended up a celebration of life". Furthermore she was actually inspired to write her own book by reading *A Can of Madness* and the fact that I published it and believed in Dolly inspired her to help other people. Dolly often says that I was the first person to believe in her. This I find extremely humbling and proud because in the last five years Dolly has helped hundreds of people around the world to express their creativity and given them a voice just as we through Chipmunkapublishing gave her a voice by publishing her book and encouraging her to be proud of who she is and what she can achieve.

As I grew Chipmunkapublishing, any skills I picked up and opportunities that came my way I wanted to pass on to Chipmunka authors so they could raise their own self esteem, improve their lives and give a voice and help more people who have been part of the mental health system for whatever reason. Five years later Chipmunka has signed up nearly 500 authors around the world and each of those authors has gone on to help other people. I call this the Chipmunka domino effect. It is part of our mental health empowerment model at Chipmunka.

Once somebody helps someone then the person that is helped often becomes stronger i.e. has a potential to do more good. When an author has their book published it may be the first time in their lives that anyone has taken their views seriously. When the author hears the news that they are going to publish their self-esteem is raised as they have something positive to focus on and they know that someone or something believes in them and believes that what they are saying is true and is actually how they feel justifiably about their condition whatever it may be.

The day of the book launch is a day of positive reinforcement. The author's family and friends will be there and they will see the author in a different light not just as someone who has had a mental illness that they cared for or didn't understand but someone who has taken a negative experience and turned it into a positive and has become a published author to help inspire other people with similar conditions and experiences. The day of the launch is also an opportunity for the author to give a talk about why they wrote the book. Therefore the author now has a new identity as a public speaker and often gives more talks as a result. Later on, the author might start getting paid to give talks as they have become an expert by experience instead of a service user or 'former mental health patient' who is not part of society.

With publication author's start to give talks to the media for the first time which can also raise their self esteem and profile giving them opportunities to write freelance articles, encourage them to write more books or find employment. I have also helped several authors receive grants so that they can promote themselves, their books and help more people. This is a win win situation as we are all working together to help the community and empower others. The stronger Chipmunka becomes and the stronger each author becomes the more people we can support, give a voice to and the more we can help society to empower people with mental health issues so mental illness becomes a thing of the past. This is a utopia that I will always strive for as it is something that I believe in and something which helps my own well being, and the more I do it the more I can help more and more people.

Bipolar, Recovery and NLP

Mental Health Empowerment

Changing the Way the World Thinks about Mental health

Mental health empowerment is a mindset. That is all. It is a perception of the mind. I began writing this book after I had learnt all the techniques that Anthony Robbins teaches. Robbins first appeared on the motivational scene in 1989 as a 25-year-old writing the highly praised self-help book Unlimited Power. Seen by his supporters as the most inspirational man on the planet and by others as an opportunist or that massive American salesman and seen by cynics as the con artist who charges people £500 - £1000 to go to a four day seminar. I first came across Robbins in 2000 when I read his material and applied his NLP methods. He is in my opinion the most articulate, practical and accessible NLP practitioner on the planet. So why mention Tony Robbins in my own book on Ultimate Well Being when describing Mental Health Empowerment. Well, because Anthony Robbins's legacy is symptomatic of a new line of thought in the world of mental health.

People with mental health issues are becoming more responsible and are slowly being given greater responsibility by the world at large. This paradigm shift as Stephen Covey would describe it if he were to focus on this has been occurring year on year for thousands of years in Western culture. The madman was always humiliated and excluded in Ancient literature in

Bipolar, Recovery and NLP

Greek Tragedy where the ultimate punishment for hubris by the gods was not murder or torture but insanity. Only in Victorian times mad people were sharing the same cells as murderers and hung because the stigma was so great. Psychiatry came along as a kind of false police service and started medicating people to control them as a form of social control and drug companies cleverly took advantage of this making hundreds of billions of pounds for their shareholders. Then NLP grew in the 70s along with the mental health survivor movement, which gained a greater identity in the twentieth century. There were interesting thinkers like RD Laing, mental health charities forming across the world and Madpride as a concept and movement had a kind of inner logic of "being proud to be mad" which in my view harps back to the old Greek adage of live thyself.

So all along the essence of mental health empowerment lies in people who are mentally ill, taking control of their own lives being responsible for them and giving back so that they can help more people. In 1992 at the age of 17, I was diagnosed with manic-depression. After several years of procrastinating and moving in and out of madness I made the decision to write my own autobiography on living with manic depression *A Can of Madness* to save my own sanity and help other people.

When I set up Chipmunkapublishing in 2002 as The Mental Health Publisher I was fortunate enough to have an insight into Mental Health Empowerment for the 21st Century and beyond. As Chipmunkapublishing documents how a generation of people with mental illness feel about their own lives and publishes books by carers, mental health charities, related organisations, employers we are facilitating Mental Health Empowerment. My work is an example of work being done by millions of people around the globe in giving a voice to people with mental health issues and breaking down the stigma. This book is not an attempt to praise what I am doing; it is an exercise to put my pulse and therefore yours and other people's pulses into breaking down the biggest taboo of all - mental illness. This book also aims to focus you on the positive transition of the chipmunka phenomenon i.e. what I describe as Mental Health Empowerment.

You may have a question. I know I do. Why is mental illness the biggest taboo of all? We are all human beings and whatever our religious or spiritual beliefs, we all know why we are going to die. We all fear death and losing our mind. On a daily basis any one us could lose our sanity as life is full of ups and downs and human beings as much as we like to think we are, are not invincible. Madness is something that is fascinating in the eye of the observer because it is something that we are all interested in but do not want to get too close to. Hence, the reason for the stigma.

The tools for the mentally ill to cure themselves have always been there and they always will be. We are now in many ways in an absurd time of self analysing in history. We might as well all be in a Woody Allen movie. We are told by governments around the world that 1 in 4 of us will have a mental illness of some kind at some time in our lives. By 2020 the World health organisation tells us that suicide will be the second most common form of death. Is this a global epidemic or just to be expected when you look at what is actually happening.

Everyone in the world could be said to have some kind of mental illness but many of them would be unaware of it as the have more pressing concerns. They need to avoid starvation, fight disease etc... We all feel up and down on a daily basis. Some of us more than others of course but we all feel this sense of imperfection - inequality as human beings. The only ones of us who don't are in contradiction to those who are e.g. those who are actually in some kind of psychosis i.e. a manic person who thinks they are god.

As psychiatry comes up with more and more mental illnesses every year, more and more people are being described as mentally ill. If this kept continuing for hundreds of years then everyone in the world would be diagnosed with a mental illness. Wouldn't that be fantastic if I was the head of the biggest pharmaceutical company in the world or even a major shareholder...? Interesting... Do not see this as cynical... It is a fact.... eventually everyone in the world could be diagnosed and if you sold the drugs that treated people you would be quid's in...

I do not see drug companies and psychiatrists having a handle on things forever for several reasons. For one so many people are aware of alternative treatments CBT (Cognitive Behavioural Therapy), NLP (Neuro- Linguistic Programming) etc... and these techniques, if used correctly are more effective than medication and do not poison your mind and body, therefore they will be more common place. There is also a lot of money to be made by generations of entrepreneurs who are into NLP, improving diet, physical exercise, gym owners etc..., healthy fruit and drink owners, giving up smoking, drinking, Buddhist retreats, self help etc... This is a huge market and new types of products will produce thousands of millionaires and hundreds of billionaires over the next fifty years.

Also taking Chipmunkapublishing as an example - we are already documenting the way tens of thousands of people with mental health issues feel about how they have been treated. If we could publish in some way 10 million books or experiences over the next 50 years then that is quite a lot of evidence that says how people have been abused, how they feel, how they got better etc... It doesn't take a rocket scientist to work out that these people and millions of people around the world who have experienced what they have will and are standing up and empowering

Bipolar, Recovery and NLP

themselves around the globe. If you thought Martin Luther King and Gandhi were an inspiration then just think about the mentally ill. They have been the most isolated group of people in the world and now they are empowering themselves so they can help the rest of the world come to terms with their own mental illness.

Being mentally ill in the past myself made me more sensitive as a person, gave me more the potential for greater good and gave me a mental toughness and will to become a success and help people that was not identifiable in my psyche before. If you struggle in life and can get over something then this gives you the potential to do more. Everyone knows that. It's a common truth.

With the Internet at our disposal people can have a voice and people's lives can change and improve. We are a consumerist generation. People can dictate what they want. There does not have to be any brand loyalty because people can buy something cheaper, better, cooler somewhere else on the web but people become involved with helping people because they know that we want to make a real difference and give people a voice. I, as an author and a CEO am just an example to someone who was once not well and then decided to give a voice to himself and others to help society.

5 ways in which Chipmunka helps authors:

Bipolar, Recovery and NLP

1)   Giving them an opportunity to have their voices heard by publishing their story
2)   Encouraging authors to speak to the media
3)   Helping authors to get their own fundraising to promote themselves and help others
4)   Giving authors an opportunity to do other things e.g. give talks, write freelance articles
5)   Encourage authors to become leaders in their own particular area of experience/expertise so that they can raise their own profile and help more people.

The way that I help others may be different to the way that you help other people as I help people through my own work i.e. the nature of my work is for a social cause. Yours may be more straightforward – having time to listen to people at work if they are upset, being good to your friends, supporting your family, donating to charity etc…

Think of 5 ways in which you help or can commit to helping other people and write a few words on each of how you help these people or how you are going to help these people.

1)

2)

3)

4)

5)

You get 1% for each reason and 1% for each explanation = 55% on your way to Ultimate Well Being.

Chapter Six

How can you make the world a better place?

Every day I make a conscious effort to make the world a better place in some way. This is why I dedicated my life to giving a voice to people with mental health issues around the world. I believe passionately that I am making a difference in some positive way and the feedback I receive from people who understand what I am doing inspires and encourages me to do even more.

It took me many years of thinking and doing to get to this stage of contentment, happiness and fulfilment. From the ages of 17-25 I was self-manifesting my manic-depression and causing a lot of pain to my family, friends, people I was in relationships with and people I came into contact with. From the ages of 25-29 I had improved a lot and was generally a good influence on people but I was still rebuilding my life to some degree and had moments of fear, disbelief and great concern.

Gradually after being focused on helping make the world a better place for so long I feel that the world or universe kind of helped me. My attitude, belief systems and ability to help others gained momentum and enabled me to be content with myself and my own life and my role within it.

We can all make the world a better place in many different ways; by believing in other people,

Bipolar, Recovery and NLP

looking after the environment, being a good neighbour, respecting others, fulfilling our potential, helping others etc…

I had very strong belief systems and did some very powerful visualisations over quite a few years where I envisaged making the world a better place. The strong visualisation techniques I used took me nearer to achieving what I wanted to achieve every day. Every moment I consciously took to find the good in others and meditated my way into finding more people who could do more good and help more people. Everything in my life approved in some way as I was focusing on these positives. The paradigm shift that occurred was remarkable. The same will happen to you too as you practise your daily incantations.

Write below in a page how you too can make the world a better place. You will not increase your well being score during this exercise although you will be learning a crucial technique to Ultimate Well Being. The happiness people in life are those that care about the Universe, the world around them and others. So in many ways, what you are writing below is the essence of ultimate Well Being therefore marinating your Well Being score. Whenever you doubt your Well Being think of helping others.

Bipolar, Recovery and NLP

How Can I Make The World A Better Place?

Bipolar, Recovery and NLP

Chapter Seven

Connecting Spiritually

After doing my visualisation techniques for two years my positive chi, as I like to call it, empowerment became automatic. I had gone through different phases and intensities of NLP for 4-5 years, which meant I was automatically happy even when I ceased practising NLP. I still had a sense of great contentment and fulfilment. This is true to this day and will carry on being true as I am fulfilled and content with the life that I lead. I have a state of equilibrium and balance that I had never had previously in my life and will remain in this zone of Ultimate Well Being.

There is not one particular moment when I realised that this had happened. I felt as if sometimes that I would try to be happy and then once my girlfriend asked me, "aren't you happy now?" And I thought about it for a moment – yes I was – so I didn't actually need to practise myself or use any techniques to be happy. This was so simple and I couldn't believe it but it was true, especially after I had probably read over 300 self-help books in the previous 10 years and then this breakthrough in consciousness and clarity of thought and contentment happened almost unwittingly. I just felt the feeling of happiness and accepted it. This is a very simple thing to actually do. It just takes a little bit of concentration, perhaps an alteration in breathing and then you find yourself at one with yourself and in a state of Ultimate Well Being. Even if you only have that feeling for a split second then see if you can get back to it. The more you practise the more you will realise that it is easily attainable. Clear your mind of everything i.e. what you are going to do, what chores you have for the day and just BE for a moment, slow down you breathing or breathe – you will be amazed how many people do not breathe. Then just focus on a feeling of contentment.

There are many meditation exercises you can do to heighten you awareness of this state and anyone can achieve this state of contentment if they just rid themselves of the irrational mind.

Once you find this feeling of contentment Ultimate Well Being – remember what it feels like, how you breathe, what your body posture is like etc… so you can get back to it at anytime when you need to. The better you can achieve this on a conscious level the easier it will happen on an unconscious level and the more that you will feel it.

Whatever you religious beliefs are, even if you have none you must have some spiritual connection with your soul, spirit, mind. Let your ego die. How many friends does the existential cynic have? Are they ever truly happy? I think not. I used to be like that. Just feel the positive energy and connect spiritually to yourself and others and your life path will be smoother and more content.

5 things that make you me connect spiritually

1)   Knowing that I am making the world a better place
2)   Knowing that I am not responsible for the mental health of others
3)   I am happy with what I do, who I am and how I feel
4)   Believing that most people are essentially good
5)   Seeing the world/universe as an amazing, awe-inspiring place.

Explanation for each – to follow

5 things that connect you spiritually

1)
2)
3)
4)
5)

Your Ultimate Well Being score increases from 55–60%. After you have listed 5 things that connect you spiritually and then increases from 60-65% when you add your reasons below.

1)

2)

3)

4)

5)

Congratulations you are now well on your way to
Ultimate Well Being. Celebrate and feel the great
feeling. Feel the sensation and celebrate.

Chapter Eight

Making the impossible possible – visualisation/emotional intelligence, perception, live your dreams.

"I am always doing that which I can not do, in order that I may learn how to do it."
Pablo Picasso

"Life moves pretty fast. If you don't stop and look around once in a while you could miss it. Ferris Bueller in *Ferris Buelller's Day Off*.

All of our lives can sometimes feel a bit like the way Matthew Broderick describes life in the film *Ferris Bueller's Day Off*. That is why in order to live an enjoyable life, the way one perceives life is extremely important.

Having high 'Emotional intelligence' is also vital in maximising one's potential and leading a fulfilled life. Daniel Goleman has written about 'Emotional Intelligence' in several self help books. Emotional Intelligence is the ability to get on with other people. The more easily one can communicate positively with other people the more positive and satisfactory one's life usually is.

Emotional Intelligence is completely different to one's I.Q. If somebody is a genius it doesn't mean that one is happy. In fact often, people who are great thinkers are often tormented with extremely unhappy lives. Recognised as one of the greatest writers of all time Proust was ill for most of his life. Nietzsche, another great writer and thinker was also ill for large periods of his life. In fact many of the world's greatest thinkers; artists, writers and politician's were tormented by living unfulfilled and unhappy lives. We all know about the apparent synergy between genius and insanity.

It makes perfect sense when Goleman argues that high Emotional Intelligence is a far more favourable attribute than having an equally high I.Q.

People who have achieved remarkable things in life have a focus and always have amazing self-belief. They are not necessarily more intelligent than other people. They may have a higher emotional intelligence, as they may be able to connect with other people on a higher level than other people. One thing that is different between the highest achievers and other people though is that the perception of people who achieve amazing things is different than other people.

Remember the visualisation techniques we learnt earlier in this book. These visualisation techniques can be used in any aspect of your life to make the impossible possible. This kind of positive reinforcement belief as I like to call it is one thing that is apparent in any instance of somebody making the impossible possible.

In 1999 Manchester United won the treble. This had never been done before in British football and may never happen again. The Manchester United players who were part of that winning season often refer to their Semi Final with Arsenal as the turning point of that season. Manchester United was doing well in the league and still in the Champions League when they faced their main rivals, Arsenal. Manchester United had not won anything so far that season. United were down to ten men towards the end of the game when Arsenal was awarded a penalty. Dennis Bergkamp's penalty was miraculously saved by Peter Schmeichel. That moment gave all the Manchester United players a new lease of life. If Arsenal had scored that penalty they were moments away from winning the tie. Instead the game turned around and Ryan Giggs was to score one of the greatest FA Cup goals of all time weaving his way through the Arsenal defence and keeping Manchester United's treble dreams alive.

On July 20, 1969, Commander Neil Armstrong became the first man on   the moon. He said the historic words, "One small step for man, and one giant leap for mankind." A camera in the Lunar Module provided live television coverage as Neil Armstrong climbed down the ladder to the surface of the moon. Here man had made the impossible possible? How had they done this? Thousands of people should take some credit. Of course, every member of the Apollo 11 crew played a major role, as did the whole of NASA, scientists who had worked on space travel, funders who had donated money. The list could go on as so many people would have directly and indirectly made the event more likely to happen. Somebody's perception was also possibly different to everybody else's, however. In President Kennedy's speech to Congress, on May 25, 1961, he expressed a concern that the United States was falling behind the Soviet Union in technology and prestige. He challenged the nation to put a man on the moon before the end of the decade. Although Kennedy had passed away, his vision for putting a man on the moon had lived on.

Success in life is almost always a matter of perception. What one's outlook is in life is often where one ends up. If I wake up in the morning and I feel relaxed, look forward to the day, see the beautiful sky and enjoy being woken up by the wonderful birds singing I am going to have a better day than if I think. "Oh no I have so much work to do, woken up again by the noisy birds", focusing on the cold and clouds and wish I had taken the day off.

It is as if every day, even every moment we have a choice as to how we want to lead our lives. Some people get trapped in a negative cycle of thinking and end up doing nothing except self-manifesting their own problems, blaming others and feeling sorry for themselves. I know because I used to be like this a long time ago before I started using NLP and writing. The kind of people with these negative perceptions will never achieve the impossible as they actually believe that they cannot achieve most things. They are the kinds of people that bring other people down as it gives them a sense of significance and makes them feel better about themselves. They are people that have negative perceptions. Everybody knows someone like this. Well the less you hang around with people with those perceptions the more you will achieve.

You can break their pattern and try to help them but mostly you will fail, as they will be placing a burden on you. If you work with people who have very low expectations of themselves then the best way for you to help them is to create a positive force field around them so their negative sense of self disappears. You will need the ability to be able to switch off when you finish work for the day so you are not overwhelmed by their negative self esteem and negative impact on the environment around you. Be careful, as you will need amazing self-belief to ensure that you keep growing if you are supporting other people at work, in your home and social life. This includes your family and friends. You can only carry so many people on your back.

You can of course help other people change their perceptions of themselves, especially if their perception of themselves is unfair or unjust. Bob Geldof's work over the last twenty years is a great example of this.

Band Aid is a British and Irish charity super group founded in 1984 by Bob Geldof and Midge Ure in order to raise money for famine relief in Ethiopia by releasing a record *"Do They Know It's Christmas?"* for the Christmas market. The single became the Christmas number one on that release and on two subsequent releases. It was produced by Trevor Horn.

Bipolar, Recovery and NLP

Bob Geldof, after watching a television news report by Michael Buerk from famine stricken Ethiopia, was so moved by the plight of starving children that he decided to try and raise money using his contacts in pop music. Geldof enlisted the help of Midge Ure from the group Ultravox to help produce a charity record. Midge Ure took Geldof's lyrics and created the melody and backing track for the record. Geldof called many of the most popular performers of the time, persuading them to give their time for free. His one criterion for selection was how famous they were in order to maximize sales of the record.

The recording studio gave Band Aid 24 hours free to record and mix the record on 25 November 1984. The recording took place between 11am and 7pm and was filmed to release as the pop video. The first track to be put down was drums by Phil Collins including the memorable opening 'African Drum' beat. Tony Hadley of Spandau Ballet was the first to record his vocal while a section sung by Status Quo was deemed unusable and replaced with the Paul Weller/Sting/Glen Gregory section. Paul Young has admitted since in a documentary that he knew his opening lines were written for David Bowie who was not able to make the recording but made a contribution to the B-side. Boy George arrived last at 6pm after Geldof woke him up by phone to have him flown over from New York on Concorde to record his solo part.

Bipolar, Recovery and NLP

The following morning Geldof appeared on the Radio 1 Breakfast Show to promote the record and promised that every penny would go to the cause. This led to a standoff with the British Government, which refused to waive the

VAT (tax) on the sales of the single. Geldof made the headlines by publicly standing up to Prime Minister Margaret Thatcher and, sensing the strength of public feeling, the government backed down and donated the tax back to the charity.

The record was released on 15 December and went straight to number 1 in the UK pop charts outselling all the other records in the chart put together. It became the fastest selling single of all time in the UK, selling a million in the first week alone. It stayed at Number 1 for five weeks, selling over 3 million copies and becoming easily the biggest selling single ever in the UK. (It has since been passed by Elton John's tribute to Diana, Princess of Wales, but it is likely to keep selling in different versions for many years to come.)

The Name *"Band Aid"* was chosen because it had a double meaning. At one level it means *a band of musicians getting together to offer aid* but, at another level, it is also an acknowledgement of the fact that such a gesture is like putting a sticking plaster on a gaping wound and does not address the full extent of the problem of world famine.

Bipolar, Recovery and NLP

The charity set up to handle the money raised is called The Band Aid Trust. This project kick started Live Aid the following year which became a global phenomenon raising over ten times as much money as the original Band Aid single.

The group has been reformed on three occasions, each time from the most successful British and Irish pop music performers of the time to record the same song at the same time of year. Co-writer Midge Ure has commented that "Every generation should have its own version".

I remember watching Live Aid from my living room at my parents' house in Gloucester in 1985. I would have been 10 years old at the time. For me it was the most moving moment of the 1980's. It made me realize how privileged I was to have a roof over my head, to be able to eat three meals a day and not to have any fatal diseases. Live Aid made me realize that I was luckier than most of the world and that I should never take that for granted. As I grew up sometimes I did take things for granted and sometimes I did not. I like to think that I learnt a real lesson that day, however. That if somebody believes in making something good for somebody else then that is a great feeling that they should hold on to and if it is heartfelt and just then other people will want to assist in strengthening a force for good.

When I attempt to define Chipmunka and what it means to me, I often think of myself as that ten-year-old watching Live Aid. What if we could have the same impact as Live Aid did in the world of mental health? Couldn't we too make the whole world stand up and listen and make the world a better place? If the equality of the world's mental health improved then people would be better able to cope with inequality and therefore the world would be a more just place. My perception of being able to make a real difference in the world's mental health enables me to have a positive outlook on well being and makes me want to continue dedicating my life to changing other people's perception on mental health issues.

Every day I receive an email, letter or phone call from somebody who says that our work at Chipmunka has really made a difference to their own life or the life of somebody very close to them, and each time I hear something as positive as this I feel like doubling my determination and capacity to help somebody else and empower or educate more people. My perception alters and I focus on the sensation of achieving more of the impossible, i.e. living in a world where there are no suicides and where there is no such thing as mental illness. Living in a world where everyone who has suffered mental ill health has gotten better and helped someone else overcome their problems. It is this attempt to achieve the impossible that motivates me to do more and inspires me to make a difference. This kind of empowerment has a positive impact on other people and they do the same. They start to help people too, and thus we have the domino effect. It is amazing how many people can be helped on a daily basis because of these types of positive belief systems.

You can do the same with your life. You can achieve the impossible. This is a choice that only you will make. You are ultimately responsible for how you feel. You cannot pass that responsibility onto somebody else. That is unfair and unjust as they have their own life to lead. You can choose to be an optimist or a pessimist. You can try and be clever and say that optimism stems from unconscious fear and pessimism stems from a lack of moral imagination but that is only being intellectual and that will not get you anywhere.

You can empower yourself and others by having an aptitude for Emotional Intelligence. This will get you half way there, but in order to make the impossible possible you have to take responsibility for your own life. You can visualise all you want but unless you feel a sense of justification for your actions i.e. a need for doing something possible, then you will not achieve it. How you perceive what you plan to do is of vital importance. You cannot set yourself a task and then alter your perception.

Many times I have daydreamed of being World Snooker Champion as I love snooker but I have never got anywhere near even being a professional snooker player. I am not good enough, but that doesn't bother me as I still love the game. When Ronnie O Sullivan was very young, approximately 5 years old, he met Steve

Bipolar, Recovery and NLP

Davis, the then world snooker champion with his father and said that one day, he too would become World Snooker Champion. Fifteen or so years later, Ronnie O Sullivan did become World Snooker Champion and retold this story. Ronnie O Sullivan deserved to be World Snooker Champion because he made it happen. Instead of daydreaming it like me he altered his perception and actually did it. Could you become World Snooker Champion too, or could I? Well that is unlikely as Ronnie O Sullivan and Steve Davis have natural ability that is far superior to most people who play snooker, but it is the combination of *physis* and *furor* as the Greeks say that makes a difference. That is natural ability and hard work. I do not get disheartened that I am not the World Snooker Champion as I love the sport and admire watching the best players at the game. I enjoy watching other people succeed and I am fascinated by trying to work out how they are so good at something that I only have an amateurish understanding of.

There have been occasions in my life when I have achieved the impossible and there will have been similar occasions in your life too. Write down five occasions in your life when you achieved something that at one moment in time you thought you would never be able to achieve and then list 5 reasons as to how you got there. No matter how small or big the achievement seems put it down. Look at my examples to help you.

Bipolar, Recovery and NLP

1)   Having a steady relationship – fell in love with a beautiful woman

2)   Achieved Ultimate Well Being - Stopped focusing on feeling mentally ill

3)   Work for myself – Saw an opportunity and took advantage of it

4)   Won Young Social Entrepreneur of The Year 2005 – passionate about the work I do and other people noticed

5)   Finished my autobiography A Can of Madness – decided to do it and did it.

6)   Passed my driving test and drive regularly – practised and felt like I deserved to drive as much as other people

7)   Repaid debts – Planning, restraint and focused on positive repercussions.

8)   Had David Cameron mention me in one of his speeches – Just happened no explanation

9)   Won Gloucester Chess Congress ahead of 244 competitors – practised, enjoyed the game and concentrated on winning each game, one at a time.

10)   Encourage other people to improve their mental health – Focused on my own model of helping myself and looked at ways other people could maximise their potential through techniques and opportunities that I used.

Bipolar, Recovery and NLP

Your Top Ten examples of achieving the impossible;

1)

2)

3)

4)

5)

6)

7)

8)

9)

10)

For each of your ten examples no matter how big or small and each reason you will receive one percent well being. This will take your percentage from 65% at the end of the previous chapter to 85%. Congratulations you are 85% of your way towards Ultimate Well Being. Jump up and down and celebrate… Go wild…And praise yourself. The world is a fantastic place… Just feel these senses of Ultimate Well Being for a few moments…. and a few moments longer…

Now turn the page and read the final chapter to graduate to 100% ultimate well being.

Chapter Nine

Being Creative

"I'm always thinking about creating. My future starts when I wake up every morning. Every day I find something creative to do with my life."
Miles Davis

"There are two ways of being creative. One can sing and dance. Or one can create an environment in which singers and dancers flourish."
Warren G. Bennis

"Creativity is inventing, experimenting, growing, taking risks, breaking rules, making mistakes, and having fun."
Mary Lou Cook

Being creative is vital to all of our well being. Having liaised with thousands and worked with hundreds of people with 'mental illness' since 2002 and having been diagnosed with manic-depression myself in 1992 at the age of 17, I know that people lose their sanity for different reasons. It may be because of overwork, drugs, drink, relationship breakdown, other reasons or a combination of different reasons. People who experience 'mental illness', especially manic-depressive, always seem to get better if they can harness their creativity in some way or other.

Bipolar, Recovery and NLP

I believe the same is true for every person. Everyone needs to harness their creativity in some way, shape or form, not just those who have a mental health related issue. They must have a creative outlet. If that creative outlet can be something that reminds them that their mad experiences can be used as a positive then that is where the real lasting change of well being can be possible. So write a book, do some art, create some music and send it in to the Chipmunkapublishing website. We are waiting to give you a voice, to encourage you to become a social entrepreneur to help others and the more you can promote yourself and believe in this mission, the more potential you will have to help others and the more we will be able to help you.

If you cannot see any kind of mental health related issue in your life or story then you are still welcome to send in your manuscript, music or art in. You may be surprised to discover that there is a mental health angle in everything.

If you are going to write a book and you do not know where to start then just think about your life for a moment. Since the age of 17 I have been absorbed in how the world perceives mental illness. When I was seventeen I was told I had manic-depression and that this was a disorder/disease that I would have for the rest of my life. Having written my own autobiography on living with manic-depression *A Can of Madness* and published nearly 250 books on mental illness in the last 5 years I now see that everyone's life is affected by mental illness. If I can make everyone in the world realise that they have an aspect of a mental health issue in their lives then Chipmunka as a publisher will have made the transition from Mental Health Survivor Publisher to Well Being Publisher. Therefore the perception will have changed. Instead of people self-manifesting their own mental illness and being stigmatised by people, the world will be more concerned with well being and improving each other's lives.

During my own recovery I have gone through different stages and controlled creativity has been present when I have made the quantum leap into well being. Below is my list of the titles of my first 5 books. I want you to come up with your 5 titles for your first 5 books. Even if you have never written a book or never envisaged writing a book, I want you to come up with 5 titles now so you can move your well being score up from 85% to 90%.

1)   A Can of Madness
2)   Curing Madness
3)   The Ultimate Guide To Well Being
4)   Mental Health Empowerment
5)   Happiness in 7 Seconds

Your 5 titles for your first 5 books

1)
2)
3)
4)

5)

We all are, or can be creative to a lesser or greater degree if we are given the opportunity. In the next few lines I will explain exactly what creativity is. Creativity always involves thinking or behaving imaginatively. Second, overall this imaginative activity is purposeful: that is, it is directed to achieving an objective. Third, these processes must generate something original. Fourth, the outcome must be of value in relation to the objective.

Creativity improves people's self-esteem, motivation and achievement.

People who are encouraged to think creatively and independently become:

> More interested in discovering things for themselves
> More open to new ideas
> Keen to work with others to explore ideas

Now we know what creativity is, let's have some fun with it. Now I want you to come up with 5 titles for recording your own music album. I'll help with coming up with titles of my own. My genre is rap. You can choose whatever musical genre you want?

1)   A Can of Madness
2)   Raps To Recovery

3)   The Maddest Rapper In The World
4)   Empowerment
5)   Mad Ghetto

List the 5 names of the albums you are thinking of recording:

1)

2)

3)

4)

5)

This brings your well being score up from 90% to 95% as long as you have put the title down for each album. If you actually go on to make the albums and they become successful, remember what inspired you to produce them and please make a donation to The Chipmunka Foundation (registered charity number 1109537). All the money will go towards helping people with mental health issues. If you cannot find a record label or do not want to set up your own website to sell it then you know where to send them in, we are waiting. Thank you for your kindness. Now one last task for that maximum score.

Although I am a writer and have recorded a rap album I am certainly not an artist. I am fortunate to know one or two extremely talented artists. The best advice one of them gave me when I asked them how I should paint was – just paint. This is what I say to people who want to write their own book and also similar to what I was advised when doing my rap album. Now I am going to challenge you and myself to come up with 5 works of art. You will see that there is already some excellent art on the Chipmunkapublishing website.

Here are my 5 titles of art. Once I write them down I commit to painting them before my fourth book comes out.

1)   A Can of Madness –
2)   The Secret Art of A Manic-Depressive
3)   Mad Art
4)   From Madness to Well Being
5)   Empowering Mad Artists Around The World

Your top 5 art masterpieces will be:

1)
2)
3)
4)
5)

Congratulations you have now increased your score from 95% to 100 percent. You now have 100 percent well being.

Bipolar, Recovery and NLP

Now how do you feel having written the 5 titles to your first 5 books? How do you feel? Pretty creative… Good. How do you feel knowing that writing those books could be used to reduce stigma on mental health and give a voice to people with mental illness, even better... Great… It's up to you if you want to write a book or not, but being creative is something that every human being should be encouraged to do. It is good for the human spirit and our sanity as long as we maintain our practical and logical side too.

There is of course more to creativity than writing, music and art but they are great examples, as each of these disciplines requires the use of different senses.

During your journey to 100% Ultimate Well being you have learnt to master many different positive states of well being. You have discovered how to measure having a healthy mind, body and soul. You have learnt what is crucial to your happiness. You have inspired yourself and become more aware of inspiring and having time for other people. You have worked on how to make the world a better place. You have connected with your spirituality and the spirituality of other people and rid yourself of your ego. You have mastered making the impossible possible by being aware of emotional intelligence and altering your perception. You have also harnessed your creativity.

Taking all this into consideration you deserve to have achieved 100% well being and there is no reason why you should not be able to maintain 100% Ultimate Well Being throughout your life. Before you sit back, relax and celebrate, spare a though for enabling other people you come into contact with in life achieving Ultimate Well Being as well. Not only is this a comforting thought but focusing on the happiness of others on a daily basis is also the key to your Ultimate Well Being. It's not rocket science, anyone can achieve it. I wish you 100% ultimate well being and the same for the people that you come into contact with. It has been a pleasure writing this book. If it has helped you in anyway, then I would love to hear about it. You can contact me through the publishing company's website at www.chipmunkapublishing.com or direct at jasonpegler@chipmunkapublishing.com. Thanks for listening. May the force of Ultimate Well Being be with you always.

Conclusion

Ultimate Well Being Contract

I make a commitment to myself to snap out of any negative thoughts that may arise and focus on Ultimate Well Being for the rest of my life.

I make a full commitment to myself to have a Healthy Mind, Body and Soul

I know what is crucial to your happiness and will ensure that I use this knowledge to maintain my happiness.

I know how to inspire myself and will therefore be at ease inspiring myself every day.

I will Inspire and have time for other people at every reasonable opportunity.

I dedicate myself to making the world a better place?

I promise to connecting myself spiritually and to let go of my ego.

I endeavour to making the impossible possible by using emotional intelligence wherever possible.

I will harness my creativity to improve my well being and enable the well being of others.

Bipolar, Recovery and NLP

I realise that signing this contract is a life long commitment to increasing my well being and that of other people.

signed by

_____

date

